Praise for *New York Times* Bestselling Author Robert Kennedy Jr.'s Book *Thimerosal*

"Kudos to Kennedy! Kennedy lucidly explains the science on Thimerosal, and then gives us a disheartening but necessary tour of the conflicts of interest in policymaking, regulation, and the media that keep this known neurotoxin in childhood vaccines. If embraced by the public and policymakers, this book can lead us to the happy end of vaccine-induced mercury poisoning in infants and young children."

—**Mary Holland**, research scholar, NYU School of Law;
coauthor, *Vaccine Epidemic*

"This book is shocking, but only because thorough and courageous investigative reporting on politically and emotionally charged topic is so rare."

—**David Austin**, associate professor, School of Psychology, Faculty of Health, Deakin University, Australia

"*Thimerosal: Let the Science Speak* educates and, hopefully, will universally inform health professionals to advise, to counsel, and to properly promote vaccines. Not just in developed countries, but in developing countries where it is most needed."

—**José G. Dórea**, Faculty of Health Sciences, Universidade de Brasília

"Robert F. Kennedy, Jr., has led in the production of an accurate and compelling documentation of the science that supports vaccine-delivered Thimerosal causation of the current autism epidemic. . . . Behind all of this is the absolute failure of our elected Congress to hold federal agencies accountable for their failure to protect the American people."

—**Boyd Haley, PhD**, professor of chemistry, University of Kentucky

"Carrying on a tradition of speaking truth to power, Robert Kennedy accurately and courageously tells what the real science really says. . . . This book is so well documented, no one can say they are well-read on this issue unless they have read this book cover to cover. It is a must-read for any citizen who understands that questioning authority is not a right of citizens in a democratic society: it is a responsibility."

—**Mary Catherine DeSoto, PhD**, professor of psychology and codirector, Psychoneuroendocrinology Lab, University of Northern Iowa

"It is unfortunate that a book recounting the history of the deliberate use of a frank toxin in medicines should be necessary. It is fortunate that Robert Kennedy, Jr., has authored that history with great attention to science, to politics, and to the consequences of the use of that toxin."

—**Julie A. Buckley, MD, FAAP**, author, *Healing Our Autistic Children*

Revised and Updated

THIMEROSAL
LET THE SCIENCE SPEAK

Revised and Updated

THIMEROSAL
LET THE SCIENCE SPEAK

The Evidence Supporting the Immediate Removal of
Mercury—a Known Neurotoxin—from Vaccines

Robert F. Kennedy, Jr.

Preface by Mark Hyman, MD
Introduction by Martha R. Herbert, PhD, MD
Foreword by U.S. Congressman Bill Posey

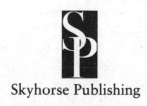

Skyhorse Publishing

Skyhorse Publishing books may be purchased in bulk at special discounts for sales promotion, corporate gifts, fund-raising, or educational purposes. Special editions can also be created to specifications. For details, contact the Special Sales Department, Skyhorse Publishing, 307 West 36th Street, 11th Floor, New York, NY 10018 or info@skyhorsepublishing.com.

Skyhorse® and Skyhorse Publishing® are registered trademarks of Skyhorse Publishing, Inc.®, a Delaware corporation.

Visit our website at www.skyhorsepublishing.com.

10 9 8 7 6 5 4

Library of Congress Cataloging-in-Publication Data is available on file.

Cover design by Brian Peterson
Cover image: Thinkstock

ISBN: 978-1-63450-442-3
Ebook ISBN: 978-1-63450-443-0

Printed in the United States of America

Contents

Foreword

Many years before my term in Congress I questioned the wisdom of injecting the mercury-based vaccine additive, Thimerosal, into children and pregnant women. When I was elected to Congress in 2008, I came to find that my predecessor, Congressman Dave Weldon, a medical doctor, shared this concern. Through working with like-minded individuals, including Mr. Robert F. Kennedy, Jr., I quickly became aware of an enduring concern among researchers, doctors, and loving parents about vaccine safety in the US and around the world. It is common sense that injecting infants with a mercury compound exposes them unnecessarily to risk.

This book is resolutely pro-vaccine and is far too valuable to be shrouded by the polarizing pro-vaccine versus anti-vaccine debate. The late 18th century work of Edward Jenner and Benjamin Waterhouse in bringing the first smallpox vaccine to the American public will be forever honored. In the same way, the contemporary work of those who introduce innovative and life-saving treatments, including vaccines, will also be remembered. This book is about making vaccines safer. Like the work of Jenner and Waterhouse, it advocates for health and wellbeing, and does so through a foundation of scientific facts and research.

Hundreds of parents from across the country have contacted me in recent years, describing their children as developing normally up to the time of receiving a particular vaccination. While the large majority of children do not have adverse reactions, we acknowledge that some children do react severely and have established a compensation program to provide for their care.

In 1999, after acknowledging that the public health community failed to do simple addition to know how much mercury-based Thimerosal young infants were receiving, the American Academy of Pediatrics (AAP) and the United States Public Health Service (USPHS) agencies recommended that Thimerosal be reduced or eliminated from vaccines. Between 1999 and 2003, Thimerosal was phased out of all routine pediatric vaccines administered in the United States. This was much welcomed and by early 2004 only small trace amounts of mercury remained in routine childhood vaccines.

In a seemingly inconceivable reversal, however, in 2004 the Centers for Disease Control and Prevention (CDC) recommended that certain infants receive the annual flu vaccine—most of which contained Thimerosal. Over the next decade the CDC's annual flu vaccine recommendations were expanded to include annual flu vaccines for infants, children, adults, and the aged. This is a significant reversal of the positive steps taken between 1999 and 2003. Had the post-2004 CDC recommendations not been taken, this book would perhaps not be necessary for the American public. (Thimerosal continues to be used throughout most of the developing world as the predominant vaccine preservative.)

The continued use of mercury, a known neurotoxin, raises particular concern for populations that are most vulnerable to neurodevelopmental harms, mainly a fetus in utero, infants, young children and the aged. When we speak of the health and safety of our children, our future generation, we speak of a societal responsibility, which we are privileged to bear.

In 2004, the Institute of Medicine (IOM) published a report refuting any link between exposure to Thimerosal and autism. This report relied heavily on several epidemiological studies, which have been criticized for involving conflicts of interest. These studies examined populations of children that were increasingly exposed to Thimerosal throughout the 1990s. Likewise, the prevalence of neurodevelopmental disorders, including autism, soared from 1 in 2,000 in the 1980s to 1 in 166 by the early 2000s. This book does not claim that Thimerosal is the only factor in these alarming prevalence rates. It does, however, call for common-sense recognition of the possible role this neurotoxin may have played in the sudden rise in the spectrum of neurodevelopmental disorders.

During the writing of this book, I was approached by a CDC researcher who felt personally led to expose instances of research misconduct within the CDC, particularly with regard to a 2004 Pediatrics article, *Age at First Measles-Mumps-Rubella Vaccination in Children With Autism and School-matched Control Subjects: A Population-Based Study in Metropolitan Atlanta*. As this book discloses, this is not the first instance of CDC conduct to come under scrutiny. Regrettably, studies on the relationship between vaccines and autism have been subject to misconduct including data manipulation and false reporting.

Many of the CDC's own studies have demonstrated a link between increased Thimerosal exposures and the development of vocal and motor tics, which are generally recognized as autism-like features. This alarming association has been downplayed to the public. Sadly, public health agencies' insistence on Thimerosal's safety has effectively inhibited objective investigations into research misconduct and conflicts of interest within health agencies and the vaccine industry.

I'm from the "Sunshine State" and believe that sunlight is the greatest disinfectant. In this book, Robert F. Kennedy, Jr. clearly sets forth the unvarnished truth on Thimerosal.

Benjamin Franklin once said, "Being ignorant is not so much a shame, as being unwilling to learn." With regard to Thimerosal in childhood vaccines, we have yet to heed Mr. Franklin's words. After reading this book, I hope you will join us in the battle to make vaccines safer for all.

US Congressman Bill Posey

Preface

Vaccinations are among the most important advances in medicine in the last century. We have eradicated smallpox from the planet and dramatically reduced death and suffering from infectious disease around the globe.

I am aggressively pro-vaccine, as are the editor and introduction contributor of this book. I am a father and family physician. I have vaccinated my children. I have been vaccinated and recommend vaccination to my patients.

Critics of this book will quickly polarize the debate. It is easy to oversimplify the issue of Thimerosal into pro-vaccine or anti-vaccine, or to confuse this issue by debating whether Thimerosal causes autism, which has not been definitively proven. This is unfortunate, and detracts from a much simpler set of questions that are ultimately the subject of this scientifically dense book.

There is no debate that mercury in any form is toxic. Scientists may debate the differences in toxicity between different forms of mercury, such as ethylmercury (which is an ingredient in Thimerosal) or methylmercury (from fish). But all would agree that mercury is a potent neurotoxin.

There is also no debate about the dramatic increase in prevalence of neurodevelopmental disorders, over the last few decades, including learning disabilities, attention deficit disorders, and autism.

There may, however, be debate on the strength of the data and science implicating mercury in this increased prevalence of brain injury in children. These questions can never be adequately answered given the challenges of doing experimental studies on human subjects over long periods of time. Obviously, no ethical review board would ever approve a study in which children were purposefully exposed to mercury in order to test its toxicity. Population studies show correlations, but never prove causation, making it impossible to draw firm conclusions.

That leaves us with a very simple, moral question, and ultimately a very personal one. Because at some point in our lives, nearly all of us will have a child or grandchild who requires vaccinations. Or we will know a pregnant woman who will have to decide whether or not to get a flu shot that might contain mercury. All of us are people and parents first, and scientists and policy makers second.

So there is only one question that really matters:

> Would you expose the unborn child or infant of a loved one to a vaccine containing mercury, a known neurotoxin, if there were other safer alternatives?

The answer to this question is simply common sense and requires no further scientific inquiry, but as Voltaire said, "common sense is not so common."

If there were no other options, if it were a question of whether to vaccinate or not to vaccinate, then of course we would choose vaccination.

But that is a false choice. There are 137 million children born each year in the world. Is our only option to subject them to a potent neurotoxin in their most delicate neurodevelopmental period? How can we best protect that future generation from preventable harm?

The arguments put forth that we cannot remove Thimerosal from vaccines are invalid. Thimerosal has already been removed from nearly all vaccines except the multidose flu vaccine in the United States. This was based on government recommendations and a call to action from many agencies and health organizations, as is well documented in this book.

However, Thimerosal still remains in nearly all the pediatric vaccines used in the developing world. There are effective alternative preservatives already in use (2-phenoxyethanol), and new ones can be developed. The Food and Drug Administration (FDA) banned mercury as a topical antiseptic (remember Mercurochrome?). And any medical products containing Thimerosal or mercury cannot be thrown in the garbage. The Environmental Protection Agency (EPA) considers them hazardous waste. Does it make any sense that even though Thimerosal is not safe to put on your skin, or to throw in the garbage, it is safe to inject into pregnant women and babies?

Cost considerations are also used as an argument to keep Thimerosal in vaccines. There is a small cost increase to use single-dose flu vaccines, but it is minor compared to the cost of neurodevelopmental disease in children. The global cost of taking Thimerosal out of all vaccines is $300 million a year, while the annual cost of autism in the United States alone is well over $100 billion. In the developing world, studies show that there is significant wastage of multidose vials, making single-dose vials comparable in cost.

There are other arguments. Some scientists we spoke to at the Department of Health and Human Services said that Thimerosal may contribute to the effectiveness of the vaccines. Any agent that increases vaccine effectiveness is referred to as an adjuvant. However, Thimerosal is approved for use only as a preservative, not as an active ingredient, and such use is illegal.

I have been involved in reviewing and contributing ideas and scientific references to this manuscript. I have also been involved in efforts to change regulatory and legislative policy to reduce potential harm from Thimerosal. I do not belong to any organization connected in any way with this issue. Nor do I have any personal or financial interest in this issue other than a scientific and moral one.

And, as a physician, my Hippocratic oath is to "first, do no harm." We should practice the precautionary principle in medicine and avoid doing harm whenever possible. And given the simple fact that mercury is toxic, I can come to no other conclusion than this: we should immediately remove Thimerosal from vaccines and all other products used in medicine.

Mark Hyman, MD
West Stockbridge, Massachusetts
June 7, 2014

Introduction: Removal of Mercury from Vaccines in the Epoch of Error Correction

This book is aggressively pro-vaccine. Its focus is not on vaccines in any general way, but only on one particular ingredient, Thimerosal, which contains ethylmercury.

Although the conversation surrounding vaccines, as with any medical issue, has many facets (especially when you consider technical issues), many people are aware of only two black-and-white options: you are either pro-vaccine, or anti-vaccine. If you are a reader who wishes to absorb and evaluate the information in this book, I ask you to consider that, at minimum, there is a third alternative: you can be pro-vaccine and at the same time seek to improve the vaccine program.[i]

This book advocates one specific step to improve vaccines: removing a known neurotoxin (mercury, in the form of Thimerosal) from the list of ingredients. To make a strong case for taking this step, the book presents voluminous evidence of:

- The toxicity of Thimerosal
- Its ineffectiveness even in the bactericidal role it is supposed to play
- Safer alternatives to Thimerosal that are already available
- A history of the calls of scientists and high-level governmental and international agencies around the world to remove Thimerosal entirely from vaccines
- Implementation of this course of action in some other countries

It argues that removing Thimerosal entirely will improve both vaccines themselves and people's trust in them.

That mercury is toxic cannot be disputed. To say otherwise is to pick a fight with the periodic table and the fundamental principles of physical chemistry. Consider the organization of electrons in atoms. Mercury is a large, heavy atom with more orbitals than lighter metals, like copper or zinc, and has a greater capacity to pick up and exchange electrons. The specific ways it can do this are not as tightly determined as in lighter atoms, making it a biochemical "wild card." Mercury is thus a metabolic poison because it can insinuate itself into situations where it doesn't belong. In particular it can substitute itself for lighter metals like zinc and selenium around which critical ancient enzyme systems are designed. This grossly cripples the specificity of enzymes and rates of reaction, and can spread chaos in the networks of metabolic processes, which try to generate workarounds to this logjam—but at great cost to biological and energetic resources, and often without success. This chaos may disrupt development as well as ongoing function throughout life.

Moreover, while claims have been made that the ethylmercury in Thimerosal is safer than the much better-studied methylmercury, these claims are based on weak, questionable evidence and poorly chosen assumptions. As reviewed in Chapters 4–6 herein, available data suggests that the toxicity of these two forms of mercury is at least comparable, and that ethylmercury may leave the blood more quickly—only to persist more stubbornly in organs and tissues of the body, particularly the brain.

Furthermore, mercury's toxicity can be even worse in the presence of aluminum, which is also an ingredient in many vaccines and has toxicity issues of its own (Chapter 11).

This all being the case, why are we still putting mercury in vaccines—or in any medical product (roughly 169 consumer products including eyedrops and nose drops still contain Thimerosal)—and how can we bring ourselves to stop doing this?

To generate the fortitude to do the right thing, it may help to put this problem in a broader context.

Although potentially hazardous substances have long been buried in the seams of the earth's mantle, leaching slowly or on occasion volcanically exploding into the living environment, human activities have contributed greatly to bringing them to the surface and putting them into circulation. Our clever, problem-solving minds have created a flood of ingenious products that increase demand for—and exposures to—these sources of potential harm.

For many years our measurement instruments were blunt enough that we only detected problems when exposures were severe. Concerns about an underbelly to our inventions were buried under elation about remarkable innovation and progress. There was little motivation to look broadly for latent or downstream effects.

Today, however, our confidence in progress is no longer so dominant, and we have entered a period of pervasive fragility. Planetary biogeochemical cycles are becoming unstable; economic vulnerabilities are persisting rather than resolving; large numbers of people are chronically ill despite enormous health care expenditures; 100,000 people a year die from unintended effects of medications used according to label;[ii] and systems science is increasingly suggesting that we need fresh approaches to health care, product development, energy, and ecosystems management.

It appears that our world is finally grasping our pileup of a huge number of errors, and we are at last entering an epoch of error correction.

What is an error? Put simply, it is a mismatch between our predictions and the outcomes. Put in systems terms, an "error" is an action that looks like a success when viewed through a narrow lens, but whose disruptive additional effects become apparent when we zoom out.

Why do predictions fail to anticipate major complications? Ironically the exquisite precision of our science may itself promote error generation. This is because precision is usually achieved by ignoring context and all the variation outside of our narrow focus, even though biological systems in particular are intrinsically variable and complex rather than uniform and simple. In fact our brains utilize this subtlety and context to make important distinctions, but our scientific methods mostly do not. The problems that come back to bite us then come from details we didn't consider.

Once an error is entrenched it can be hard to change course. The initial investment in the error, plus fear of the likely expense (both in terms of time and money) of correcting the error, as well as the threat of damage to the reputations of those involved—these all serve as deterrents to shifting course. Patterns of avoidance then emerge that interfere with free and unbiased conduct of scientific investigations and public discourse. But if the error is not corrected, its negative consequences will continue to accumulate. When change eventually becomes unavoidable, it will be a bigger, more complicated, and expensive problem to correct—with further delay making things still worse.

Some errors happen out of naïveté and then perpetuate themselves—the introduction of non-native species, such as rabbits in Australia that lack local predators, need not be repeated for the problem to perpetuate itself. Some catastrophes, such as the British Petroleum oil spill in the Gulf of Mexico, are local but with widely dispersed consequences, and they dramatize the need for upgrading workflows and standards to prevent similar catastrophes in the future. Some disasters occur through a combination of errors—for example, in the case of Hurricane Katrina and the flooding of New Orleans, the combination of institutional failures and a global warming–driven increase in the power and frequency of storms. These catastrophes and disasters are often worsened by a series of unfortunate actions and/or inaction.

When it comes to mercury, not only is it clearly toxic, even at very low exposures,[iii iv v] but our bodies derive no physiological benefit from it whatsoever. Nevertheless, one out of six children in the United States is born with levels of mercury high enough to be put at risk for neurological complications like learning disabilities, motor skill impairments, and short-term memory loss.[vi]

We can be exposed to mercury by eating fish (particularly those predators high on the food chain), being downwind of coal-fired power plants and other coal-fired industrial processes such as cement kilns, being near mines, being downwind of trash incinerators that burn hazardous and medical waste, breaking mercury-containing devices such as older thermometers, and having dental amalgams. People, including infants and pregnant mothers, can also be exposed to mercury through vaccines. In the United States, this exposure comes mainly from influenza vaccines. Although Thimerosal was removed from mandatory childhood vaccines in the United States, cumulative exposure is still high due to regular Thimerosal-containing flu shot administration starting in pregnancy and infancy. In other countries, however, particularly in developing countries (Chapters 2 and 3), more types of vaccines may contain mercury, and at higher levels.

To reduce the population's exposure to mercury from non-vaccine sources requires policy, educational, and technical changes targeting wide swaths of the population and many different industries and communities. It is a protracted process that will be slowed by significant industry pushback. In addition, the oceans, atmosphere, waterways, and areas of land that have been contaminated with mercury will be very difficult to clean up comprehensively.

To take mercury out of vaccines is a different matter. It is used as a preservative in multidose vials, even though it doesn't actually do that job so well (Chapter 10), and we have safe and effective alternatives (Chapter 12). Companies making vaccines could either change the preservative or shift to single-dose vials, which actually will not increase societal costs as much as has been claimed, because of wastage associated with multidose vials (see Chapter 12 and the book's recommendations). The big point here is that there are a finite and modest number of entities that need to make a discrete and specific change—and then the job of getting mercury out of vaccines will be done.

You may ask why we should take mercury out of vaccines if there's no definitive proof that vaccines or the mercury in them causes autism. To this I will answer: that is not the right question. The right question is, *why do we persist in putting a potent toxin into a vital medical product when we don't really need to?*

Complex chronic illnesses are generally multifactorial—genetic weak spots may create vulnerability—but a pileup of noxious exposures and stressors is what wears the system down. I include autism in the broad category of complex chronic disease because of the thousands of papers now in the scientific literature documenting pathophysiology such as oxidative stress, dysfunction of mitochondrial bioenergetics, and immune/inflammatory responses that greatly overlap with what we are finding in other chronic illnesses.[vii][viii] For all of these conditions the tipping point is not just the environmental insult itself, but the way it overwhelms the system, which has been pushed close to the edge by a prior accumulation of environmental insults that have been progressively degrading the physiological systems in our bodies and brains. The shift into an illness state may be gradual, or it may occur at some particular point when the physiological systems cannot compensate anymore and shift their functioning to a less resource- and energy-demanding (and thereby less efficient) state. I predict that ultimately we will determine that it is not any one or a few environmental risk factors that uniquely tip people over into chronic illness, but rather the total, degradative load (or "allostatic load") of exposures, stressors, and low-nutrient-density food that tips most people over the edge into illness from latent vulnerabilities.[ix x xi xii]

From the vantage point of a total (allostatic) load model of chronic disease, basic management and prevention principles include reducing noxious exposures and stressors as much as possible, and also increasing nutritional and lifestyle supports.[xiii] Every little bit counts—and in the case of mercury, it is so toxic that even a little bit can go a long way in dragging the system down. As a metabolic "wild card" mercury does not have a one-to-one relationship with specific illnesses; but rather, by disturbing fundamental developmental processes and acting as a metabolic poison, it degrades the integrity of the system and aggravates people's vulnerabilities. In particular, it poisons critical core regulatory and protective pathways (including methylation, DNA repair, and thioredoxin)[xiv xv xvi xvii xviii xix xx]—and, when such systems are dysfunctional, many things suffer. Even at low doses it can interfere with chemical processes in brain and body, lead to gross and subtle neuromotor problems and subtle or dramatic cognitive impairment,[xxi] promote autoimmune conditions such as rheumatoid arthritis and multiple sclerosis,[xxii] and bias the system toward being more fragile and vulnerable to future challenges.

Even so, while our physiology has environmentally vulnerable spots where mercury can contribute to this process of system overload and degradation, those same physiological processes are also vulnerable to myriad other noxious influences.[xxiii] From both the total (allostatic) load and the precautionary points of view, mercury is among a broad range of noxious exposures that degrade body and brain health. Such exposures should therefore be totally avoided, if possible.[xxiv] Different people may have different weak points, making epidemiology of particular diseases an insensitive way to pick up the range of mercury's impacts.

With all of this in mind, the bottom line is that *by exposing the population to unnecessary mercury in vaccines, we are gambling with population health through the same intervention that we use to protect it.*

The painful truth is that our country and planet face a rocky road in years to come—unstable weather patterns, fires, natural disasters, risks of novel infectious diseases, risks of food and water shortages, health problems exacerbated by these environmen tal challenges, and prospects of recurrent economic constriction. Under these circumstances, why would we want to expose our population to yet another noxious stressor that could further deplete our resilience and interfere with our ability to think straight—when it is totally unnecessary?

Based upon all of this, it is clear now that mercury is something to which no one should be deliberately exposed. As such, it is an error to include it in vaccines or indeed in any therapeutics—and in these domains it is an error within our grasp to correct, and prudent to do so. We tend to take a long time to correct errors[xxv]—it took seventy-five years to get the lead out of gasoline.[xxvi] [xxvii] Let's do a better job this time. So many considerations and pieces of evidence are compiled in this one comprehensive volume. I hope and implore that it moves us all to do whatever it takes—make whatever adjustments necessary—to correct this error, because it CAN be corrected—indeed MUST be corrected—so let's just DO IT. THEN we can focus more effectively on the harder problems lying ahead.

Martha R. Herbert, PhD, MD

Notes

[i] Poland GA, Kennedy RB, McKinney BA, Ovsyannikova IG, Lambert ND, Jacobson RM, et al. Vaccinomics, adversomics, and the immune response network theory: individualized vaccinology in the 21st century. Seminars in immunology. 2013;25(2):89-103. doi: 10.1016/j.smim.2013.04.007. PubMed PMID: 23755893; PubMed Central PMCID: PMC3752773.

[ii] Lazarou J, Pomeranz BH, Corey PN. Incidence of adverse drug reactions in hospitalized patients: a meta-analysis of prospective studies. JAMA. 1998;279(15):1200-5. PubMed PMID: 9555760.

[iii] US National Institute of Environmental Health Sciences. Mercury.http://www.niehs.nih.gov/health/topics/agents/mercury/.

[iv] US Food and Drug Administration, US Environmental Protection Agency. What You Need to Know About Mercury in Fish and Shellfish (Brochure). March, 2004:http://www.fda.gov/food/resourcesforyou/consumers/ucm110591.htm.

[v] Agency for Toxic Substances and Disease Registry CfDC. Toxic Substances Portal - Mercury. April, 1999:http://www.atsdr.cdc.gov/toxfaqs/tf.asp?id=113&tid=24.

[vi] US National Institute of Environmental Healthy Sciences. Child Development and Environmental Toxins.http://www.niehs.nih.gov/health/assets/docs_a_e/child_development_and_environmental_toxins_508.pdf.

[vii] Rossignol DA, Frye RE. A review of research trends in physiological abnormalities in autism spectrum disorders: immune dysregulation, inflammation, oxidative stress, mitochondrial dysfunction and environmental toxicant exposures. Mol Psychiatry. 2012;17(4):389-401. doi: 10.1038/mp.2011.165. PubMed PMID: 22143005; PubMed Central PMCID: PMC3317062.

[viii] Khansari N, Shakiba Y, Mahmoudi M. Chronic inflammation and oxidative stress as a major cause of age-related diseases and cancer. Recent patents on inflammation & allergy drug discovery. 2009;3(1):73-80. PubMed PMID: 19149749.

[ix] Herbert M. Autism: From Static Genetic Brain Defect to Dynamic Gene-Environment Modulated Pathophysiology. In: Krimsky S, Gruber J, editors. Genetic Explanations: Sense and Nonsense. Cambridge, MA: Harvard University Press; 2013. p. 122-46.

[x] Herbert MR, Weintraub K. The Autism Revolution: Whole Body Strategies for Making Life All It Can Be. New York, NY: Random House with Harvard Health Publications; 2012.

[xi] McEwen BS. Stress, adaptation, and disease. Allostasis and allostatic load. Ann N Y Acad Sci. 1998;840:33-44. Epub 1998/06/18. PubMed PMID: 9629234.

xii Knox SS. From 'omics' to complex disease: a systems biology approach to gene-environment interactions in cancer. Cancer Cell Int. 2010;10:11; http://www.cancerci.com/content/0/1/. Epub 2010/04/28. doi: 1475-2867-10-11 [pii]. 10.1186/1475-2867-10-11. PubMed PMID: 20420667; PubMed Central PMCID: PMC2876152.

xiii Herbert MR. Everyday Epigenetics: From Molecular Intervention to Public Health and Lifestyle Medicine. North American Journal of Medicine and Science. 2013;6(3):167-70 (open access).

xiv Carvalho CM, Chew EH, Hashemy SI, Lu J, Holmgren A. Inhibition of the human thioredoxin system. A molecular mechanism of mercury toxicity. J Biol Chem. 2008;283(18):11913-23. doi: 10.1074/jbc.M710133200. PubMed PMID: 18321861.

xv Arner ES, Holmgren A. Physiological functions of thioredoxin and thioredoxin reductase. European journal of biochemistry / FEBS. 2000;267(20):6102-9. PubMed PMID: 11012661.

xvi Pilsner JR, Lazarus AL, Nam DH, Letcher RJ, Sonne C, Dietz R, et al. Mercury-associated DNA hypomethylation in polar bear brains via the LUminometric Methylation Assay: a sensitive method to study epigenetics in wildlife. Molecular ecology. 2010;19(2):307-14. doi: 10.1111/j.1365-294X.2009.04452.x. PubMed PMID: 20002585.

xvii Ariza ME, Holliday J, Williams MV. Mutagenic effect of mercury (II) in eukaryotic cells. In vivo. 1994;8(4):559-63. PubMed PMID: 7893984.

xviii Goodrich JM, Basu N, Franzblau A, Dolinoy DC. Mercury biomarkers and DNA methylation among Michigan dental professionals. Environ Mol Mutagen. 2013;54(3):195-203. doi: 10.1002/em.21763. PubMed PMID: 23444121; PubMed Central PMCID: PMC3750961.

xix Hanna CW, Bloom MS, Robinson WP, Kim D, Parsons PJ, vom Saal FS, et al. DNA methylation changes in whole blood is associated with exposure to the environmental contaminants, mercury, lead, cadmium and bisphenol A, in women undergoing ovarian stimulation for IVF. Hum Reprod. 2012;27(5):1401-10. doi: 10.1093/humrep/des038. PubMed PMID: 22381621; PubMed Central PMCID: PMC3329190.

xx Al Bakheet SA, Attafi IM, Maayah ZH, Abd-Allah AR, Asiri YA, Korashy HM. Effect of long-term human exposure to environmental heavy metals on the expression of detoxification and DNA repair genes. Environmental pollution. 2013;181:226-32. doi: 10.1016/j.envpol.2013.06.014. PubMed PMID: 23872045.

xxi Grandjean P, Landrigan PJ. Neurobehavioural effects of developmental toxicity. Lancet Neurol. 2014;13(3):330-8. doi: 10.1016/S1474-4422(13)70278-3. PubMed PMID: 24556010.

xxii Silbergeld EK, Silva IA, Nyland JF. Mercury and autoimmunity: implications for occupational and environmental health. Toxicol Appl Pharmacol. 2005;207(2 Suppl):282-92. doi: 10.1016/j.taap.2004.11.035. PubMed PMID: 16023690.

xxiii Herbert MR. Contributions of the environment and environmentally vulnerable physiology to autism spectrum disorders. Curr Opin Neurol. 2010;23(2):103-10. Epub 2010/01/21. doi: 10.1097/WCO.0b013e328336a01f. PubMed PMID: 20087183.

xxiv Liu J, Lewis G. Environmental toxicity and poor cognitive outcomes in children and adults. Journal of environmental health. 2014;76(6):130-8. PubMed PMID: 24645424.

xxv Grandjean P, Choi A. The delayed appearance of a mercurial warning. Epidemiology. 2008;19(1):10-1. doi: 10.1097/EDE.0b013e31815c481a. PubMed PMID: 18091412.

xxvi Kitman JL. The Secret History of Lead. The Nation. 2000 (March 20):http://www. thenation.com/article/secret-history-lead.

xxvii United Nations Environmental Program. Phasing Lead Out of Gasoline: An Examination of Policy Approaches in Different Countries. Stevenage, Hertfordshire, UK: Earthprint (University of London); 1999.

Author's Introduction

People who advocate for safer vaccines should not be marginalized or denounced as anti-vaccine. I am pro-vaccine. I had all six of my children vaccinated. I believe that vaccines have saved the lives of hundreds of millions of humans over the past century and that broad vaccine coverage is critical to public health. But I want our vaccines to be as safe as possible.

Indeed, the greatest threats to the kind of widespread vaccine coverage needed to protect global health are public doubt about vaccine safety and mistrust of vaccine regulators. And we cannot heal that mistrust by simply dismissing legitimate questions about Thimerosal as the fruit of mindless paranoia. For example, solid peer-reviewed science supports the well-documented popular skepticism about the safety of the mercury-laden vaccine preservative Thimerosal.

As this book shows, there is a broad consensus among research scientists that Thimerosal is a dangerous neurotoxin that should be immediately removed from medicines. Several hundred peer-reviewed scientific publications by the world's leading research scientists, public health agencies, universities, and teaching hospitals have confirmed that Thimerosal is a potent neurotoxin that has never been proven safe for medical use and for which cost-effective alternatives exist.

Indeed, the evidence of Thimerosal's neurotoxicity is so overwhelming and the lack of any safety data so complete that anyone who is willing to read science and who believes in the capacity for scientific methods to determine empirical truths must conclude that Thimerosal causes serious brain damage.

I am rabidly pro-science. For thirty years as a litigator and environmental advocate, I have fought to make rigorous science the driver of public policy in the global warming arena, in the tobacco wars, and in my many battles with pesticide and chemical companies as well as in many dozens of legal skirmishes ranging from the Hudson River to Alaska's Cook Inlet, from the West Virginia coal fields to the Louisiana oil patch, from the Caribbean island of Vieques to Puget Sound. I have fought these battles on issues including acid rain, ozone, coal ash, particulates, PCBs, lead, mercury, hydrocarbons, pesticides, and numerous other poisons that have been the subject of the hundreds of cases I've argued against polluters and their crooked scientists.

For many years, I've been puzzled by the bland and apparently baseless insistence by public health regulators and members of the press that it is safe to inject mercury—one of the world's most neurotoxic elements—into young children and pregnant women. Over the past three years, I've engaged a crack team of respected scientific researchers to review the voluminous peer-reviewed literature related to Thimerosal and human health. Not surprisingly, that team was unable to find even a single publication that credibly demonstrates Thimerosal's safety. Meanwhile, reams of toxicological, pharmacological, epidemiological, animal, and human studies have implicated Thimerosal in a range of neurological disorders. In fact, there is a virtually unanimous scientific consensus among the hundreds of research scientists who have published peer-reviewed articles in the field that Thimerosal is immensely toxic to brain tissue and should not be injected into children.

Nevertheless, today, we continue to expose millions of babies and pregnant women in this country and elsewhere to one of the world's most potent neurotoxins, even though far safer and more economic alternatives exist. Most US vaccine makers, for example, have already switched to Thimerosal-free injections in pediatric vaccines administered to American children. And the vaccine industry had pleaded with the CDC to allow it to switch to non-toxic alternatives in the remaining Thimerosal-preserved vaccines. The CDC's refusal to allow the transition is baffling. I assembled this book to make that task easier for the agency and to dissuade the press from accepting the tired claim that anyone who questions Thimerosal safety is "anti-science" and "anti-vaccine."

Robert F. Kennedy, Jr.

Executive
Summary

The public widely believes that Thimerosal, a controversial, mercury-containing preservative used in some vaccines since the 1930s, was eliminated from the vaccine supply a decade ago.[1][2][3] However, Thimerosal is still being used in significant and perhaps dangerous quantities, despite the fact that:

1. There is convincing evidence of Thimerosal's harm to human health, particularly in vulnerable populations of infants and young children to whom health providers have administered Thimerosal most heavily.
2. Concerns over vaccine safety, including exposure to Thimerosal, continue to have a negative impact on vaccination rates, public trust, and, thus, public health.[4][5][6]
3. Evidence has not shown Thimerosal to be a consistently effective preservative, and safer, better preservative alternatives are readily available.

Public health agencies and government officials have repeatedly declared Thimerosal-preserved vaccines to be safe. Among the most important examples of these statements is a widely known report from the Institute of Medicine (IOM) published in 2004. The report purported to refute any link between Thimerosal exposure and autism. However, this conclusion was based almost entirely on epidemiological studies, which are unable to prove causation. Furthermore, the epidemiological studies have many flaws, and their authors possess significant conflicts of interest.[7]

Despite the official line on Thimerosal's safety, an earlier report from the IOM in 2001, as well as from other public health agencies, government officials, and scientists, have raised significant concerns about Thimerosal-preserved vaccines.[8][9] Overall, the official statements from governmental health organizations have neither reflected nor acknowledged a vast, accumulating, and compelling body of research contradicting safety contentions.[10][11][12][13][14][15] Evidence from epidemiological, animal, cell culture, and clinical studies in the United States and from abroad suggests that the mercury in Thimerosal can in fact cause brain injury in children.

The quality and strength of the data vary; however, when taken as a whole, the evidence for potential harm cannot be ignored. We can call for more data, more studies, and more trials, though we recognize that long-term outcome studies covering decades are unlikely ever to be done. Nevertheless, we believe there is already more than sufficient data to determine probable risk and to call for a global effort to switch from Thimerosal to a safer preservative or to single-dose vials that do not require preservatives.

Exposure to Thimerosal increased beginning in 1989 and rose sharply during the early 1990s as new vaccines were added to

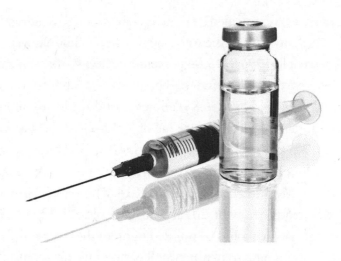

the US childhood vaccine schedule. This increased exposure to mercury via vaccines coincided closely with increased case reports of neurodevelopmental disorders, including a dramatic increase in autism spectrum disorder (ASD) cases and a rise in attention deficit hyperactivity disorder (ADHD).[16][17] According to various studies, the prevalence of ASDs rose in the US from a historical rate of approximately 1 in 2,000 through the 1980s to as high as 1 in 166 children by the early 2000s.[18][19] Attention problems reported by pediatricians' offices rose from 1.4 percent of patients in 1979 to 9.2 percent by 1996, according to one study, with other studies also documenting a steady upward movement in rates of ADD and ADHD from 1970s' baselines.[20][21][22]

Although Thimerosal now only appears in trace amounts in vaccines on the US childhood immunization schedule, the potential threat to children's neurological health continues today in the form of seasonal flu vaccines, preserved with Thimerosal, that are administered to pregnant women and babies.[23][24][25][26][27] Recent CDC figures confirm

ADHD prevalence has remained as high as nearly 1 in 10 children.[28][29] The prevalence of any developmental disability in US children went up from 12.84 percent in 1996 to 15.04 percent by 2008.[30] ASD statistical rates, for their part, have soared higher still. In March 2012, the reported prevalence (as of 2008, in 8 year olds) stood at 1 in 88 children; in March 2013, the prevalence figure (as of 2011–2012, between the ages of 6 and 17 years) came in at a staggering 1 in 50 children, with 1 in 31 boys affected, though this report was based on a less-reliable survey of parents. Most recently, in March 2014, a more reliable figure of 1 in 68 was reported (as of 2010, in 8 year olds).[31][32][33][34][35] (For clarification purposes, it should be pointed out that the common claim of autism rates continuing to climb after Thimerosal's phaseout from the routine childhood vaccination schedule in 2003 has not, as yet, been borne out. Most of the children assessed in the recently published prevalence surveys were born in the late 1990s and early 2000s, and thus subject to Thimerosal exposure rates from that time.)

Thimerosal is not likely to be solely responsible for the documented spike in neurodevelopmental disorders in recent decades. For ASD, for instance, a number of other contributing genetic and environmental factors are under investigation. Even so, the evidence suggesting a link between Thimerosal and a large percentage of neurodevelopmental disorders, as this document will detail, mandates action. There are nearly four million children born every year in the United States and about 137 million children born annually around the world, and many of them appear to be at risk of injury from the Thimerosal in vaccines.[36][37]

In the interest of reducing potential health risks, assuaging public fears, and increasing domestic and global vaccination rates, this book's editors, and a substantial cohort of other experts, assert that Thimerosal should be removed from all vaccines. This book aims to compile and evaluate all germane research on Thimerosal. It will examine Thimerosal's historical and ongoing use in vaccines while documenting the real extent of its potential hazards and disadvantages.

This document is organized as follows.

Part One reviews the known dangers of mercury exposure, the history of Thimerosal use in the United States, studies showing that Thimerosal is harmful, and recommendations by scientists and various organizations for the elimination of Thimerosal from medical products.

Part Two demonstrates that Thimerosal is not an effective preservative and explains that a shift away from Thimerosal-preserved, multidose vaccine vials to single-dose vials (which do not require preservatives) can make economic as well as moral sense, both domestically and abroad.

Part Three explores the scientific literature concerning potential relationships between Thimerosal exposure and autism.

Part Four reviews the methodological flaws and conflicts of interest that undermine the credibility of the oft-cited scientific literature disavowing links between Thimerosal and neurological damage. Part Four also relates the inappropriate and biased actions taken by governmental agencies and their agency representatives defending Thimerosal and suppressing research into its potential dangers.

Part Five discusses the failure of the media to accurately and responsibly cover the Thimerosal controversy.

Based on this book's analysis, we are calling for policy and industry shifts that will lead to Thimerosal's removal from all remaining vaccines within a year. Vaccines are unquestionably one of the greatest achievements in medical science. They have prevented countless terrible illnesses. We hope that the elimination of an unnecessary mercury-containing ingredient in vaccines will ease future doubts about vaccine safety. Restoring faith in the vaccine regimen while maintaining or increasing vaccination rates is critical in the United States and especially in developing nations, where Thimerosal-containing childhood vaccines are still very much in use.

SUMMARY OF KEY FINDINGS AND RECOMMENDATIONS

Addressing the Risk of Thimerosal in Vaccines

The acknowledgment of the potential risk from Thimerosal by governmental health agencies as this document calls for would represent a significant public policy shift that is admittedly fraught with legitimate concerns, which include:

- Reducing public confidence in the safety of vaccines for children and for adults.
- A subsequent impact on vaccine compliance, and thus declines in vaccination rates.
- The cost of switching from Thimerosal-preserved vaccines to alternative vaccines or single-dose, preservative-free vaccines.

While these are fair concerns, what follows in brief are the facts that justify, allow, and compel a transition to a safe, effective, and cost-effective alternative vaccine strategy.

Thimerosal-Containing Vaccine Facts

- Although correlation does not prove causation, the increase in the number of Thimerosal-containing children's vaccines in the late 1980s and early 1990s coincided closely with a sudden jump in neurodevelopmental disorder diagnoses and deficits such as autism and attention problems.[38][39]

- Before 1989, the maximal Thimerosal dose by age two was 200 micrograms, which works out to 100 micrograms of mercury because Thimerosal is half ethylmercury by weight.[40][41][42][43] By 1999, the potential mercury exposure by age two had more than doubled to 237.5 micrograms, with a two month old receiving 62.5 micrograms or 125 times the Environmental Protection Agency's (EPA) safe reference dose (RfD) of 0.1 microgram per kilogram per day for methylmercury, a different, better-studied form of organic mercury than ethylmercury.[44][45][46]

- In 1999, based on recommendations from the American Academy of Pediatrics (AAP) and the United States Public Health Service (USPHS) agencies, which include the Centers for Disease Control and Prevention (CDC), the Food and Drug Administration (FDA), the National Institutes of Health (NIH), and the Health Resources and Services Administration (HRSA), removal of Thimerosal from the childhood vaccine schedule as a precautionary measure began. Yet Thimerosal has inexplicably remained in multidose flu vaccines still to the present day.[47][48]

- Today, CDC guidelines recommend annual flu vaccines for pregnant women and everyone over six months of age.[49] Based on these current flu shot recommendations, the average child could be exposed to as much as 187.5 micrograms of mercury by his or her eighth birthday.[50] In effect, the CDC has switched the main source of American children's Thimerosal exposure from early childhood vaccines to Thimerosal-preserved flu shots, with exposure beginning in utero.
- A single Thimerosal-preserved flu vaccine contains 25 micrograms of ethylmercury. If the EPA RfD for ingested methylmercury is applied to this injected ethylmercury figure, an individual would have to weigh more than 250 kilograms (551 pounds) for the 25 microgram exposure to be considered safe. Young children are commonly given half doses of Thimerosal-preserved flu shots nowadays, working out to approximately 14 times a safe daily exposure for a 20-pound (9-kilogram) individual.
- Rates of ASD and other neurodevelopmental disorders and deficits have continued to rise, perhaps in association with the exposure to Thimerosal through flu vaccines administered during early childhood and to pregnant women.

Toxicology: Ethylmercury vs. Methylmercury

- Mercury is a known and unquestioned neurotoxicant.[51] Most toxicology studies have been done on the form of mercury known as methylmercury, which is typically found in fish. However, there is substantial data that implicate ethylmercury, the type found in Thimerosal, as a similarly or perhaps even more potent biological toxin.

• Faster clearance from the blood of ethylmercury is used to argue for its lessened exposure risk compared to methylmercury.[52] Yet studies show that while ethylmercury quickly clears the blood, it is not excreted from the body and is instead preferentially deposited and sequestered in organs and tissues, including the brain.[53 54 55 56 57]

• Mercury easily passes through the placenta to the fetus, and some evidence has suggested ethylmercury might pass even more readily than methylmercury.[58 59 60 61 62 63 64]

Flawed Studies and the 2004 IOM Report

The 2004 IOM report stated that no causal link between autism and Thimerosal could be made, and that further research should focus on more promising lines of investigation about the etiology of autism.[65] This pronouncement was taken by government agencies, the media, and most researchers at face value. Yet the five epidemiologic papers that were primarily relied upon by the IOM to reach its conclusion contain many serious methodological flaws, and some of their authors have serious conflicts of interest. These flaws and conflicts are all exhaustively documented in Part Three, with some of the key points being:

• The Verstraeten 2003 study from the CDC underwent multiple revisions, such as excluding subgroups of children, before publication. With each revision, the relative risks for autism and some other neurodevelopmental disorders decreased. The final study showed no consistent significant associations between Thimerosal exposure and neurodevelopmental outcomes.[66]

- In the early runs of the data in the Verstraeten study, those children receiving the highest mercury dose of greater than 25 micrograms were, by one month of age, twice as likely to have speech/language delays, five-and-a-half times as likely to develop tics, anywhere from four to more than six times as likely to have attention-deficit disorder (ADD), from seven-and-a-half to more than eleven times as likely to have autism, and eight times as likely to have attention-deficit hyperactivity disorder (ADHD).[67 68]

- Verstraeten, who left the CDC to work for a major pharmaceutical company and maker of Thimerosal-preserved vaccines, himself reported that the findings published in 2003 were not negative, but neutral, and that further study was warranted.[69 70 71 72]

- Three of the IOM-accepted studies relied in whole or in part on Danish population autism statistics, which showed that autism levels increased after Thimerosal was removed from vaccines in 1992. This evidence strongly suggested that Thimerosal was not linked to autism. However, the IOM did not properly account for confounding factors in the data, such as the counting of both outpatient and inpatient cases after 1995 that expanded the number of children known to be affected, the adopted use of a broader definition of autism in 1994, and the exclusion prior to 1992 of the largest Danish clinic treating autism, which cared for 20 percent of autism cases.[73 74 75 76 77 78 79]

- Some of the researchers involved in the Danish studies and other European research accepted by the IOM had serious conflicts of interest by working directly for vaccine makers or receiving funding from national vaccine agencies, such as the CDC.[80 81 82 83 84 85 86 87 88 89 90 91]

In summary, the conclusions of the IOM report from 2004 should be viewed with extreme caution and skepticism and not as the final word on the theory of Thimerosal exposure causing autism (as well as other neurological injuries) in a significant portion of the affected population.

Policy Statements against Thimerosal

Numerous reports have called for the removal of Thimerosal from vaccines despite official statements otherwise offering reassurances about its safety. Concerns and statements have been made over the years as previously noted by the IOM, CDC, FDA, NIH, AAP, as well as the US Congress, the American Academy of Family Physicians (AAFP), the US Department of Agriculture (USDA), the European Medicines Agency, and the California Environmental Protection Agency (Cal/EPA). These expressions of concern are detailed in Chapter 9. This following sampling of statements reflects some of the widespread uncertainty regarding the safety of Thimerosal.

- In 1982, the FDA recommended that Thimerosal be banned from topical over-the-counter products.[92 93] In August of 1998, an FDA internal Point Paper recommended that for "investigational vaccines indicated for maternal immunization, the use of single-dose vials should be required to avoid the need of preservative in multidose vials. Of concern here is the potential neurotoxic effect of mercury, especially when considering cumulative doses of this component in early infancy."[94][95]

- In 2001, the IOM advised that "full consideration be given to removing Thimerosal from any biological or pharmaceutical product to which infants, children, and pregnant women are exposed."[96]
- In May 2003, the Committee on Government Reform of the US Congress found that "the committee, upon a thorough review of the scientific literature and internal documents from government and industry did find evidence that Thimerosal did pose a risk" and "[o]ur public health agencies' failure to act is indicative of institutional malfeasance for self-protection and misplaced protectionism of the pharmaceutical industry."[97]
- In 2004, the Cal/EPA stated, "The scientific evidence that . . . Thimerosal causes reproductive toxicity is clear and voluminous . . . [and] includes severe mental retardation or malformations in human offspring who were poisoned when their mothers were exposed to ethylmercury or Thimerosal while pregnant."[98]

Alternatives to Thimerosal-Preserved Vaccines

Finding alternatives to Thimerosal as a preservative in flu vaccines in the United States and in childhood vaccines around the world is critical. The facts suggest that safer, more effective preservatives exist and that cost considerations arguing against the removal of Thimerosal are unfounded.

- Currently, many childhood vaccines are given in single-dose vials that do not require a preservative.[99]
- An alternative preservative, 2-PE (2-phenoxyethanol), which is used in a childhood polio vaccine, was demonstrated to be 70 times less toxic than Thimerosal to human cells in a 2010 study.[100] [101]
- Thimerosal has also been shown to be less effective as a preservative than 2-PE.[102] [103]
- The cost of switching to single-dose vials for all vaccines globally is estimated at $300 million annually.[104] [105] The cost of autism in the United States alone, however, has recently been estimated at $137 billion annually.[106] [107] [108]
- According to a 2003 study, the per dose production cost of a single-dose vial is about 25 cents compared to 10 cents for a multidose vial. Yet that study estimated that 60 percent of multidose vials' contents is lost due to wastage, offsetting the multidose cost benefits.[109]
- This study also reported that health workers have shown reluctance opening multidose vials for vaccinating only a few children, leading to lower overall vaccination rates.
- Notably, the pharmaceutical industry has expressed a willingness and ability in the past to quickly shift away from Thimerosal preservation. Shortly after the July 1999 statement from the AAP/USPHS calling for Thimerosal's removal from childhood vaccines, two major vaccine manufacturers wrote letters to the CDC indicating that they could supply enough Thimerosal-free versions of their HepB and DTaP (diphtheria, tetanus, and acellular pertussis) products to meet the total vaccine demand. The

CDC, however, rejected this offer.[110] [111] [112] [113] [114] [115] [116] The FDA allowed the vaccine industry to market its existing Thimerosal-containing stocks, the last lots of which did not run out until 2003.[117] [118] [119] [120] [121]

Recommendations

- The immediate removal of Thimerosal from all vaccines globally, which has precedent in the United States (except for flu vaccines) with the post-1999 AAP/USPHS statement phaseout.

- The reevaluation of the cost-effectiveness of multidose vials considering reports of 60 percent wastage and missed vaccination opportunities because of the reluctance of health care workers to open multidose vials to vaccinate only a few children.

- The consideration of switching to single-dose vials, the use of 2-PE as an alternative preservative, and research into new and different preservative options.

Notes

1 http://www.putchildrenfirst.org/media/f.5.pdf.

2 http://www.cdc.gov/vaccinesafety/Concerns/thimerosal/index.html.

3 http://www.cdc.gov/vaccinesafety/concerns/thimerosal/thimerosal_timeline.html.

4 Kennedy A, Lavail K, Nowak G, Basket M, Landry S. Confidence about vaccines in the United States: understanding parents' perceptions. *Health Aff* (Millwood). 2011 Jun;30(6):1151-9.

5 http://online.wsj.com/article/SB10001424052702303863404577284001227981464.html.

6 http://www.cdc.gov/mmwr/preview/mmwrhtml/mm6133a2.htm.

7 Immunization Safety Review Committee, Board on Health Promotion and Disease Prevention, Institute of Medicine. *Immunization Safety Review: Vaccines and Autism.* National Academies Press. Washington, DC. May 2004.

8 Kathleen Stratton, Alicia Gable, and Marie C. McCormick, eds.; Immunization Safety Review Committee, Board on Health Promotion and Disease Prevention, Institute of Medicine. *Immunization Safety Review: Thimerosal-Containing Vaccines and Neurodevelopmental Disorders.* The National Academies Press. Washington, DC. October 1, 2001.

9 See Chapter 9 of this book for further references.

10 http://www.nytimes.com/2005/06/25/science/25autism.html?pagewanted=all.

11 http://articles.latimes.com/2010/mar/13/science/la-sci-autism13-2010mar13.

12 http://www.nytimes.com/2007/09/27/health/27vaccine.html?_r=1.

13 http://www.sfgate.com/news/article/California-study-finds-no-link-between-vaccine-3233360.php.

14 http://www.usatoday.com/news/health/2009-08-23-swine-flu-qna_N.htm.

15 http://www.newscientist.com/article/mg21728990.200-poison-pill-not-all-mercury-is-toxic.html.

16 Baker JP. Mercury, vaccines, and autism: one controversy, three histories. *Am J. Public Health.* 2008; 98:244–253.

17 Fombonne E. Epidemiology of pervasive developmental disorders. *Pediatr Res.* 2009 Jun;65(6):591-8.

18 Rutter M. Incidence of autism spectrum disorders: Changes over time and their meaning. *Acta Paediatrica.* 2005 Jan; 94(1): 2-15.

19 Fombonne E. Epidemiology of pervasive developmental disorders. *Pediatr Res.* 2009 Jun;65(6): 591-8.

[20] Kelleher KJ, McInerny TK, Gardner WP, Childs GE, Wasserman RC. Increasing identification of psychosocial problems: 1979-1996. *Pediatrics*. 2000 Jun;105(6):1313-21.

[21] http://www2.aap.org/pros/pdfs/Pearls/Pearl%20CBS%20-%20Increasing%20ID%20 of%20Psychosoc%20Probs.pdf.

[22] Safer DJ, Krager JM. A survey of medication treatment for hyperactive/inattentive students. *JAMA*. 1988 Oct 21;260(15):2256-8.

[23] http://www.fda.gov/BiologicsBloodVaccines/SafetyAvailability/VaccineSafety/ UCM096228.

[24] http://www.cdc.gov/mmwr/preview/mmwrhtml/rr5908a1.htm.

[25] http://www.cdc.gov/flu/about/season/index.htm.

[26] http://www.cdc.gov/flu/pdf/protect/vis-flu.pdf.

[27] http://www.cdc.gov/vaccines/parents/downloads/parent-ver-sch-0-6yrs.pdf.

[28] http://www.cdc.gov/mmwr/preview/mmwrhtml/mm5944a3.htm.

[29] http://www.cdc.gov/ncbddd/adhd/data.html.

[30] Boyle CA, Boulet S, Schieve LA, Cohen RA, Blumberg SJ, Yeargin-Allsopp M, Visser S, Kogan MD. Trends in the prevalence of developmental disabilities in US children, 1997-2008. *Pediatrics*. 2011 Jun;127(6):1034-42. doi: 10.1542/peds.2010-2989. Epub 2011 May 23.

[31] http://www.cdc.gov/media/releases/2012/p0329_autism_disorder.html.

[32] http://www.cdc.gov/media/releases/2013/a0320_autism_disorder.html.

[33] http://www.nytimes.com/2013/03/21/health/parental-study-shows-rise-in-autism-spectrum-cases.html?_r=0.

[34] http://beta.congress.gov/congressional-record/2013/04/26/extensions-of-remarks-section/ article/E576-1.

[35] http://www.cdc.gov/mmwr/preview/mmwrhtml/ss6302a1.htm?s_cid=ss6302a1_w.

[36] http://www.cdc.gov/nchs/fastats/births.htm.

[37] http://www.who.int/whr/2005/media_centre/facts_en.pdf.

[38] Baker JP. Mercury, vaccines, and autism: one controversy, three histories. *Am J. Public Health*. 2008; 98:244–253.

[39] Fombonne E. Epidemiology of pervasive developmental disorders. *Pediatr Res*. 2009 Jun;65(6):591-8.

[40] http://www.chop.edu/service/vaccine-education-center/vaccine-schedule/history-of-vaccine-schedule.html.

[41] http://www.cdc.gov/vaccines/pubs/vacc-timeline.htm.

[42] Committee on Infectious Diseases and Committee on Environmental Health, American Academy of Pediatrics. Thimerosal in vaccines—an interim report to clinicians. *Pediatrics*. 1999 Sep;104(3 Pt 1):570-4.

[43] Baker JP. Mercury, vaccines, and autism: one controversy, three histories. *Am J. Public Health*. 2008; 98:244–253.

[44] http://www.cdc.gov/mmwr/preview/mmwrhtml/00056261.htm.

l

[45] http://www.cdc.gov/growthcharts/data/set1clinical/cj41l017.pdf.

[46] http://www.epa.gov/hg/exposure.htm.

[47] http://www.cdc.gov/vaccinesafety/concerns/thimerosal/.

[48] Joint statement of the American Academy of Pediatrics (AAP) and the United States Public Health Service (USPHS). *Pediatrics.* 1999 Sep;104(3 Pt 1):568-9.

[49] http://www.cdc.gov/mmwr/preview/mmwrhtml/rr6207a1.htm.

[50] http://www.fda.gov/BiologicsBloodVaccines/SafetyAvailability/VaccineSafety/UCM09 6228.

[51] http://www.epa.gov/hg/health.htm.

[52] Pichichero ME, Cernichiari E, Lopreiato J, Treanor J. Mercury concentrations and metabolism in infants receiving vaccines containing thiomersal: a descriptive study. *Lancet.* 2002 Nov 30; 360(9347):1737-1741.

[53] Burbacher T, Shen D, Liberato N, Grant K, Cernichiari E, Clarkson T. Comparison of blood and brain mercury levels in infant monkeys exposed to methylmercury or vaccines containing thimerosal. *Environ Health Perspect.* 2005; 113(8):1015-1021.

[54] Harry GJ, Harris MW, Burka LT. Mercury concentrations in brain and kidney following ethylmercury, methylmercury and Thimerosal administration to neonatal mice. *Toxicol Lett.* 2004 Dec 30;154(3):183-9.

[55] http://adventuresinautism.blogspot.com/2008/03/mark-blaxill-and-boyd-haley-respond-to.html.

[56] Holmes AS, Blaxill MF, Haley BE. Reduced levels of mercury in first baby haircuts of autistic children. *Int J Toxic.* 2003;111(4):277-285.

[57] Blanuša M1, Orct T, Vihnanek Lazarus M, Sekovanić A, Piasek M. Mercury disposition in suckling rats: comparative assessment following parenteral exposure to thiomersal and mercuric chloride. J Biomed Biotechnol. 2012;2012:256965. doi: 10.1155/2012/256965. Epub 2012 Jul 26.

[58] Goldman LR, Shannon MW. AAP committee on Environmental Health technical report: mercury in the environment: implications for pediatricians. *Pediatrics.* 2001 Jul 1; 108: 197-205.

[59] Slikker W Jr. Developmental neurotoxicity of therapeutics: survey of novel recent findings. *Neurotoxicology.* 2000;21:50.

[60] Ayoub D, Yazbak F. Influenza vaccination during pregnancy: a critical assessment of the recommendations of the Advisory Committee on Immunization Practices (ACIP). *J Am Phys Surg.* 2006; 11(2):41-47.

[61] http://www.epa.gov/iris/subst/0073.htm.

[62] Fujita M, Takabatake E. Mercury levels in human maternal and neonatal blood, hair and milk. *Bull Environ Contam Toxicol.* 1977 Aug;18(2):205-9.

[63] Ukita T, Takeda Y, Sato Y, Takahashi T. Distribution of 203Hg labeled mercury compounds in adult and pregnant mice determined by whole-body autoradiography. *Radioisotopes.* 1967;16:439-448.

⁶⁴ Léonard A, Jacquet P, Lauwerys RR. Mutagenicity and teratogenicity of mercury compounds. *Mutat Res.* 1983 Jan; 114(1):1-18.

⁶⁵ Immunization Safety Review Committee, Board on Health Promotion and Disease Prevention, Institute of Medicine. *Immunization Safety Review: Vaccines and Autism.* National Academies Press. Washington, DC. May 2004.

⁶⁶ Verstraeten T, Davis RL, DeStefano F, Lieu TA, Rhodes PH, Black SB, Shinefield H, Chen RT. Safety of Thimerosal-Containing Vaccines: A Two-Phased Study of Computerized Health Maintenance Organization Databases. *Pediatrics.* 2003 Nov; 112(5): 1039-1048.

⁶⁷ Thomas Verstraeten, "It just won't go away," email to Robert Davis and Frank DeStefano, December 17, 1999.

⁶⁸ SafeMinds. *Generation Zero—Thomas Verstraeten's First Analyses of the Link Between Vaccine Mercury Exposure and the Risk of Diagnosis of Selected Neuro-Developmental Disorders Based on Data from the Vaccine Safety Datalink: November-December 1999.* September 2004.

⁶⁹ National Academy of Science, Institute of Medicine, Immunization Safety Review Committee. *Thimerosal-Containing Vaccines and Neurodevelopmental Outcomes.* Public Meeting. Cambridge, Massachusetts. Monday, July 16, 2001.

⁷⁰ Committee on Infectious Diseases and Committee on Environmental Health, American Academy of Pediatrics. Thimerosal in vaccines—an interim report to clinicians. *Pediatrics.* 1999 Sep;104(3 Pt 1):570-4.

⁷¹ http://www.gsk.com/products/our-vaccines.html.

⁷² Verstraeten T. Thimerosal, the Centers for Disease Control and Prevention, and GlaxoSmithKline. *Pediatrics.* 2004 Apr;113(4):932.

⁷³ Stehr-Green P, Tull P, Stellfeld M, Mortenson PB, Simpson D. Autism and thimerosal-containing vaccines: lack of consistent evidence for an association. *Am J Prev Med.* 2003 Aug;25(2):101-6.

⁷⁴ Madsen KM, Lauritsen MB, Pedersen CB, Thorsen P, Plesner AM, Andersen PH, Mortensen PB. Thimerosal and the occurrence of autism: negative ecological evidence from Danish population-based data. *Pediatrics.* 2003 Sep;112(3 Pt 1):604-6.

⁷⁵ Hviid A, Stellfeld M, Wohlfahrt J, Melbye M. Association between thimerosal-containing vaccine and autism. *JAMA.* 2003 Oct 1;290(13):1763-6.

⁷⁶ Madsen KM, Hviid A, Vestergaard M, Schendel D, Wohlfahrt J, Thorsen P, Olsen J, Melbye M. A population-based study of measles, mumps, and rubella vaccination and autism. *N Engl J Med.* 2002 Nov 7;347(19):1477-82.

⁷⁷ Blaxill, Mark; SafeMinds. *Danish Thimerosal-Autism Study in Pediatrics: Misleading and Uninformative on Autism-Mercury Link.* 2003 Sep *available at* http://www.SafeMinds.org/research/Blaxill-DenmarkAutismThimerosalPediatrics.pdf.

⁷⁸ Lauritsen MB, Pedersen CB, Mortensen PB. The incidence and prevalence of pervasive developmental disorders: a Danish population-based study. *Psychol Med.* 2004 Oct;34(7):1339-46.

⁷⁹ Trelka JA, Hooker BS. More on Madsen's analysis. *J Am Phys Surg.* 2004; 9(4):101.

[80] Rimland B. Association between thimerosal-containing vaccine and autism. *JAMA*. 2004 Jan 14;291(2):180; author reply 180-1.

[81] Stehr-Green P, Tull P, Stellfeld M, Mortenson PB, Simpson D. Autism and Thimerosal-containing vaccines lack of consistent evidence for an association. *Am J Prev Med*. 2003; 25(2): 101-106.

[82] http://www.putchildrenfirst.org/chapter5.html.

[83] http://www.putchildrenfirst.org/media/5.9.pdf.

[84] http://www.reuters.com/article/2011/04/13/us-crime-research-funds-idUS-TRE73C8JJ20110413.

[85] http://www.justice.gov/usao/gan/press/2011/04-13-11.html.

[86] http://www.huffingtonpost.com/robert-f-kennedy-jr/time-for-cdc-to-come-clea_b_16550.html.

[87] http://www.ageofautism.com/2010/03/poul-thorsens-mutating-resume.html.

[88] Transcript. Immunization Safety Review Committee, Vaccines and Autism. February 9, 2004. Institute of Medicine of the National Academy of Sciences. Washington DC *available at* http://www.putchildrenfirst.org/media/6.16.pdf.

[89] Committee on Safety of Medicines Declaration of Interests. *Medicines Act 1968 Advisory Bodies Annual Reports 2001*. *available at* http://wayback.archive.org/web/20040408205314/http://www.mca.gov.uk/aboutagency/regframework/csm/csmdoi01.pdf.

[90] http://pediatrics.aappublications.org/content/114/3/584.abstract/reply.

[91] http://www.bmj.com/content/335/7618/480?tab=responses.

[92] United States. Mercury in medicine report. *Congressional Record*. Washington: GPO, May 21, 2003: 1011-1030.

[93] US National Archives and Records Administration, Office of the Federal Register. Status of Certain Additional Over-the-Counter Drug Category II and III Active Ingredients. Federal Register 63, no. 77 (22 April 1998): 19799.

[94] United States. Mercury in medicine report. *Congressional Record*. Washington: GPO, May 21, 2003: 1011-1030.

[95] Geier DA, Sykes LK, Geier MR. A review of Thimerosal (Merthiolate) and its ethylmercury breakdown product: specific historical considerations regarding safety and effectiveness. *J Toxicol Environ Health B Crit Rev*. 2007 Dec;10(8):575-96.

[96] Kathleen Stratton, Alicia Gable, and Marie C. McCormick, eds.; Immunization Safety Review Committee, Board on Health Promotion and Disease Prevention, Institute of Medicine. *Immunization Safety Review: Thimerosal-Containing Vaccines and Neurodevelopmental Disorders*. The National Academies Press. Washington, DC. October 1, 2001.

[97] United States. Mercury in medicine report. *Congressional Record*. Washington: GPO, May 21, 2003: 1011-1030.

[98] http://oehha.ca.gov/prop65/CRNR_notices/pdf_zip/hgbayer1.pdf.

[99] http://www.fda.gov/BiologicsBloodVaccines/SafetyAvailability/VaccineSafety/UCM096228.

[100] http://www.fda.gov/downloads/BiologicsBloodVaccines/Vaccines/ApprovedProducts/UCM133479.pdf.

[101] Geier DA, Jordan SK, Geier MR. The relative toxicity of compounds used as preservatives in vaccines and biologics. *Med Sci Monit.* 2010 May;16(5):SR21-7.

[102] Khandke L, Yang C, Fan J, Han H, Rashidbaigi KKA, Green BA, Jansen KU. *Development of a Multidose for Prevnar 13™. Vaccine Technology III.* John G. Auniņš, Barry C. Buckland, Kathrin U. Jansen, Paula Marques Alves, eds., ECI Symposium Series, Volume P13. 2010.

[103] Khandke L, Yang C, Krylova K, Jansen KU, Rashidbaigi A. Preservative of choice for Prev(e)nar 13™ in a multidose formulation. *Vaccine.* 2011 Sep 22;29(41):7144-53. doi: 10.1016/j.vaccine.2011.05.074. Epub 2011 Jun 7.

[104] King K, Paterson M, Green SK. Global justice and the proposed ban on thimerosal-containing vaccines. *Pediatrics.* 2013 Jan;131(1):154-6. doi: 10.1542/peds.2012-2976. Epub 2012 Dec 17.

[105] http://www.who.int/immunization_delivery/systems_policy/IPAC_2012_April_report.pdf.

[106] http://www.autismspeaks.org/science/science-news/%E2%80%98costs-autism%E2%80%99-summit.

[107] http://www.autismspeaks.org/science/science-news/autism%E2%80%80%99s-costs-nation-reach-137-billion-year.

[108] http://www.cdc.gov/media/releases/2012/t0329_Autism_Telebriefing.html.

[109] Drain PK., Nelson CM, Lloyd JS. Single dose versus multidose vaccine vials for immunization programmes in developing countries. *Bull World Health Organ.* 2003;81(10):726-31. Epub 2003 Nov 25.

[110] Adel Mahmoud, letter to Jeffrey Koplan, July 7, 1999.

[111] Adel Mahmoud, letter to David Satcher, July 7, 1999.

[112] Adel Mahmoud, letter to Jeffrey Koplan, September 8, 1999.

[113] Adel Mahmoud, letter to Walter Orenstein, September 8, 1999.

[114] John Jabara, letter to Jeffrey Koplan, July 21, 1999.

[115] http://www.gsk.com/about-us/our-history.html.

[116] Jeffrey Koplan, letter to John Labara, November 26, 1999.

[117] http://www.fda.gov/ohrms/dockets/dailys/04/aug04/080404/04p-0349-cp00001-01-vol1.pdf.

[118] http://www.safeminds.org/about/history-and-accomplishments.html.

[119] http://www.cdc.gov/vaccinesafety/concerns/thimerosal/thimerosal_timeline.html.

[120] http://www.autismresourcefoundation.org/info/info.2002.html.

[121] http://health.state.ga.us/pdfs/prevention/immunization/Thimerosal%20Timeline.pdf.

THIMEROSAL
LET THE SCIENCE SPEAK

PART ONE:

THIMEROSAL'S DANGERS TO HUMAN HEALTH AND THE BRAIN

Chapter 1:
A Brief History of
Thimerosal and the
Dangers of Mercury

Humankind has known about the toxic effect of mercury going back to ancient Greek, Roman, Egyptian, Chinese, and Hindu civilizations.[122] [123] Medical practitioners found mercury useful in the manner of other biologically poisonous, metallic elements such as arsenic and silver. An 11th-century Persian scholar, for example, reported mercury's effectiveness against lice and scabies.[124] Many examples of mercury's chronic harm to humans also appear in history. For example, the Romans sent prisoners to work in mercury mines, where the sentenced often died of poisoning.

Before the invention of modern antibiotics and antiseptics, physicians experimented with "germicides," including acids and mercury-containing compounds, to try to stave off microbial pathogens. Thimerosal was born of these efforts in the early 20th century.

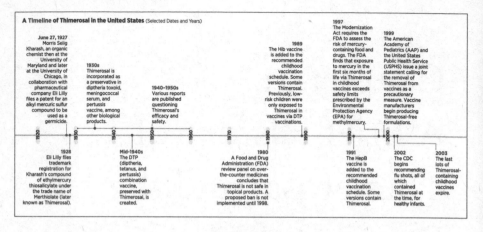

A Timeline of Thimerosal in the United States (Selected Dates and Years)

FIGURE 1

Trademarked in 1928 by pharmaceutical company Eli Lilly as Merthiolate, the white powder consists of 49.55 percent mercury by weight in the form of ethylmercury bound to thiosalicylate.[125] (Note: Other common names for Thimerosal include Merthiolate and, in Europe, Thiomersal.[126] [127] Yet other names are Merfamin, Merthiolate sodium, Mertorgan, Merzonin, Merzonin sodium, Timerosal, Thimerosalate, and, principally in Europe, Thiomersalate.[128] [129] For clarity and consistency, we will use "Thimerosal" throughout this text, with the capital letter denoting that Thimerosal is a trade name, though a lowercased spelling is commonly used.)

In the following decades, Thimerosal would make its way into various antiseptic products, including nasal sprays, eyewashes, vaginal spermicides, and diaper rash treatments.[130] [131] Starting in the 1930s, pharmaceutical companies began to use Thimerosal in vaccines for the intended purpose of preventing bacterial contamination, a well-documented threat to vaccine recipients.

Investigators for Eli Lilly tested Thimerosal on tissue cultures, in animals, and, to an extent, in humans. Yet these early studies failed to demonstrate Thimerosal's safety and efficacy in a manner that could be considered unimpeachable. (This book will explore the matter of Thimerosal's questionable efficacy in Part Two.)

Eli Lilly investigators H. M. Powell and W. A. Jamieson reported in 1931 that various animals seemed to tolerate high doses of Thimerosal. Rabbits, for example, tolerated on the order of 25 milligrams per kilogram of body weight—comparatively much higher than those ever used in vaccines. However, many of those animals given higher doses did die of evident mercury poisoning just days later.

Also notable in these early animal toxicity studies and many later research efforts was that the researchers failed to assess or perform socialization behaviors and cognition tests. In other words, though the animals may have survived Thimerosal exposure, their social behavior might have been altered as a result of mercury-induced brain damage.

In this same study, Powell and Jamieson also reported on the first injection of Thimerosal into humans. In 1929, during an epidemic of meningococcal meningitis in Indianapolis, K. C. Smithburn administered Thimerosal to twenty-two ill patients at Indianapolis City Hospital.[132] The Thimerosal had no apparent therapeutic benefit, and all the patients died, seven of them within one day of Thimerosal administration.[133]

Yet, despite the deaths of all of these patients, Powell and Jamieson described the experiment as a success. The authors reported that their patients seemed to tolerate the high dosages of the 1 percent Thimerosal solution. The drug was administered intravenously at a volume of up to 50 cubic centimeters per injection (equating to an exposure of 25,000 micrograms of mercury), and the most-exposed patient received a total of 180 cubic centimeters over five doses. As the researchers noted, none of the patients showed shock or allergic anaphylaxis reactions upon administration of the Thimerosal. But, then again, neither of these side effects is associated with toxic mercury exposure, which can take months before presenting symptoms. Apparently, because of the abbreviated survival period, the longest that Powell and Jamieson were able to observe a patient was only sixty-two days after the administration of Thimerosal.[134]

Importantly, the Powell and Jamieson study neglected to mention that the patients given Thimerosal by Smithburn were not healthy individuals. It is possible, therefore, that any short-term neurological or other deleterious effects of the Thimerosal would have been masked by or attributed to the patients' meningitis infections.[135]

Eli Lilly used the Smithburn, Powell, and Jamieson results for decades as evidence of Thimerosal's safety.[136] Subsequent research on Thimerosal, and mercury in general, though, has cast doubt on those apparently favorable early conclusions.

Different Forms of Mercury			
	Organic	Inorganic	Metallic/Elemental
Chemical description	Bound to carbon	Bound to elements such as chlorine, sulfur or oxygen; known as "mercury salts"	Not bound to other elements
Appearance	As Thimerosal, a white or slightly yellow powder	White powders or crystals, though mercuric sulfide (cinnabar) is red and turns black when exposed to light	Shiny silver metal that is liquid at room temperature
Common human exposure routes	Methylmercury in seafood; ethylmercury in Thimerosal	Exposures at levels of concern not common, but found in some batteries, homeopathic remedies, and skin-bleaching creams	Dental amalgams; air pollution from mining, manufacturing, coal, and waste burning

FIGURE 2

6

Investigators now recognize that mercury in all its forms is a potential neurodevelopmental poison. The three broad forms of mercury are organic, inorganic, and elemental.[137] The "organic" category contains methylmercury, a mercury compound found in seafood, as well as ethylmercury, an ingredient in Thimerosal. Certain elemental and organic mercury compounds are known to be potent neurotoxins.[138]

Mercury can severely disrupt the normal neurodevelopmental processes in the human brain, causing problems in migration and division of neurons, as well as cell degeneration and ultimately cell death.[139][140][141][142] In particular, mercury has a high binding affinity for the element selenium, which in the human body is found in proteins that protect cells from damaging free radicals of oxygen. The brain relies on selenium-containing proteins for this antioxidant protection more so than other tissues, so the selenium shortfalls that mercury creates help explain why mercury is neurotoxic at very low levels.[143][144][145]

The so-called oxidative stress that results from insufficient antioxidant protection disrupts gene expression. All cells contain the same genetic information in their DNA, so in order to produce the vastly different cell types in our bodies, from blood to bone, these genes must be only selectively "turned on," or expressed. One of the chief mechanisms for regulating gene expression is known as methylation, which is the binding of a methyl group to a location on a DNA molecule. Methylation inhibits the expression of a nearby gene. This sort of regulation is known as epigenetic regulation, as it involves the modification of DNA without an alteration of the underlying genetic information. Oxidative stress brought on by mercury exposure prevents proper methylation, and thus interferes with epigenetic regulation, which can lead to improper development in an organism.[146] [147] Other recent findings have also shown that the type of cells that allow synchronization of neural networks during attention, called parvalbumin-expressing interneurons, do not develop if their supply of selenium is disrupted or if they experience oxidative stress.[148]

Studies have shown that developing brains are particularly susceptible to mercury.[149] [150] Studies in 1986 and 1989 examined children in a New Zealand population exposed prenatally to mercury through maternal fish consumption. When evaluated at four and six years of age, the children with moderate-to-high exposures (as measured through the proxy of mercury content in their mothers' hair of greater than six parts per million) had significant decreases in test performance.[151] [152] [153]

In 1997, Philippe Grandjean, now affiliated with the University of Southern Denmark and the Harvard School of Public Health, and colleagues published a study based on a population in the Faroe Islands, near Denmark. This population traditionally has high mercury exposures because of a diet rich in pilot whale meat. The researchers found that children with prenatal exposure to mercury displayed cognitive deficits in language, attention, memory and—though less pronounced—in visuospatial and motor functions.[154] The study overall suggested that mercury has widespread effects on brain function.[155]

Further work with the Faroe Islands cohort produced a relevant 2004 study. This research noted that delays in auditory responses—an indicator of brain damage—resulting from prenatal mercury exposure persisted in subjects at least into their early teens, again indicating that some neurotoxic effects from mercury are "irreversible."[156] A review article in 2012 stated that "emerging evidence indicates [methylmercury] may have adverse effects on the neurologic and other body systems at common low levels of exposure," and that "in children, prenatal exposure may be more deleterious than postnatal exposure for most, but likely not all, neurodevelopmental measures."[157]

Other recent findings in this vein come from a study with Inuit children in Arctic Quebec. The 2012 study reported a correlation between children's mercury exposure concentrations in the womb (from their mothers' fish-heavy diets) and later classroom assessments consistent with attention-deficit hyperactivity disorder

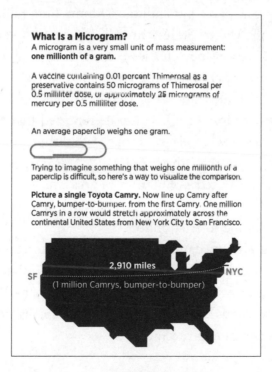

What Is a Microgram?
A microgram is a very small unit of mass measurement: one millionth of a gram.

A vaccine containing 0.01 percent Thimerosal as a preservative contains 50 micrograms of Thimerosal per 0.5 milliliter dose, or approximately 25 micrograms of mercury per 0.5 milliliter dose.

An average paperclip weighs one gram.

Trying to imagine something that weighs one millionth of a paperclip is difficult, so here's a way to visualize the comparison.

Picture a single Toyota Camry. Now line up Camry after Camry, bumper-to-bumper, from the first Camry. One million Camrys in a row would stretch approximately across the continental United States from New York City to San Francisco.

SF — 2,910 miles — NYC
(1 million Camrys, bumper-to-bumper)

FIGURE 3

(ADHD).[158] Another 2012 study on subjects recruited in New Bedford, Massachusetts, also associated prenatal exposure to mercury (again through the proxy of maternal hair mercury levels) with a greater risk of ADHD-related behaviors, and at levels as low as one microgram per gram, or one part per million.[159]

Additional important research in this area is the work that has drawn connections between exposure to mercury during fetal development and apparently permanent reductions in a child's intelligence. In a 2005 study, Leonardo Trasande of New York University found that between 316,588 and 637,233 children each year have cord blood mercury levels greater than 5.8 micrograms per liter, or 5.8 parts per million. (About four million children are born in the United States annually.[160]) According to Trasande, that 5.8 micrograms per liter level is the lowest concentration at which adverse neurodevelopmental effects were demonstrated in the New Zealand and Faroe Islands studies, and is associated with a persistent loss of IQ. Trasande reported that the IQ losses linked to mercury exposure range from three-quarters of an IQ point to more than three points.[161] Trasande calculated that these mercury-affected population figures are sufficient to cause diminished lifetime economic productivity for each birth year cohort, amounting to $8.7 billion.[162]

Given the evident damage that mercury can cause to human tissues, particularly the brain, and the less-than-straightforward manner in which Thimerosal's safety was assessed in early literature, we now turn to the more historically recent use of Thimerosal-containing vaccines.

Notes

[122] http://www.dartmouth.edu/~toxmetal/toxic-metals/mercury/mercury-history.html.

[123] http://www.mercuryinschools.uwex.edu/curriculum/hg_in_world.htm.

[124] Abd-El-Aziz AS, Carraher CE Jr, Pittman CU Jr, Sheats JE, Zeldin M, eds. *Macromolecules Containing Metal and Metal-Like Elements, Volume 3: Biomedical Applications*. Wiley-Interscience. 2004.

[125] Baker JP. Mercury, vaccines, and autism: one controversy, three histories. *Am J. Public Health*. 2008; 98:244–253.

[126] http://www.vaccine-tlc.org/docs/Thimerosal%20Material%20Safety%20Data%20Sheet.pdf.

[127] http://www.ncbi.nlm.nih.gov/pubmed?term=thiomersal.

[128] http://www.safcglobal.com/etc/medialib/docs/Sigma/Product_Information_Sheet/1/t5125pis.Par.0001.File.tmp/t5125pis.pdf.

[129] http://www.who.int/immunization/sage/meetings/2012/april/timerosol_problems_costs_solution_de_chile.pdf.

[130] Geier DA, Sykes LK, Geier MR. A review of Thimerosal (Merthiolate) and its ethylmercury breakdown product: specific historical considerations regarding safety and effectiveness. *J Toxicol Environ Health B Crit Rev*. 2007 Dec;10(8);575-96.

[131] Geier DA, King PG, Hooker BS, Dórea JG, Kern JK, Sykes LK, Geier MR. Thimerosal: Clinical, epidemiologic and biochemical studies. Clin Chim Acta. 2015 Apr 15;444:212-220. doi: 10.1016/j.cca.2015.02.030. Epub 2015 Feb 21.

[132] Smithburn KC, Kempf GE, Zerfas LG, Gilman LH. Meningococcic meningitis: a clinical study of one hundred and forty-four cases. *J Am Med Assoc*. 1930; 95:776–780.

[133] United States. Mercury in medicine report. *Congressional Record*. Washington: GPO, May 21, 2003: 1011-1030.

[134] Powell HM, Jamieson, WA. Merthiolate as a germicide. *Am J Hyg*. 1931;13:296–310.

[135] Geier DA, Sykes LK, Geier MR. A review of Thimerosal (Merthiolate) and its ethylmercury breakdown product: specific historical considerations regarding safety and effectiveness. *J Toxicol Environ Health B Crit Rev*. 2007 Dec;10(8):575-96.

[136] United States. Mercury in medicine report. *Congressional Record*. Washington: GPO, May 21, 2003: 1011-1030.

[137] http://www.cdc.gov/vaccinesafety/updates/thimerosal_faqs_mercury.htm.

[138] Clarkson TW, Nordberg GF, Sager PR. Reproductive and developmental toxicity of metals. *Scand J Work Environ Health*. 1985 Jun; 11 (3 Spec No):145-54.

[139] Bland C, Rand MD. Methylmercury induces activation of Notch signaling. *Neurotoxicology*. 2006 Dec;27(6):982-91.

[140] Crump KS, Kjellström T, Shipp AM, Silvers A, Stewart A. Influence of prenatal mercury exposure upon scholastic and psychological test performance: benchmark analysis of a New Zealand cohort. *Risk Anal*. 1998 Dec; 18(6):701-713.

[141] Barrie S. Environmental factors contributing to the development of autism spectrum disorder—a large database retrospective study; Aug. 27, 2010 *available at* http://issuu.com/personalizedmedicine/docs/carestudyd6.

[142] Costa M, Christie NT, Cantoni O, Zelikoff JT, Wang XW, Rossman TG. DNA damage by mercury compounds: An overview. *Proc. of Advances for Mercury Toxicology. Advances in Mercury Toxicology*. Suzuki T., ed. Plenum Press, New York. 1991; 255-273.

[143] Chen C, Yu H, Zhao J, Li B, Qu L, Liu S, Zhang P, Chai Z. The roles of serum selenium and selenoproteins on mercury toxicity in environmental and occupational exposure. *Environ Health Perspect*. 2006 Feb;114(2):297-301.

[144] Carvalho CM, Chew EH, Hashemy SI, Lu J, Holmgren A. Inhibition of the human thioredoxin system: a molecular mechanism of mercury toxicity. *J Biol Chem*. 2008 May 2;283(18):11913-23. doi: 10.1074/jbc.M710133200. Epub 2008 Mar 4.

[145] Branco V, Canário J, Lu J, Holmgren A, Carvalho C. Mercury and selenium interaction in vivo: effects on thioredoxin reductase and glutathione peroxidase. *Free Radic Biol Med*. 2012 Feb 15;52(4):781-93. doi: 10.1016/j.freeradbiomed.2011.12.002. Epub 2011 Dec 13.

[146] Waly MI, Hornig M, Trivedi M, Hodgson N, Kini R, Ohta A, Deth R. Prenatal and postnatal epigenetic programming: implications for GI, immune, and neuronal function in autism. *Autism Res Treat*. 2012;2012:190930. doi: 10.1155/2012/190930. Epub 2012 Jun 19.

[147] Deth R, Hodgson N, Trivedi M, Muratore C, Waly M. Autism: a neuroepigenetic disorder. *Autism Science Digest*. Issue 03 *available at* http://www.scribd.com/doc/78560867/Autism-A-Neuroepigenetic-Disorder-Deth-R-et-al#download.

[148] Pitts MW, Raman AV, Hashimoto AC, Todorovic C, Nichols RA, Berry MJ. Deletion of selenoprotein P results in impaired function of parvalbumin interneurons and alterations in fear learning and sensorimotor gating. *Neuroscience*. 2012 Apr 19;208:58-68. doi: 10.1016/j.neuroscience.2012.02.017. Epub 2012 Feb 21.

[149] Mahaffey KR. Methylmercury: a new look at the risks. *Public Health Rep*. 1999 Sep-Oct;114(5):396-9, 402-13.

[150] Committee on the Toxicological Effects of Methylmercury, Board on Environmental Studies and Toxicology, National Research Council. *Toxicological Effects of Methylmercury*. National Academy Press, Washington, DC. 2000.

[151] Kjellström T, Kennedy P, Wallis S, Mantell C. *Physical and Mental Development of Children with Prenatal Exposure to Mercury from Fish. Stage 1, Preliminary Tests at Age 4 (Report 3080)*. Stockholm: National Swedish Environmental Protection Board; 1986.

[152] Kjellström T, Kennedy P, Wallis S. *Physical and Mental Development of Children with Prenatal Exposure to Mercury from Fish. Stage 2, Interviews and Psychological Tests at Age 6 (Report 3642).* Stockholm: National Swedish Environmental Protection Board; 1989.

[153] Committee on the Toxicological Effects of Methylmercury, Board on Environmental Studies and Toxicology, National Research Council. *Toxicological Effects of Methylmercury.* National Academy Press, Washington, DC. 2000.

[154] http://www.hsph.harvard.edu/faculty/philippe-grandjean/.

[155] Grandjean P, Weihe P, White RF, Debes F, Araki S, Yokoyama K, Murata K, Sørensen N, Dahl R, Jørgensen PJ. Cognitive deficit in 7-year-old children with prenatal exposure to methylmercury. *Neurotoxicol Teratol.* 1997 Nov-Dec;19(6):417-28.

[156] Murata K, Weihe P, Budtz-Jørgensen E, Jørgensen PJ, Grandjean P. Delayed brainstem auditory evoked potential latencies in 14-year-old children exposed to methylmercury. *J Pediatr.* 2004 Feb;144(2):177-83.

[157] Karagas MR, Choi AL, Oken E, Horvat M, Schoeny R, Kamai E, Cowell W, Grandjean P, Korrick S. Evidence on the human health effects of low-level methylmercury exposure. *Environ Health Perspect.* 2012 Jun;120(6):799-806. doi: 10.1289/ehp.1104494. Epub 2012 Jan 24.

[158] Boucher O, Jacobson SW, Plusquellec P, Dewailly E, Ayotte P, Forget-Dubois N, Jacobson JL, Muckle G. Prenatal methylmercury, postnatal lead exposure, and evidence of attention deficit/hyperactivity disorder among Inuit children in Arctic Québec. *Environ Health Perspect.* 2012 Oct;120(10):1456-61. doi: 10.1289/ehp.1204976. Epub 2012 Aug 16.

[159] Sagiv SK, Thurston SW, Bellinger DC, Amarasiriwardena C, Korrick SA. Prenatal exposure to mercury and fish consumption during pregnancy and attention-deficit/hyperactivity disorder-related behavior in children. *Arch Pediatr Adolesc Med.* 2012 Dec;166(12):1123-31. doi: 10.1001/archpediatrics.2012.1286.

[160] http://www.cdc.gov/nchs/fastats/births.htm.

[161] http://pediatrics.med.nyu.edu/genpeds/our-faculty/leonardo-trasande.

[162] Trasande L, Landrigan PJ, Schechter C. Public health and economic consequences of methyl mercury toxicity to the developing brain. *Environ Health Perspect.* 2005 May;113(5):590-6.

Chapter 2:
The Increase in Thimerosal-Containing Children's Vaccines Coincided with a Rise in Neurodevelopmental Disorders

Although correlation does not prove causation, the increase in the number of Thimerosal-containing children's vaccines in the late 1980s and early 1990s coincided closely with a sudden jump in neurodevelopmental disorder diagnoses and deficits such as autism and attention problems.[163] [164]

Since the early 1970s, children in the United States had generally received only three types of vaccinations. These vaccinations were administered in a total of eight injections in the first eighteen months of life, rising to ten injections by age six. The three vaccines in use were diphtheria, tetanus, and pertussis (DTP), oral polio vaccine (OPV), and measles, mumps, and rubella (MMR).[165] [166] Only the DTP vaccine contained Thimerosal, at a preservative level of 0.01 percent per 0.5 milliliters, which works out to 50 micrograms of Thimerosal per shot.[167] Given that Thimerosal is about 50 percent mercury by weight, children were historically exposed to about 100 micrograms of mercury in their first eighteen months and about 125 micrograms by first grade or so.

Starting in the 1970s and into the early 1980s, vaccine manufacturers began facing an onslaught of lawsuits from families claiming their children had suffered serious injuries from vaccines, especially DTP. The vaccine market grew volatile, with manufacturers going out of business or threatening to cease production.[168] [169] Fears also emerged of a resurgence in childhood diseases.[170] As a result, Congress created a federal product liability program to ensure vaccine supply and to provide a forum for injured individuals to seek compensation from the government, not vaccine makers. The legislation, the National Childhood Vaccine Injury Act of 1986 (Public Law 99-660), established the National Vaccine Injury Compensation Program (VICP, better known as the "Vaccine Court").[171] It was shortly thereafter that the early infant immunization schedule began to expand considerably.

Then, in 1989, responding to recommendations by the Department of Health and Human Services' Advisory Committee on Immunization Practices (ACIP), state public health officials around the United States began increasing the types and total number of vaccinations required for school attendance.[172] [173] Some of these vaccines contained Thimerosal, depending on the manufacturer.[174] A single dose of Haemophilus b conjugate vaccine (HbCV, or Hib) was added to the schedule in 1989, and in 1991 a four-shot Hib regimen was recommended in the first fifteen months of life.[175] [176] The three-shot hepatitis B (HepB) vaccine was also approved in 1991.[177] DTaP (diphtheria, tetanus, and acellular pertussis), versions of which contained Thimerosal, began replacing some of the fourth DTP shots children received at fifteen months of age from about 1992 onward. In 1997, the ACIP recommended DTaP for all four of the previously prescribed DTP shots.[178] [179] [180]

By 1999, the new vaccination schedules called for children before the age of two to receive nineteen vaccine injections to protect against eleven infectious diseases, and eleven of the injections were preserved with Thimerosal.[181] [182] Even premature, low-birthweight babies received a Thimerosal-preserved HepB shot within twelve hours of birth if the mother tested positive for hepatitis B.[183] [184] Children entering first grade were supposed to have received twenty-two injections, twelve of which could have included Thimerosal at a preservative level.[185] The HepB vaccine contained 25 micrograms of Thimerosal, while DTaP and Hib contained around 50 micrograms. The corresponding mercury levels were therefore between 12.5 and 25 micrograms of mercury per 0.5 milliliter vaccine dose.

Accordingly, children born in the 1990s could have been injected with up to 237.5 micrograms of mercury from vaccines by their second birthday. Some children received an additional 37.5 microgram dose of mercury from three Thimerosal-preserved influenza shots as well.[186] Historically, prior to 1989, children had received about 100 micrograms of mercury by their second birthdays, and only in 25 microgram increments spread over four doctor's visits. The 1990s schedules, however, exposed children to as much as 62.5 micrograms of mercury from three vaccines during a single doctor visit at two, four, six, and/or fifteen months of age.[187] Taking the scenario of a two-month-old, typical 5-kilogram (11-pound) child, he or she would have been injected with 125 times the Environmental Protection Agency's safe "reference dose" (RfD) estimate of 0.1 microgram of methylmercury per kilogram of body weight per day.[188] [189] (RfD, which has been established by the EPA for methylmercury but not for ethylmercury, will be discussed further in Chapter 4.)

These increases in mercury intake could very well have multiplied the risk of neurological damage for American children, as an ensuing rise in neurological disorders appears to bear out. In May 1999, school nurse Patti White, RN of the Missouri Central District School Nurse Association, offered her perspective on the possible health impacts of the Thimerosal-containing HepB vaccine in testimony before Congress:

> The elementary grades are overwhelmed with children who have symptoms of neurological and/or immune system damage: epilepsy, seizure disorders, various kinds of palsies, autism, mental retardation, learning disabilities, juvenile-onset diabetes, asthma, vision/hearing loss, and a multitude of new conduct/behavior disorders. We [school nurses] have come to believe the hepatitis B vaccine is an assault on a newborn's developing neurological and immune system. Vaccines are supposed to be making us healthier. However, in twenty-five

17

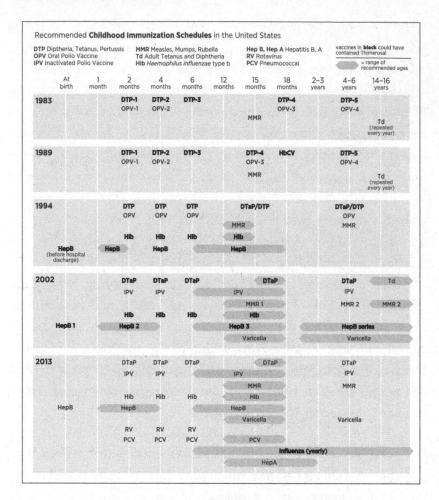

FIGURE 4

years of nursing I have never seen so many damaged, sick kids. Something very, very wrong is happening to our children.[190]

White's assertion is supported by some compelling figures, as first conveyed in the Executive Summary. Attention problems,

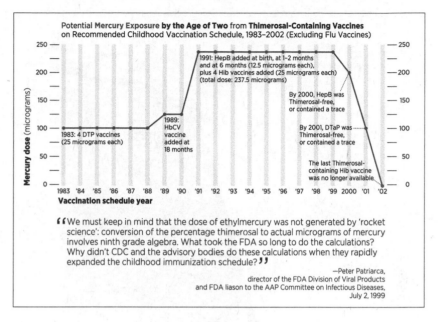

Potential Mercury Exposure **by the Age of Two** from **Thimerosal-Containing Vaccines** on Recommended Childhood Vaccination Schedule, 1983–2002 (Excluding Flu Vaccines)

*f f*We must keep in mind that the dose of ethylmercury was not generated by 'rocket science': conversion of the percentage thimerosal to actual micrograms of mercury involves ninth grade algebra. What took the FDA so long to do the calculations? Why didn't CDC and the advisory bodies do these calculations when they rapidly expanded the childhood immunization schedule? *J J*

—Peter Patriarca,
director of the FDA Division of Viral Products
and FDA liason to the AAP Committee on Infectious Diseases,
July 2, 1999

FIGURE 5

including ADD and ADHD, reported by pediatrician's offices rose from 1.4 percent of patients in 1979 to 9.2 percent by 1996, according to a 2000 study.[191] Recent data from the CDC obtained and compiled by the *New York Times* suggest that as of 2011 and 2012, 11 percent of school-age children had received an ADHD diagnosis, representing a 16 percent increase since 2007 and a 41 percent rise over the past decade.[192] From 1996 to 2008, the prevalence of developmental disabilities in US children such as those White spoke about went up more than 17 percent, from 12.84 percent of the population to 15.04 percent.[193]

With regard to autism and autism spectrum disorders (ASDs), studies have documented a major jump in recent decades in prevalence,

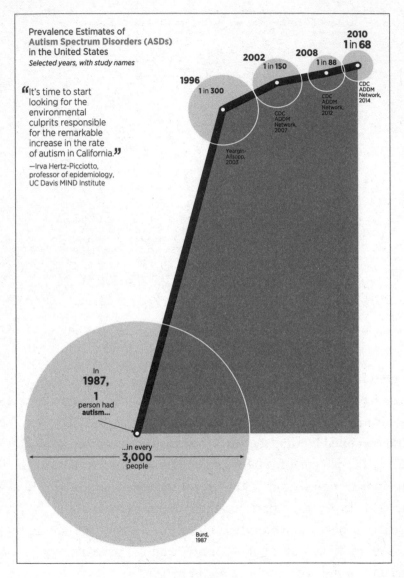

FIGURE 6

or the number of reported cases present in a given population at a certain time. Across various countries, including the United States, starting in the late 1960s through the 1990s, studies pegged the prevalence rate for autism at about 1 in 2,000 children.[194][195] Some studies of populations outside the United States began documenting a rise in prevalence in the late 1980s. Studies then conducted in the United States in the late 1990s and early 2000s also revealed a startling jump from earlier figures. In metropolitan Atlanta in 1996 and then in Brick Township, New Jersey, in 1998—the latter study conducted because of residents' concerns about seemingly high community ASD rates—prevalence estimates turned out to be 1 in 300 and 1 in 150 children for ASDs, respectively.[196][197] By 2004, the American Academy of Pediatrics (AAP) and the CDC placed the rate of ASDs in children at 1 in 166 as of 2000. At that time, there were about half a million people up to age twenty-one with an ASD in the United States, with 26,000 new cases each year.[198]

The numbers have continued to climb. In 2007, the CDC's new estimate for the rate of ASDs rose to 1 in 150 (based on 2002 data), then to 1 in 110 in 2009 (based on 2006 data), to 1 in 88 (based on 2008 data), and, most recently, in March 2014, to a truly alarming 1 in 68 children (based on 2010 data).[199][200][201] (The children assessed in these last four reports from the Autism and Developmental Disabilities Monitoring (ADDM) Network were eight years old, so the prevalence rates reflect possible exposures from many years prior to data collection.) Intriguingly, a 2010 study by Environmental Protection Agency (EPA) scientists identified 1988 to 1989 as the approximate "changepoint" year when cases of autism began to dramatically increase, according to data sets from California as well as a worldwide composite of studies—the same period, in the United

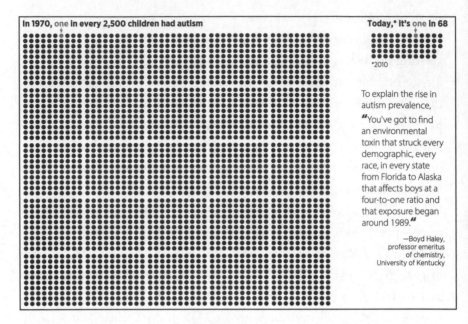

In 1970, one in every 2,500 children had autism

Today,* it's one in 68

*2010

To explain the rise in autism prevalence, "You've got to find an environmental toxin that struck every demographic, every race, in every state from Florida to Alaska that affects boys at a four-to-one ratio and that exposure began around 1989."

—Boyd Haley,
professor emeritus
of chemistry,
University of Kentucky

FIGURE 7

States at least, when the vaccine schedule expanded and Thimerosal exposure began increasing.[202]

In 1997, concern over the toxicity of mercury led Congress to pass a law called the Food and Drug Administration Modernization Act, which required the FDA to review the use of mercury in pediatric vaccines, foods, and other products. The FDA found that the mercury level in the childhood vaccine schedule surpassed safety guidelines set by the EPA.[203][204][205]

As a result, in July 1999, the AAP and the US Public Health Service (USPHS) agencies, which include the CDC, the FDA, the National Institutes of Health (NIH), and the Health Resources and Services Administration (HRSA), recommended that vaccine makers reduce or eliminate Thimerosal in vaccines.[206][207] The joint statement read in part:

> The recognition that some children could be exposed to a cumulative level of mercury over the first 6 months of life that exceeds one of the federal guidelines on methylmercury now requires a weighing of two different types of risks when vaccinating infants. On the one hand, there is the known serious risk of diseases and deaths caused by failure to immunize our infants against vaccine-preventable infectious diseases; on the other, there is the unknown and probably much smaller risk, if any, of neurodevelopmental effects posed by exposure to Thimerosal. The large risks of not vaccinating children far outweigh the unknown and probably much smaller risk, if any, of cumulative exposure to Thimerosal-containing vaccines over the first 6 months of life. Nevertheless, because any potential risk is of concern, the US Public Health Service (USPHS), the American Academy of Pediatrics (AAP), and vaccine manufacturers agree that thimerosal-containing vaccines should be removed as soon as possible.[208]

The Institute of Medicine (IOM) and European regulatory agencies made similar recommendations.[209][210]

Vaccine producers accordingly began taking steps in 1999 to reduce Thimerosal levels in children's vaccines, and the first vaccines with reduced levels began to appear that year.[211][212] However, some vaccines still contained trace amounts of Thimerosal, which is defined as one microgram of mercury per dose or less.[213][214][215] Some of the Thimerosal-reduced vaccines, namely Pediarix DTaP and Engerix HepB, eventually became Thimerosal-free in 2007.[216][217][218]

Despite requests by groups such as the Coalition for Mercury-Free Drugs and SafeMinds to recall all Thimerosal-preserved vaccines, the FDA allowed the vaccine industry to market its existing stocks, the last lots of which did not run out until 2003.[219][220][221][222][223] This slow withdrawal prompted criticism in a 2003 congressional report as well:

> Rather than acting aggressively to remove thimerosal from children's vaccines, the FDA and other agencies within the Department of Health and Human Services (HHS) adopted an incremental approach that allowed children to continue to be exposed to ethylmercury from vaccines for more than two additional years [after 2000]. In fact, in 2001, the Centers for Disease Control and Prevention (CDC) refused even to express a preference for thimerosal-free vaccines, despite the fact that thimerosal had been removed from almost every childhood vaccine produced for use in the United States.[224]

Shortly after the July 1999 statement from the AAP/USPHS, two major vaccine manufacturers indicated to the CDC that they could supply enough Thimerosal-free versions of their products to meet the total vaccine demand. These letters appear on the following pages. Merck wrote to CDC and other national health officials that the company could accelerate its capability to manufacture its new Thimerosal-free HepB vaccine, Recombivax HB.[225][226][227][228] SmithKline Beecham (now GlaxoSmithKline), meanwhile, wrote the CDC saying it could meet the US market's needs for DTaP with Thimerosal-free Infanrix through the remainder of 1999 and the first half of 2000.[229][230] CDC director Jeffrey Koplan wrote SmithKline Beecham back expressing that the CDC would "continue to provide the States with a choice among currently licensed brands of DTaP vaccine."[231] In other words, even when presented with broad Thimerosal-free immunization options from willing manufacturers, the CDC declined to implement mercury-free vaccines (see examples of the letters beginning on page 27).

Even as pharmaceutical companies reduced levels of Thimerosal and removed it altogether from most pediatric vaccines in America, based on the precautionary principle, the firms did not pursue the elimination of Thimerosal in developing countries. Part of the reason appears to be economics. According to the World Health Organization (WHO), Thimerosal-preserved, multidose vaccines remain the less expensive option compared to nonpreserved, single-dose vaccines. WHO also points out that Thimerosal-preserved multidose vaccines are presently and readily available, while potential new formulations preserved with alternatives to Thimerosal, such as 2-phenoxyethanol (2-PE) used for inactivated polio vaccine or phenol used for typhoid vaccine and pneumococcal vaccine, would require new (and likely costly) clinical evaluations for safety and efficacy, as well as regulatory approval.[232][233][234][235] UNICEF (the United Nations Children's Fund), which purchases 40 percent of all vaccines used in developing countries, supplied 300 million doses of Thimerosal-containing vaccines in 2010, such as a Thimerosal-containing version of Merck's Recombivax HB to prevent hepatitis B.[236][237][238][239]

Whether for economic or for other reasons, tens of millions of children in the world's poorest nations continue to be injected each year with vaccines containing Thimerosal, a chemical that studies suggest could be linked to neurodevelopmental disorders.

Adel A. F. Mahmoud, M.D., Ph.D.
President
Merck Vaccines

Merck & Co., Inc.
One Merck Drive
P.O. Box 100
Whitehouse Station NJ 08889-0100
Tel 908 423 4316
Fax 908 735 1232

July 7, 1999 – via facsimile 404-639-7111

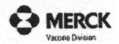 MERCK
Vaccine Division

Jeffrey P. Koplan, M.D., M.P.H.
Director
Centers for Disease Control and Prevention
1500 Clifton Road
Atlanta, Georgia 30333

Dear Dr. Koplan:

I am pleased to share with you the following statement:

Merck recognizes that public trust in the safety of vaccines used in the National Immunization Program is critical to that program's success. Therefore, Merck has assessed its capability to accelerate the manufacture of thimerosal-free vaccines. Beginning in early September 1999 and contingent upon FDA approval of a manufacturing supplement for Merck's hepatitis B vaccine, RECOMBIVAX HB®, the Company believes it could provide sufficient thimerosal-free vaccine (although supplies will be tight) to accomplish the following public health objectives:

- *Vaccinate all high-risk infants (those born to Hepatitis B Surface Antigen positive mothers) with thimerosal-free hepatitis B vaccine at birth, one and six months of age;*

- *Vaccinate all low-risk infants (those born to Hepatitis B Surface Antigen negative mothers) at birth with thimerosal-free hepatitis B vaccine, followed by a thimerosal-free combination vaccine for hepatitis B and Hib (COMVAX®), at 2, 4, and 12-15 months of age.*

Please let me know if additional information is needed.

Best regards,

Adel Mahmoud

SB
SmithKline Beecham
Pharmaceuticals

July 31,1999

Dr. Jeffrey Koplan, Director
Centers for Disease Control and Prevention
1600 Clifton Rd., NE
Atlanta, GA 30333
(404) 639-7111 (fax)

Dear Dr. Koplan,

SmithKline Beecham Pharmaceuticals (SB) as a manufacturer of vaccines has been involved in discussions recently surrounding thimerosal in vaccines, and is aware of and sensitive to the related statements issued by the American Academy of Pediatrics (AAP), U.S. Surgeon General, the Department of Health and Human Services, and the Centers for Disease Control and Prevention (CDC). As a manufacturer, we agree that, despite the absence of any scientific data that thimerosal causes adverse effects, whenever possible "thimerosal-containing vaccines should be removed as soon as possible", as is recommended in the July 7 Joint Statement of the AAP and the U.S. Public Health Service (PHS). For this reason we wish to inform you that SB is in a position to supply Infanrix (Diptheria and Tetanus Toxoids and Acellular Pertussis Vaccine Adsorbed), the only U.S. licensed DTPa vaccine that does not use thimerosal as a preservative, in enough quantities to supply the estimated U.S. market needs for at least the remainder of 1999 and the first half of 2000. By that time, other thimerosal free DTPa products, including SB's pentavalent DTPa/HB/IPV, will likely be available, pending FDA approval.

We have significantly increased our inventories of Infanrix in light of the fact that DTPa vaccines are currently a major contributor to the amount of thimerosal which may be given in the pediatric recommended vaccination schedule. Not only are there cumulatively five doses of DTPa vaccine administered to children under 7 years of age, but also three of those doses are recommended in the first 6 months of life. Furthermore, thimerosal-containing DTPa vaccines have the highest concentration of thimerosal among currently recommended vaccines with 25mcg of mercury per dose, more than twice the amount of hepatitis B vaccines. Consequently, infants who receive the first three doses of DTPa vaccine during the first six months of life are exposed cumulatively to 75mcg of mercury, nearing the threshold established by the U.S. Environmental Protection Agency (EPA) of 80mcg of mercury. By contrast, infants receiving Infanrix for the primary series (and a non-thimerosal containing Hib vaccine), can receive all other recommended vaccines, irrespective of manufacturer, and still not exceed the cumulative levels of mercury under the EPA reference guidelines.

Several weeks ago, SmithKline Beecham was approached by the vaccine contracting department at the CDC inquiring about our ability to supply the entire U.S. DTPa market with Infanrix and the potential for an exclusive DTPa contract, until other non-thimerosal DTPa vaccines were licensed. In reviewing our inventory levels, SmithKline Beecham is now in the position to move forward with such a contract. We believe the exclusive availability of Infanrix DTPa moves the AAP, CDC and PHS much closer to their stated objectives of thimerosal free vaccines in the U.S. We look forward to discussing this possibility with you further in the days to come

Sincerely,

John Jabara, Vice President and Director
Vaccines Business Unit, U.S.

RECEIVED
AUG 6 1999
96 B5
CDC EXEC SEC

. Code
. Update Ep.
. NIP/Ostroff sig

28

DEPARTMENT OF HEALTH & HUMAN SERVICES   Public Health Service

---

Centers for Disease Control
and Prevention (CDC)
Atlanta GA 30333

NOV 26 1999

Mr. John Jabara
Vice President and Director
Vaccines Business Unit, U.S.
SmithKline Beecham Pharmaceuticals
One Franklin Plaza
P.O. Box 7929
Philadelphia, Pennsylvania 19101

Dear Mr. Jabara:

I am responding to your letters to Mr. Kevin Thurm, Deputy Secretary to the Department of Health and Human Services (HHS), Dr. David Satcher, Assistant Secretary for Health and Surgeon General (HHS), and to me concerning SmithKline Beecham (SKB) Pharmaceuticals' increased inventories of a thimerosal-free Diphtheria and Tetanus Toxoid and Acellular Pertussis Vaccine (DTaP), which are capable of meeting domestic market needs through the first half of calendar year 2000.

The Centers for Disease Control and Prevention's (CDC) National Immunization Program staff has communicated this updated information regarding your supply to the 64 immunization projects. CDC also plans to monitor DTaP ordering patterns and continue to provide the States with a choice among currently licensed brands of DTaP vaccine.

CDC appreciates the contributions of SKB Pharmaceuticals and other vaccine manufacturers in our Nation's ongoing efforts to effectively and safely reach the immunization goals for our children and youth.

Sincerely,

Jeffrey P. Kaplan, M.D., M.P.H.
Director

29

Notes

[163] Baker JP. Mercury, vaccines, and autism: one controversy, three histories. *Am J. Public Health*. 2008; 98:244–253.

[164] Fombonne E. Epidemiology of pervasive developmental disorders. *Pediatr Res*. 2009 Jun;65(6):591-8.

[165] http://www.chop.edu/service/vaccine-education-center/vaccine-schedule/history-of-vaccine-schedule.html.

[166] http://www.cdc.gov/vaccines/pubs/vacc-timeline.htm.

[167] Committee on Infectious Diseases and Committee on Environmental Health, American Academy of Pediatrics. Thimerosal in vaccines—an interim report to clinicians. *Pediatrics*. 1999 Sep;104(3 Pt 1):570-4.

[168] http://www.historyofvaccines.org/content/articles/vaccine-injury-compensation-programs.

[169] http://www.homelandsecuritynewswire.com/supreme-court-ruling-renders-vaccine-manufacturers-immune-lawsuits.

[170] http://www.gpo.gov/fdsys/pkg/CHRG-107hhrg77527/html/CHRG-107hhrg77527.htm.

[171] http://www.hrsa.gov/vaccinecompensation/index.html.

[172] http://www.cdc.gov/mmwr/preview/mmwrhtml/00038256.htm.

[173] Hinman AR, Orenstein WA, Schuchat A; Centers for Disease Control and Prevention (CDC). Vaccine-preventable diseases, immunizations, and MMWR—1961-2011. *MMWR Surveill Summ*. 2011 Oct 7;60 Suppl 4:49-57.

[174] Committee on Infectious Diseases and Committee on Environmental Health, American Academy of Pediatrics.Thimerosal in vaccines—an interim report to clinicians. *Pediatrics*. 1999 Sep;104(3 Pt 1):570-4.

[175] http://www.cdc.gov/vaccines/schedules/images/schedule1989s.jpg.

[176] http://www.cdc.gov/mmwr/preview/mmwrhtml/00041736.htm.

[177] http://www.cdc.gov/mmwr/preview/mmwrhtml/00033405.htm.

[178] http://wonder.cdc.gov/wonder/prevguid/m0041836/m0041836.asp.

[179] http://www.cdc.gov/mmwr/preview/mmwrhtml/00048610.htm.

[180] Fine, A. *Diphtheria, Tetanus and Acellular Pertussis (DTaP): A Case Study*. Background paper prepared for the Committee on the Evaluation of Vaccine Purchase Financing in the United States. April 2003 *available at* http://iom.edu/~/media/Files/Activity%20Files/Disease/VaccineFinancing/FineBackgroundPaper.pdf.

[181] http://www.cdc.gov/vaccines/pubs/vacc-timeline.htm.

[182] http://www.cdc.gov/vaccines/recs/schedules/child-schedule.htm.

[183] American Academy of Pediatrics Committee on Infectious Diseases. Update on timing of hepatitis B vaccination for premature infants and for children with lapsed immunization. *Pediatrics.* 1994 Sep;94(3):403-4.

[184] http://www.cdc.gov/mmwr/pdf/rr/rr5102.pdf.

[185] http://www.cdc.gov/mmwr/preview/mmwrhtml/00056261.htm.

[186] Ball LK, Ball R, Pratt RD. An assessment of thimerosal use in childhood vaccines. *Pediatrics.* 2001 May;107(5):1147-54.

[187] http://www.cdc.gov/mmwr/preview/mmwrhtml/00056261.htm.

[188] http://www.cdc.gov/growthcharts/data/set1clinical/cj41l017.pdf.

[189] http://www.epa.gov/hg/exposure.htm.

[190] http://www.vaccinationcouncil.org/2009/05/21/school-nurses-speak-out-on-hepatitis-b-vaccine/.

[191] Kelleher KJ, McInerny TK, Gardner WP, Childs GE, Wasserman RC. Increasing identification of psychosocial problems: 1979-1996. *Pediatrics.* 2000 Jun;105(6):1313-21.

[192] http://www.nytimes.com/2013/04/01/health/more-diagnoses-of-hyperactivity-causing-concern.html?pagewanted=all&_r=0.

[193] Boyle CA, Boulet S, Schieve LA, Cohen RA, Blumberg SJ, Yeargin-Allsopp M, Visser S, Kogan MD. Trends in the prevalence of developmental disabilities in US children, 1997-2008. *Pediatrics.* 2011 Jun;127(6):1034-42. doi: 10.1542/peds.2010-2989. Epub 2011 May 23.

[194] Fombonne E. The epidemiology of autism: a review. *Psychol Med.* 1999 Jul;29(4):769-86.

[195] Newschaffer CJ, Curran LK. Autism: an emerging public health problem. *Public Health Rep.* 2003 Sep-Oct; 118(5): 393–399.

[196] Yeargin Allsopp M, Rice C, Karapurkar T, Doernberg N, Boyle C, Murphy C. Prevalence of autism in a US metropolitan area. *JAMA.* 2003 Jan 1;289(1):49-55.

[197] Bertrand J, Mars A, Boyle C, Bove F, Yeargin-Allsopp M, Decoufle P. Prevalence of autism in a United States population: the Brick Township, New Jersey, investigation. *Pediatrics.* 2001 Nov;108(5):1155-61.

[198] http://www.cdc.gov/ncbddd/autism/documents/autismcommunityreport.pdf.

[199] http://www.cdc.gov/ncbddd/autism/addm.html.

[200] http://www.cdc.gov/media/releases/2012/p0329_autism_disorder.html.

[201] http://www.cdc.gov/media/releases/2013/a0320_autism_disorder.html.

[202] McDonald ME, Paul JF. Timing of increased autistic disorder cumulative incidence. *Environ Sci Technol.* 2010 Mar 15;44(6):2112-8.

[203] Baker JP. Mercury, vaccines, and autism: one controversy, three histories. *Am J Public Health.* 2008; 98:244–253.

[204] Offit PA, Jew RK. Addressing parents' concerns: do vaccines contain harmful preservatives, adjuvants, additives, or residuals? *Pediatrics.* 2003 Dec;112(6 Pt 1):1394-7.

205 http://www.fda.gov/RegulatoryInformation/Legislation/FederalFoodDrugand-CosmeticActFDCAct/SignificantAmendmentstotheFDCAct/FDAMA/default.htm.

206 http://www.cdc.gov/vaccinesafety/concerns/thimerosal/.

207 http://www.usphs.gov/aboutus/agencies/hhs.aspx.

208 Joint statement of the American Academy of Pediatrics (AAP) and the United States Public Health Service (USPHS). *Pediatrics.* 1999 Sep;104(3 Pt 1):568-9.

209 http://www.cdc.gov/mmwr/preview/mmwrhtml/mm4826a3.htm.

210 http://www.fda.gov/BiologicsBloodVaccines/QuestionsaboutVaccines/UCM070430.

211 http://www.fda.gov/BiologicsBloodVaccines/SafetyAvailability/VaccineSafety/UCM096228.

212 http://www.fda.gov/downloads/BiologicsBloodVaccines/Vaccines/ApprovedProducts/UCM244609.pdf.

213 http://www.fda.gov/BiologicsBloodVaccines/SafetyAvailability/VaccineSafety/UCM096228.

214 Baker JP. Mercury, vaccines, and autism: one controversy, three histories. *Am J. Public Health.* 2008; 98:244–253.

215 Halsey NA, Goldman L. Balancing risks and benefits: *Primum non nocere* is too simplistic. *Pediatrics.* 2001 Aug;108(2):466-7.

216 http://www.fda.gov/BiologicsBloodVaccines/Vaccines/ApprovedProducts/default.htm.

217 http://www.health.state.mn.us/divs/idepc/immunize/safety/tcontent.pdf.

218 http://www.nvic.org/Downloads/FDA-Response-to-Thimerosal-Petition.aspx.

219 http://www.fda.gov/ohrms/dockets/dailys/04/aug04/080404/04p-0349-cp00001-01-vol1.pdf.

220 http://www.safeminds.org/about/history-and-accomplishments.html.

221 http://www.cdc.gov/vaccinesafety/concerns/thimerosal/thimerosal_timeline.html.

222 http://www.autismresourcefoundation.org/info/info.2002.html.

223 http://health.state.ga.us/pdfs/prevention/immunization/Thimerosal%20Timeline.pdf.

224 United States. Mercury in medicine report. *Congressional Record.* Washington: GPO, May 21, 2003: 1011-1030.

225 Adel Mahmoud, letter to Jeffrey Koplan, July 7, 1999.

226 Adel Mahmoud, letter to David Satcher, July 7, 1999.

227 Adel Mahmoud, letter to Jeffrey Koplan, September 8, 1999.

228 Adel Mahmoud, letter to Walter Orenstein, September 8, 1999.

229 John Jabara, letter to Jeffrey Koplan, July 21, 1999.

230 http://www.gsk.com/about-us/our-history.html.

231 Jeffrey Koplan, letter to John Labara, November 26, 1999.

232 http://www.who.int/immunization/newsroom/thiomersal_questions_and_answers/en/index.html.

[233] http://www.who.int/immunization/sage/meetings/2012/april/USFDA_perspective_thimerosal_alternatives.pdf.

[234] http://www.who.int/immunization/sage/meetings/2012/april/thiomersal_summary_sessions_1_2.pdf.

[235] http://www.merck.com/product/usa/pi_circulars/p/pneumovax_23/pneumovax_pi.pdf.

[236] http://www.unicef.org/mdg/poverty.html.

[237] http://www.unicef.org/supply/files/UNICEF_Supply_Annual_Report_2010_web.pdf.

[238] http://www.who.int/csr/disease/hepatitis/whocdscsrlyo20022/en/index4.html#vaccines.

[239] http://www.merck.com/product/usa/pi_circulars/r/recombivax_hb/recombivax_pi.pdf.

Chapter 3:
Despite Reductions in Thimerosal in US Childhood Vaccines, Potential Exposure Remains High

It would be a mistake to believe that only poor children in developing nations are still being exposed to Thimerosal.[240] Most Americans are surprised to learn that many flu vaccines still contain Thimerosal, according to a 2006 survey funded by putchildrenfirst.org, a parent-led vaccine safety advocacy group.[241] For a variety of reasons, children's total Thimerosal exposure remains quite high, despite the phaseout of Thimerosal-preserved vaccines from the childhood vaccination schedule.

One reason this exposure remains high is that Thimerosal at a standard preservative level of 0.01 percent or trace levels is still found in childhood diphtheria and tetanus toxoids (DT) vaccines, a childhood DTaP vaccine (Tripedia), a childhood DTaP+Hib vaccine (TriHIBit), two booster tetanus and diphtheria toxoids (Td) vaccines (Sanofi Pasteur's Decavac and a MassBiologics Laboratories' product), and the single dose formulation of Novartis's flu shot.[242][243][244][245] All told, as of April 2009, Thimerosal was still present in approximately 169 FDA-approved prescription and over-the-counter drugs, including nasal sprays and antibiotics.[246][247][248]

Even as Thimerosal doses were being reduced or removed from many standard children's vaccines, the CDC began recommending flu shots for healthy infants between six and twenty-three months of age. The CDC issued these recommendations, updating the agency's 2001 recommendations on flu vaccines, in April 2002. At that time, all FDA-approved flu shot vaccines (inactivated influenza virus) were either Thimerosal-preserved or had trace amounts of Thimerosal.[249][250][251][252]

The CDC's reasons for lowering the age of flu vaccinations for children are questionable, because very little scientific evidence actually exists that indicates that flu vaccinations are effective at preventing children under two years of age from contracting influenza. Several studies appearing in *The Lancet, JAMA,* and *Pediatrics International* and by the Cochrane Collaboration have essentially concluded that the efficacy of an inactivated virus vaccine was no better than a placebo.[253][254][255][256][257][258] In fact, research suggests that flu shots are not very effective at preventing flu-like illnesses in healthy adults, either. On the order of one hundred adults need to be vaccinated, a 2010 study

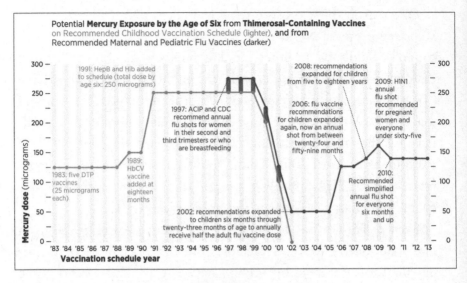

FIGURE 8

found, to prevent flu-like illness in just one person in an average flu season.[259]

Nonetheless, the latest CDC recommendations for the 2013 to 2014 flu season still call for every person six months of age or older to receive an annual flu vaccination.[260] In effect, the CDC has switched the main source of American children's Thimerosal exposure from early childhood vaccines to Thimerosal-preserved flu shots.

Five out of the nine brands approved for children under eighteen are still Thimerosal-preserved or contain trace amounts of Thimerosal as of the 2013 to 2014 flu season. The multidose vials from CSL Limited, ID Biomedical Corporation of Quebec (distributed by GlaxoSmithKline), Novartis, and Sanofi Pasteur for Afluria, FluLaval and Flulaval Quadrivalent, Fluvirin, and Fluzone, respectively, contain a preservative level of Thimerosal equaling 25 micrograms or less of mercury per 0.5 milliliter of vaccine; Novartis also markets a single-use, prefilled syringe with a trace of Thimerosal.[261 262]

The rise in the share of Thimerosal from flu vaccines began in 1997, when ACIP and the CDC first recommended the shots for pregnant women in their second and third trimesters, as well as those who were breastfeeding.[263 264 265] In 2002, the CDC extended the recommendation to all children six through twenty-three months of age, and in 2004, recommended that women in all stages of pregnancy be vaccinated.[266 267] Two years later, in 2006, the recommendation was extended to children twenty-four to fifty-nine months of age, with two staggered doses for the child's first vaccination; in 2008, it was extended to children five to eighteen years of age.[268 269]

Then another vaccine was added to the mix. In 2009, along with the seasonal influenza vaccine, the CDC began recommending the 2009 H1N1 vaccine for everyone under sixty-five, including pregnant women and children.[270] The CDC also raised the possibility of giving young children two doses.[271] Following this CDC regimen, pregnant women could receive two 0.5 milliliter doses of a Thimerosal-preserved influenza vaccine during their pregnancy, which contained H1N1 starting in 2010, while children under nine years of age could each receive up to a 0.5 milliliter dose containing 25 micrograms of Thimerosal per year.[272 273 274] Adherence to the CDC recommendations were high: About 43 percent of pregnant women—nearly half of the pregnant population, in other words—received the H1N1 vaccine during the 2009 to 2010 flu season, according to unpublished data from the CDC appearing in the *American Journal of Obstetrics & Gynecology*.[275]

In 2010, to reduce complexity and ensure that adults who might be at increased risk of flu complications received vaccinations, the CDC recommended that everyone ages six months or older obtain a flu shot.[276] Complying individuals between eighteen and forty-nine years old—previously outside the recommended age range—could now be exposed to about an 800 microgram greater maximum exposure to mercury over that time span of thirty-three years. In this way, the CDC's expanding flu shot recommendations have substantially increased the potential exposure to mercury from vaccines over a lifetime for both children and adults.

While the coverage rates for the flu vaccine for children and pregnant women are not as high as for the childhood pediatric vaccine schedule in the 1990s and through current day, the rates have nevertheless become substantial.[277] For the 2012 to 2013 flu season, flu vaccine coverage stood at 56.6 percent for children ages six months to seventeen years, according to the CDC—a rise of 5 percentage points from the previous flu season.[278] The final statistics, made available in September 2013, did not break down this large age range any further. But preliminary survey results had estimated that more than two-thirds (68.1 percent) of children aged six months to four years were vaccinated; for the five-to-twelve-year age bracket, the figure was 57.2 percent.[279] Back in the early years of the expanding flu shot recommendations, such as in 2003 and 2004, the CDC gauged the childhood influenza vaccination coverage rate at under 1 in 5, but this figure has risen steadily over the years to today's majority coverage.[280 281 282 283] For pregnant women, the influenza vaccination coverage rate in 1997 was estimated at just 11 percent, rising to 19 percent by 2008, and in recent years has climbed closer to 40 percent.[284 285]

Flu shot–derived Thimerosal is a potential danger to a developing fetus, according to various studies. Organic mercury (including ethyl- and methylmercury) can readily cross into the brain and placenta, as acknowledged in reports from the early 2000s from Lynn Goldman and Michael Shannon, William Slikker, Jr., and David Ayoub and F. Edward Yazbak.[286][287][288] In regard to methylmercury, studies have found that the fetal blood level of mercury (as indicated by mercury levels in umbilical cord blood) typically exceeds the level in the mother's blood.[289] A Japanese study from 1997 showed that the cord blood methylmercury concentration can reach 4.4 times that of the mother.[290] Another Japanese study from 1967 suggested that—at least in mice—ethylmercury proportionally accumulates more in fetal tissue compared to maternal tissue, particularly in the central nervous system.[291][292]

Other studies have weighed in on the possibility of harm. A 2000 study by Gregory Stajich measured mercury levels in preterm and term infants prior to and after receiving vaccines. The study documented a "significant increase" in mercury levels in both groups of infant. The study's abstract further noted that "post-vaccination mercury levels were significantly higher in preterm infants as compared with term infants. Because mercury is known to be a potential neurotoxin to infants, further study of its pharmacodynamics is warranted."[293] A study following in 2002 by Michael Pichichero—which will be discussed in detail in the next chapter and that claimed to support Thimerosal's safety—found Thimerosal blood levels as high as 20 nanomoles per liter in two-month-olds administered shots of Thimerosal-preserved DTaP and HepB this exposure to 37.5 micrograms of ethylmercury from the two shots, however, rises to 62.5 micrograms when a Thimerosal-containing Hib shot is included, as was recommended at the two-month visit starting in the 1990s.[294]

These last two studies' findings become especially relevant given that a 2005 study showed Thimerosal can be toxic to developing human neurons at levels as low as a 4.35 nanomolar concentration—below the 29 nanomolar concentration that is considered the safe limit for mercury in umbilical cord blood.[295] [296]

A 2012 study by Australian scientists Ian Brown and David Austin examined the potential mercury exposure for a fetus whose mother receives a single Thimerosal-preserved flu shot. Even completely unrealistically assuming that the placenta blocks fully 99 percent of the available mercury, only for the final two gestational weeks would the mercury exposure for the fetus, based on its weight, not exceed the EPA's RfD for methylmercury. Optimistically assuming that the placenta may block perhaps 90 percent of the mercury, a fetus at that the start of the second trimester would still receive about one hundred times the EPA's RfD.[297]

The alarming implications of this study are supported by an epidemiological study carried out in 2012 by an independent researcher, Gary Goldman, based in California. Goldman queried the Vaccine Adverse Event Reporting System (VAERS)—a database we will explain further later in this book—for fetal-loss reports for three consecutive flu seasons after administration of maternal flu vaccines. "Fetal-loss reports" refer to spontaneous abortions or stillbirths. The flu seasons in question were 2008 to 2009, 2009 to 2010, and 2010 to 2011. For the 2009 to 2010 flu season, pregnant women were advised to obtain an H1N1 vaccination in addition to their regular seasonal flu shot. Multidose versions of the H1N1 vaccine contained Thimerosal.[298] From VAERS, Goldman found that incidence of fetal-loss reports per one million pregnant women who were vaccinated spiked dramatically in 2009 to 2010. The incidence rates were as follows: 2008 to 2009—6.8; 2009 to 2010—77.8; 2010 to 2011—12.6.[299]

Given these documented hazards, we will now analyze and measure Thimerosal exposure in the past decade through today compared to the 1990s. As explained previously, American children who were fully vaccinated according to the standard childhood vaccination schedule between 1991 and 1999, and who happened to be injected with vaccines that all contained Thimerosal, would have received as much as 475 micrograms of Thimerosal by age two. That equates to an exposure to 237.5 micrograms of mercury.[300 301 302 303] By six years of age, the children would have received a final DTaP shot possibly containing Thimerosal for an additional 50 micrograms of Thimerosal, and thus 25 micrograms of mercury, totaling off at 525 micrograms of Thimerosal and 262.5 micrograms of mercury.[304]

Let us now compare that to children who grew up in the last decade receiving just Thimerosal-containing, multidose flu vaccines. Children born in 2003 whose parents began following the CDC's flu recommendations in 2002, for instance, could conceivably have been exposed to 50 micrograms of Thimerosal in utero. Next, children could have received one 25-microgram dose of Thimerosal at six months of age, followed by two other 25-microgram doses between the ages of one and two and then two and three, per receiving the vaccine on an annual basis. After three years of age, children are administered a full adult dose of vaccine, which can contain 50 micrograms of Thimerosal, for an exposure of 150 micrograms from ages four through six. The total for children born in 2002, then, could come to 225 micrograms of

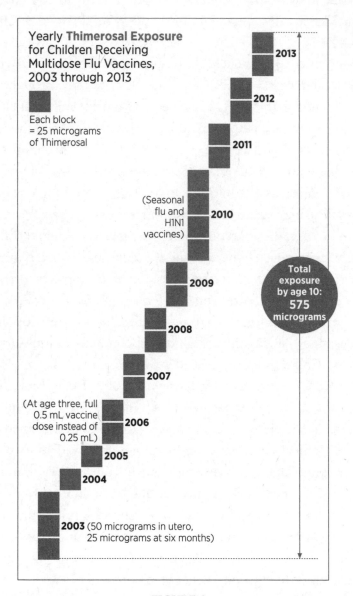

FIGURE 9

Thimerosal, and 112.5 micrograms of mercury, through their first six years of life.[305] [306]

Children born more recently, however, could have received an additional 50 micrograms of Thimerosal on top of that amount from the H1N1 vaccine in the 2009 to 2010 flu season.[307] [308] [309] In fact, if parents of children born today follow CDC flu shot recommendations to the letter, even those who now receive no Thimerosal from other early childhood vaccines, but receive Thimerosal-preserved flu shots, will have a potential total dose of about 187.5 micrograms of mercury between the time they are six months old and their eighth birthday. That number approaches the 237.5 micrograms of mercury that those vaccinated in the 1990s received from the early childhood schedule by age two.

Though the mercury exposure from vaccines is no longer as acute as it once was, it begins in utero, a critical period for neurological development, and it extends throughout a lifetime, carrying with it the potential risk for adverse neurological consequences. Under the CDC's 2013 recommendations, eight-year-old children still face the possibility of an additional exposure of 25 micrograms of mercury every year for the rest of their lives should they receive a Thimerosal-containing multidose flu shot and if the preservative remains in use. Presuming a seventy-eight-year life expectancy and an annual flu shot, this scenario would add up to a total lifetime maximum exposure of about 1,937.5 micrograms (1.9375 milligrams) of mercury.[310] [311]

Every year, well over one hundred million Americans receive a flu vaccine. The figure for the 2012 to 2013 flu season approached 140 million adults and children.[312] Of the 145 million doses projected to have been available in 2012, the CDC estimated that 59 percent were Thimerosal-preserved. The remaining 41 percent was a mix of inactivated flu shots plus a live-virus vaccine nasal spray, called Flumist, which does not contain Thimerosal. Flumist, however, is not approved for pregnant women, thus increasing the chances that they will receive a Thimerosal-containing flu vaccine.[313][314] For the most recent 2013 to 2014 flu season, of the high-end estimated 145 million flu vaccine doses made available, the picture has substantially improved: only 39 percent of the doses is Thimerosal-preserved. Several new "quadrivalent" vaccines, with components of four flu viruses rather than the typical three (trivalent), became available. As in years past, though, every multidose vial manufactured for the 2013 to 2014 flu season contains Thimerosal.[315]

HMOs and state and local health departments apparently generally opt for the multidose vaccines, which contain a preservative level of Thimerosal and are less expensive than single-dose shots.[316][317][318][319][320] The CDC has stated these vaccines are safe to be injected into human beings.[321][322] This would not seem consistent with the EPA guidelines advising for "safe end-of-life management"—that is, safe disposal—of Thimerosal-containing vaccines as a mercury-containing commercial medical product.[323][324] The mercury levels in some Thimerosal-containing vaccines are high enough to have the vaccines, if unused and set to be discarded, classified as hazardous waste. A 2007 document from the Wisconsin Department of Natural Resources Bureau of Waste and Materials Management details how to properly dispose of excess vaccines containing Thimerosal. It points out that vaccines preserved with 0.01 percent Thimerosal—which would include DTP/DTaP and Hib back in the 1990s and early 2000s, as well as current multidose flu vials—have about 50 milligrams of mercury per liter. That level exceeds the 0.2 milligrams per liter regulatory level for mercury to be characterized as hazardous waste. Accordingly, excess Thimerosal-containing vaccines must either be shipped back to the manufacturer (if unexpired) or transported to a hazardous waste collection facility, lest the mercury be released into the environment.[325] Yet government regulators allow this chemical to be injected into pregnant women and children during their most vulnerable developmental stages. It does not appear that summary statements of the supposedly better economics of Thimerosal-preserved multidose vaccines over single-dose vaccines have taken into account these hidden transportation and environmental hazard mitigation costs.

The CDC, as noted previously, did not express a preference for Thimerosal-free formulations for pediatric vaccines in the early 2000s, even though at least two major manufacturers advised that they could supply enough preservative-free vaccine to meet demand. Similarly, when it has come to Thimerosal-containing flu vaccine formulations, the CDC has again not taken a stance that would encourage a transition away from preserved multidose vials.

In April 2004, Damien A. Braga, the US president of Aventis Pasteur (now Sanofi Pasteur), wrote to Julie Gerberding, director of the CDC, regarding the possibility that the CDC might imminently recommend that pediatric populations receive preservative-free flu vaccines.[326] Braga expressed support for such a transition in a "carefully planned" and not an "abrupt" fashion, as with the 1999 USPHS/AAP policy statement, and in order to "maintain continued public confidence" in the pediatric as well as the adult national influenza immunization program. Braga wrote: "Aventis Pasteur supports the development of a timetable to ensure an

45

orderly transition to a policy that expresses preference for preservative-free influenza vaccine for infants."[327] Despite these overtures, Gerberding responded that in making its new recommendations that children ages six to twenty-three months receive routine flu shots, the CDC through ACIP "did not express a preference for any type of licensed influenza vaccine over another for this age group."[328]

The case remained the same in 2006, when the CDC again expanded flu shot recommendations. Sanofi Pasteur was prepared to double its production of Thimerosal-free children's flu vaccines, reflecting demand for such formulations from some parents, doctors, and medical groups. Neither the CDC nor state health departments, however, requested that it do so. A CDC spokesperson at the time told this book's author that the agency still did not "have a preference for Thimerosal-free vaccines."[329] Gerberding, it should be noted, wrote in her letter to Braga:

> CDC is committed to working with the Food and Drug Administration, other partners, and manufacturers, such as Aventis Pasteur, to assure the continued reduction or removal of thimerosal from influenza vaccine targeted for children and pregnant women as expeditiously as possible without causing interruption in the flu vaccine supply for the upcoming flu season.

A decade later, children and pregnant women continue to be injected with Thimerosal via flu vaccines.

Notes

240 http://www.unicef.org/supply/files/UNICEF_Supply_Annual_Report_2010_web.pdf.

241 http://www.putchildrenfirst.org/media/f.5.pdf.

242 http://www.fda.gov/BiologicsBloodVaccines/SafetyAvailability/VaccineSafety/UCM096228.

243 http://www.fda.gov/downloads/biologicsbloodvaccines/vaccines/approvedproducts/ucm101580.pdf.

244 http://www.fda.gov/downloads/BiologicsBloodVaccines/Vaccines/ApprovedProducts/UCM246215.pdf.

245 https://www.novartisvaccinesdirect.com/Pdf/Fluvirin-PI-2010-2012_approved.pdf.

246 http://www.fda.gov/RegulatoryInformation/Legislation/FederalFoodDrugand-CosmeticActFDCAct/SignificantAmendmentstotheFDCAct/FDAMA/ucm100219.htm?utm_source=fdaSearch&utm_medium=website&utm_term=mercury&utm_content=9.

247 http://www.fda.gov/ohrms/dockets/dockets/04p0349/04p-0349-ref0001-38-Tab-34-CDER-Drug-Info-vol7.pdf.

248 http://www.fda.gov/ohrms/dockets/98fr/042999b.txt.

249 http://www.cdc.gov/mmwr/preview/mmwrhtml/rr5103a1.htm.

250 http://www.cdc.gov/ncidod/diseases/flu/fluvirus.htm.

251 http://www.cdc.gov/mmwr/preview/mmwrhtml/rr5004a1.htm.

252 http://www.fda.gov/BiologicsBloodVaccines/SafetyAvailability/VaccineSafety/UCM096228.

253 Jefferson T, Smith S, Demicheli V, Harnden A, Rivetti A, Di Pietrantonj C. Assessment of the efficacy and effectiveness of influenza vaccines in healthy children: systematic review. *Lancet*. 2005 Feb 26-Mar 4; 365(9461): 773-780.

254 Smith S, Demicheli V, Di Pietrantonj C, Harnden AR, Jefferson T, Matheson NJ, Rivetti A. Vaccines for preventing influenza in healthy children. *Cochrane Database Syst Rev.* 2006 Jan 25; (1): CD004879.

255 Jefferson T, Rivetti A, Harnden A, Di Pietrantonj C, Demicheli V. Vaccines for preventing influenza in healthy children. *Cochrane Database Syst Rev.* 2008 Apr 16;(2):CD004879. doi: 10.1002/14651858.CD004879.pub3.

256 Hoberman A, Greenberg DP, Paradise JL, Rockette HE, Lave JR, Kearney DH, Colborn DK, Kurs-Lasky M, Haralam MA, Byers CJ, Zoffel LM, Fabian IA, Bernard BS, Kerr JD.

Effectiveness of inactivated influenza vaccine in preventing acute otitis media in young children: a randomized controlled trial. *JAMA.* 2003 Sep 24;290(12):1608-16.

[257] Maeda T, Shintani Y, Nakano K, Terashima K, Yamada Y. Failure of inactivated influenza A vaccine to protect healthy children aged 6-24 months. *Pediatr Int.* 2004 Apr;46(2):122-5.

[258] http://www.cochrane.org/.

[259] http://summaries.cochrane.org/CD001269/vaccines-to-prevent-influenza-in-healthy-adults.

[260] http://www.cdc.gov/mmwr/preview/mmwrhtml/rr6207a1.htm.

[261] http://www.cdc.gov/flu/about/season/index.htm.

[262] http://www.cdc.gov/mmwr/preview/mmwrhtml/rr6207a1.htm.

[263] Mak TK, Mangtani P, Leese J, Watson JM, Pfeifer D. Influenza vaccination in pregnancy: current evidence and selected national policies. *Lancet Infect Dis.* 2008 Jan;8(1):44-52.

[264] http://www.cdc.gov/mmwr/preview/mmwrhtml/00047346.htm.

[265] Boksa P. Maternal infection during pregnancy and schizophrenia. *J Psychiatry Neurosci.* 2008;33(3):183-5.

[266] http://www.cdc.gov/mmwr/preview/mmwrhtml/rr5103a1.htm.

[267] http://www.cdc.gov/flu/protect/vaccine/qa_vacpregnant.htm.

[268] http://www.cdc.gov/mmwr/preview/mmwrhtml/rr5510a1.htm.

[269] http://www.cdc.gov/mmwr/preview/mmwrhtml/rr5707a1.htm.

[270] http://www.cdc.gov/mmwr/preview/mmwrhtml/rr5808a1.htm.

[271] http://www.cdc.gov/mmwr/preview/mmwrhtml/rr5810a1.htm.

[272] http://www.cdc.gov/flu/about/qa/vaccine-selection.htm.

[273] http://www.cdc.gov/h1n1flu/.

[274] http://www.fda.gov/NewsEvents/Newsroom/PressAnnouncements/ucm172772.htm.

[275] Moro PL, Broder K, Zheteyeva Y, Revzina N, Tepper N, Kissin D, Barash F, Arana J, Brantley MD, Ding H, Singleton JA, Walton K, Haber P, Lewis P, Yue X, Destefano F, Vellozzi C. Adverse events following administration to pregnant women of influenza A (H1N1) 2009 monovalent vaccine reported to the Vaccine Adverse Event Reporting System. *Am J Obstet Gynecol.* 2011 Nov;205(5):473.e1-9. doi: 10.1016/j.ajog.2011.06.047. Epub 2011 Jun 21.

[276] http://www.cdc.gov/mmwr/preview/mmwrhtml/rr5908a1.htm.

[277] http://www.cdc.gov/vaccines/stats-surv/nis/articles.htm.

[278] http://www.cdc.gov/flu/fluvaxview/coverage-1213estimates.htm.

[279] http://www.cdc.gov/flu/pdf/fluvaxview/kennedy_2013_summit_slides2.pdf.

[280] http://www.cdc.gov/mmwr/preview/mmwrhtml/mm5504a3.htm?s_cid=mm5504a3_e.

[281] http://www.cdc.gov/mmwr/preview/mmwrhtml/mm5539a1.htm.

[282] http://www.cdc.gov/mmwr/preview/mmwrhtml/mm5637a2.htm.

[283] http://www.cdc.gov/flu/professionals/vaccination/trends/age-groups.htm.

[284] http://www.cdc.gov/flu/pdf/professionals/nhis89_08fluvaxtrendtab.pdf.

[285] http://www.cdc.gov/mmwr/preview/mmwrhtml/mm6138a2.htm?s_cid=mm6138a2_w.

[286] Goldman LR, Shannon MW. AAP committee on Environmental Health technical report: mercury in the environment: implications for pediatricians. *Pediatrics.* 2001 Jul 1; 108: 197-205.

[287] Slikker W Jr. Developmental neurotoxicity of therapeutics: survey of novel recent findings. *Neurotoxicology.* 2000;21:50.

[288] Ayoub D, Yazbak F. Influenza vaccination during pregnancy: a critical assessment of the recommendations of the Advisory Committee on Immunization Practices (ACIP). *J Am Phys Surg.* 2006; 11(2):41-47.

[289] http://www.epa.gov/iris/subst/0073.htm.

[290] Fujita M, Takabatake E. Mercury levels in human maternal and neonatal blood, hair and milk. *Bull Environ Contam Toxicol.* 1977 Aug;18(2):205-9.

[291] Ukita T, Takeda Y, Sato Y, Takahashi T. Distribution of 203Hg labeled mercury compounds in adult and pregnant mice determined by whole-body autoradiography. *Radioisotopes.* 1967;16:439-448.

[292] Ayoub D, Yazbak F. Influenza vaccination during pregnancy: a critical assessment of the recommendations of the Advisory Committee on Immunization Practices (ACIP). *J Am Phys Surg.* 2006; 11(2):41-47 at 44.

[293] Stajich GV, Lopez GP, Harry SW, Sexson WR. Iatrogenic exposure to mercury after hepatitis B vaccination in preterm infants. *J Pediatr.* 2000 May;136(5):679-81.

[294] Pichichero MF, Cernichiari E, Lopreiato J, Treanor J. Mercury concentrations and metabolism in infants receiving vaccines containing thiomersal: a descriptive study. *Lancet.* 2002 Nov 30; 360(9347):1737-1741.

[295] Parran DK, Barker A, Ehrich M. Effects of thimerosal on NGF signal transduction and cell death in neuroblastoma cells. *Toxicol Sci.* 2005 Jul;86(1):132-40.

[296] Hurley AM, Tadrous M, Miller ES. Thimerosal-containing vaccines and autism: a review of recent epidemiologic studies. *J Pediatr Pharmacol Ther.* 2010 Jul;15(3):173-81.

[297] Brown I, Austin D. Maternal transfer of mercury to the developing embryo/fetus: is there a safe level? *Toxicological & Environmental Chemistry.* 2012; 94:8, 1610-1627.

[298] http://www.cdc.gov/h1n1flu/vaccination/thimerosal_qa.htm.

[299] Goldman G. Comparison of VAERS fetal-loss reports during three consecutive influenza seasons: was there a synergistic fetal toxicity associated with the two-vaccine 2009/2010 season? *Hum Exp Toxicol.* 2012 Sep 27. [Epub ahead of print].

[300] http://www.cdc.gov/mmwr/preview/mmwrhtml/00041736.htm.

[301] http://www.cdc.gov/mmwr/preview/mmwrhtml/00033405.htm.

[302] http://www.fda.gov/BiologicsBloodVaccines/SafetyAvailability/VaccineSafety/UCM096228.

[303] Ball LK, Ball R, Pratt RD. An assessment of thimerosal use in childhood vaccines. *Pediatrics.* 2001 May;107(5):1147-54.

[304] http://www.cdc.gov/mmwr/preview/mmwrhtml/00056261.htm.

305 http://www.cdc.gov/mmwr/preview/mmwrhtml/mm5102a4.htm.

306 http://www.fda.gov/BiologicsBloodVaccines/SafetyAvailability/VaccineSafety/ UCM096228.

307 http://www.cdc.gov/h1n1flu/vaccination/thimerosal_qa.htm.

308 http://www.cdc.gov/h1n1flu/.

309 http://www.fda.gov/NewsEvents/Newsroom/PressAnnouncements/ucm172772.htm.

310 http://www.cdc.gov/flu/protect/vaccine/vaccines.htm.

311 http://www.cdc.gov/mmwr/preview/mmwrhtml/rr5908a1.htm.

312 http://www.cdc.gov/flu/fluvaxview/coverage-1213estimates.htm.

313 https://web.archive.org/web/20130719215501/http://www.cdc.gov/flu/about/qa/vaxsupply.htm.

314 http://www.cdc.gov/flu/about/qa/vaxsupply.htm#table.

315 http://www.cdc.gov/mmwr/preview/mmwrhtml/rr6207a1.htm.

316 http://www.huffingtonpost.com/robert-f-kennedy-jr/a-poisonous-move-for-kids_b_16899.html.

317 http://www.nvic.org/VaccineSafetyTips.aspx.

318 http://www.everydayhealth.com/allergy-specialist/swine-flu-vaccines-thimerosal.aspx.

319 http://www.immunizemaryland.org/pdfs/resources/2010-2011%20MD%20Flu%20Season%20Wrap-Up%20Materials_FINAL.pdf.

320 http://pediatrics.about.com/cs/immunizations/a/find_a_flu_shot.htm.

321 http://www.cdc.gov/flu/protect/vaccine/thimerosal.htm#safe.

322 http://www.sfgate.com/health/article/Mercury-laced-shots-OK-for-kids-CDC-says-2799655.php.

323 http://www.epa.gov/hg/mgmt_options.html#Medical.

324 http://www.epa.gov/hg/spills/index.htm#disposal.

325 http://web.archive.org/web/20091122091534/http://dnr.wi.gov/org/aw/wm/publications/anewpub/WA841.pdf.

326 http://en.sanofi.com/our_company/history/history.aspx.

327 Damien A. Braga, letter to Julie Louise Gerberding, April 20, 2004.

328 Julie Louise Gerberding, letter to Damien A. Braga, June 18, 2004.

329 http://www.huffingtonpost.com/robert-f-kennedy-jr/a-poisonous-move-for-kids_b_16899.html.

Chapter 4:
The Comparable Dangers of Ethylmercury and Methylmercury

A major reason for public confusion regarding the potential danger of mercury in Thimerosal is that this mercury is not the same type regularly encountered in seafood.[330] Government recommendations advising pregnant women and young children to limit their consumption of seafood high in mercury are well known. The element, which occurs naturally and from sources of industrial pollution, is consumed by fish and stored in their tissues. Mercury accumulates especially in larger, long-lived, predatory fish, such as sharks and swordfish.[331][332]

The type of mercury found in seafood is called methylmercury; the type that is used in Thimerosal is called ethylmercury.[333]

Government health agencies, such as the CDC, maintain that ethylmercury is less toxic than methylmercury because it is broken down and excreted more quickly. Accordingly, as the CDC states on its website, ethylmercury is much less likely to "accumulate in the body and cause harm."[334] The World Health Organization states that the half-life of ethylmercury—that is, the length of time half of a given dose remains in the body—is "short (less than one week) compared to methyl mercury (1.5 months), making exposure to ethylmercury in blood comparatively brief."[335]

The scientific literature, however, does not unanimously support these statements. Multiple studies conducted recently and dating back decades contradict the notion that ethylmercury is less toxic than methylmercury. Aside from laboratory experiments, the comparable danger posed by the two types of mercury was also plainly evidenced in the 1950s, 1960s, and 1970s, when ethylmercury- and methylmercury-containing fungicides poisoned human populations.[336]

Poisoning epidemics first brought the menace of methylmercury to light. A major event was the Minamata Bay disaster in Japan. Widespread human consumption of mercury-contaminated fish from the industrially polluted Minamata Bay in the late 1950s and early 1960s poisoned 121 people and killed 46. After a second outbreak in a separate location, nearly 3,000 people were eventually certified as having been poisoned.[337 338]

An epidemic in Iraq in the early 1970s from methylmercury fungicide–tainted grain also helped alert the public to the threat of this form of mercury.[339] The consumption of homemade bread prepared with mercury fungicide–tainted seed led to more than 6,500 hospital cases of poisoning and 459 deaths.[340]

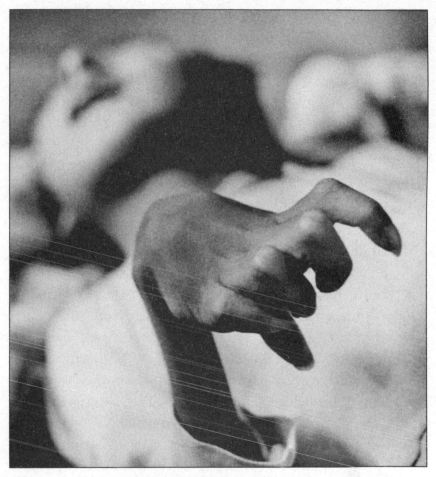

This photo is of the gnarled hand of a sufferer of Minamata disease, Tomoko Uemura. The Japanese girl was poisoned in the womb by methylmercury. American photojournalist W. Eugene Smith took the photo. Credit: Aileen Archive

In 1995, based on such epidemics as well as the Faroe Island and New Zealand studies and other research, the EPA established a safe "reference dose" (RfD). An RfD is defined as "an estimate of a daily exposure to the human population (including sensitive subgroups) that is likely to be without an appreciable risk of adverse effects when experienced during a lifetime," according to the EPA.[341]

The EPA adopted for methylmercury an RfD of 0.1 microgram of mercury per kilogram of the individual's body weight per day.[342][343] Other health agencies set their own recommended limits for methylmercury exposure, such as the FDA in 1979, the World Health Organization in 1989 and the US Agency for Toxic Substances and Disease Registry (ATSDR) in 1999. The highest of these limits was the WHO's, at 0.47 microgram per kilogram of body weight per day.[344][345]

Based on continued concerns about methylmercury exposure, gaps in the scientific data regarding mercury toxicity and conflicting RfD recommendations, in 1999 the US Congress directed the EPA to contract with the nonprofit, independent National Research Council (NRC) to prepare recommendations on an updated and appropriate RfD. The EPA commissioned the National Academy of Sciences (NAS) and the NRC to carry out a study on toxicological effects of methylmercury compounds. The goal was to review the process used by the EPA to establish national safety standards. The committee evaluated the literature, which demonstrated methylmercury compounds' high toxicity to brain tissue, even at minute levels. The NAS ultimately agreed with the EPA's originally conceived RfD, which remains in place today.[346]

An RfD has never been established for ethylmercury, presumably because there is not a common environmental exposure or route of ingestion as with the methylmercury in seafood. Ethylmercury, however, unlike methylmercury, is injected into the human body as part of Thimerosal.

A single Thimerosal-preserved flu vaccine contains 25 micrograms of ethylmercury. If the EPA RfD for ingested methylmercury is applied to this injected ethylmercury figure, an individual would have to weigh more than 250 kilograms (551 pounds) for the 25 microgram exposure to be considered safe. Young children are commonly given half-doses of Thimerosal-preserved flu shots nowadays, working out to approximately fourteen times a safe daily exposure for a 20-pound (9-kilogram) individual. Back in the 1990s, a two-month-old child could have received 62.5 micrograms from three vaccines in a single doctor's visit. Assuming the child weighed about 5 kilograms (11 pounds), he or she would have received 125 times the EPA RfD for methylmercury.

At least one study has suggested that the methylmercury RfD should be set lower for infants and also for fetuses. In 1995, Steven Gilbert and Kimberly Grant-Webster wrote:

Available information on the developmental neurotoxic effects of MeHg [methylmercury], particularly the neurobehavioral effects, indicates that the fetus and infant are more sensitive to adverse effects of MeHg. It is therefore recommended that pregnant women and women of childbearing age be strongly advised to limit their exposure to potential sources of MeHg. Based on results from human and animal studies on the developmental neurotoxic effects of methylmercury, the accepted reference dose should be lowered to 0.025 to 0.06 MeHg [microgram]/kg/day.[347]

What might this mean for a fetus nowadays? We'll take the low end of that estimate and apply it to an average 1.15-kilogram

(2.54-pound) fetus at the start of the third trimester.[348] A fetus exposed to 25 micrograms of mercury via a Thimerosal-preserved flu shot administered to its pregnant mother would be subject to 870 times the proposed lower reference dose.

It should be pointed out, of course, that eating a 6-ounce can of tuna also "overexposes" a child to mercury based on an RfD of 0.1 microgram per kilogram of body weight per day. According to an FDA study, a 6-ounce can of tuna contains on average about 17 micrograms of methylmercury, though this level can vary significantly.[349] As many studies have indicated, however, and which we will review, it is a false equivalency to apply the RfD for methylmercury to ethylmercury. There are other considerations regarding the tuna example. A 2005 paper pointed out that the methylmercury consumed when eating a tuna sandwich has already reacted with proteins and other protective substances in the fish, such as selenium and glutathione. This "bound" methylmercury should not be as toxic, therefore, as an equivalent amount of unprocessed mercury injected into muscle or subcutaneously.[350]

Newer research supports older data that "safe" levels of ethylmercury exposure might indeed be lower than the EPA's RfD. A 2012 Italian study, for instance, showed that ethylmercury-containing Thimerosal diminished the viability of human cells in the lab at a concentration one-fiftieth that of methylmercury.[351] Japanese research on rats in 1968 showed that ethylmercury compounds, such as ethylmercuric chloride from which Thimerosal is made, clear the body more slowly than the mercury compounds mercuric chloride and phenylmercuric chloride.[352] A book chapter in 1972 by Staffan Skerfving, an emeritus professor at Lund University in Sweden, reviewed literature on methylmercury versus ethylmercury, noting several instances where compounds of the latter appeared more toxic than the former in animal studies.[353] For example, ethylmercury chloride killed off half of a test population of mice—a classic "LD50" (lethal dose) study—within a week at a concentration of 12 milligrams of mercury per kilogram of body weight; methylmercury chloride's LD50, meanwhile, lethal to half the mice was 14 milligrams.[354][355]

Further examples abound. Pig studies by Tryphonas and Nielsen in 1973 showed that ethylmercury "proved much more toxic" than methylmercury.[356] Meanwhile, another 1973 study that emerged from a 1971 international conference found the toxicity of ethylmercury compounds comparable to or even greater than that of methylmercury, as well as more persistent in the brain. An advisory committee at the conference reported that the International Committee on Maximum Allowable Concentration for Mercury and Its Compounds grouped ethylmercury with methylmercury, and observed that accounts of human intoxication with ethylmercury have usually described neurological and other symptoms similar to those of methylmercury. The report noted that in studies of patients transfused with a commercial product of human plasma containing 0.01 percent Thimerosal, as well as in studies of mice injected with an ethylmercury solution, the increased level of inorganic mercury added to the mercury already existing in the body resulted in a "longer biological half-life of total mercury than that reported for methylmercury injection."[357]

The WHO's conclusion that ethylmercury is safer because of its "short" half-life may be based on observations that ethylmercury disappears from blood samples quicker than methylmercury. This tendency may be evidence not of ethylmercury's comparative safety, but of its greater danger if, as science has suggested, ethylmercury is not leaving the body but simply migrating more rapidly to the organs, including the brain. Indeed, studies have shown that an ethylmercury compound's short residence in the blood stems from its ability to more easily pass into the organs, where it can remain for long periods and possibly cause injury. For example, A. M. J. N. Blair in 1975 dosed squirrel monkeys intranasally with saline or Thimerosal daily for six months, finding that, compared to the saline group, mercury concentrations in the Thimerosal group were significantly raised in the brain, liver, muscle, and kidney, though not in the blood. Although there were no signs of toxicity in the animals, Blair concluded that the "accumulation of mercury from chronic use of thiomersal-preserved medicines is viewed as a potential health hazard for man."[358]

In 1985, Laszlo Magos showed that the neurotoxicity of both mercury types was broadly comparable. Higher levels of inorganic mercury were found in the kidneys and brains of rats that were fed ethylmercury, though more brain damage was seen in the methylmercury-fed rats. Lower concentrations occurred in those same organs of organic and total mercury in the ethylmercury-treated rats.[359] A short 2002 review in *Molecular Psychiatry* agreed with Magos' work, noting "there appears to be little difference in the neurotoxicity of [methylmercury] and [ethylmercury]," while noting at the time of publication that the anecdotal evidence of autistic children having an "abnormal body burden" of mercury had yet to be explored in the peer-reviewed literature.[360] (Part Three will review relevant subsequent studies on this topic.)

Beyond a possibly greater capacity to have inorganic mercury accumulate in organs, Thimerosal also passes more easily from a mother's bloodstream through the placenta into a developing baby than does methylmercury. That was the evaluation made in a 1983 review study by A. Leonard.[361] In addition, a 1995 study demonstrated that both ethylmercury and methylmercury cause mutagenic changes at similar concentrations in bacterial cells.[362]

With these and other studies as background, an important study in humans took place in the early 2000s. The study, by Michael Pichichero of the University of Rochester Medical Center and published in *The Lancet* in 2002, lent some apparent scientific credence to the idea that ethylmercury is safer than methylmercury.[363] [364] The study assessed mercury levels in the blood, urine, and feces of forty infants ages six months or younger three to twenty-eight days after they had received Thimerosal-preserved vaccines (DTaP, HepB, and in some cases Hib). For comparison, twenty-one similar infants who received Thimerosal-free vaccines were also evaluated. Although infants who received Thimerosal-preserved vaccines had higher levels of mercury in their blood, urine, and feces than did the infants who received Thimerosal-free vaccines, the authors concluded that the levels of mercury detected were not greater than what is considered safe. Most of the mercury from the injected Thimerosal seemed to have left the children's bloodstreams more rapidly than methylmercury found in the blood of those eating fish in previous studies; the researchers estimated a half-life of seven days for ethylmercury in the blood. Pichichero concluded that ethylmercury, therefore, did not remain in children's bodies long enough to possibly cause damage.

In a number of respects, though, this well-known study was seriously flawed. For example, every child in the study was tested only once. The infants were not followed for any length of time, so there was no possibility of seeing a change in the children's mercury levels, or whether any mercury poisoning effects occurred in later years.[365] The study also did not indicate whether any of the children had low levels of the antioxidant glutathione, a substance that helps clear mercury from the body. Glutathione deficiency has been associated with sensitivity to Thimerosal, according to studies by Gotz Westphal, and a 2007 study by Geier and Geier found deficiencies in glutathione pathways in a small group of children with autism who had received Thimerosal-preserved vaccines.[366 367 368 369] The Pichichero study's cohort size of just sixty-one infants was too small to likely include individuals with an autism spectrum disorder (based on an estimated prevalence in the early 2000s of 1 in 166), who again as studies have suggested are poor excreters of mercury. Furthermore, Pichichero, who helped develop the HiB vaccine and previously received grants and honoraria as a consultant for Eli Lilly and other vaccine makers, did not declare these potential conflicts of interest in a statement in his paper, as would seem to be required by *The Lancet's* peer review rules.[370 371 372 373 374]

Notable concerns about the study were voiced in a 2003 letter to *The Lancet* by Neal Halsey, of the Institute for Vaccine Safety at Johns Hopkins Bloomberg School of Public Health, and Lynn Goldman, also of the Bloomberg School of Public Health. Halsey and Goldman pointed out that Pichichero and colleagues "did not measure the peak blood concentrations that occurred within hours after the injections." The concentration listed for one child in the study of 20.55 nanomoles per liter was obtained five days post-vaccination. Assuming Pichichero's own estimate of an ethylmercury half-life in the blood of seven days, the peak blood concentration for this child was 29.4 nanomoles per liter—exceeding the conventional safety threshold of 29.0 nanomoles per liter, and casting doubt on the study's claim that "no children had a concentration of blood mercury exceeding 29 nmol/L." The child in question had received 37.5 micrograms of ethylmercury rather than the possible maximum exposure of 62.5 micrograms. In the latter scenario, the child's peak blood mercury concentration would have hit 48.3 nanomoles per liter. Another child in the study registered a 7 nanomole per liter blood concentration 21 days post-vaccination; extrapolating backwards, this child's peak mercury level might have reached 42 nanomoles per liter. Halsey and Goldman's letter further pointed out that the children in the study—some already with no margin of safety for further mercury exposure—seemed to have come from a population with low background environmental and maternal exposure to methylmercury.[375]

Soon after Pichichero's study came out, new evidence emerged that ethylmercury lingers in the body. The then-director of SafeMinds, Mark Blaxill, and Boyd Haley, then-chairman of the chemistry department at the University of Kentucky, reviewed Pichichero's data, and in an unpublished letter submitted to *Pediatrics* came to a very different conclusion. Pichichero and colleagues had measured the excretion levels of mercury in the stools of 22 healthy infants exposed to Thimerosal-containing vaccines. A range was found for the infants aged two and six months of 23 to 141 nanograms per gram of stool (dry weight). Blaxill and Haley wrote: "The authors interpreted these levels, mere parts per billion, as positive evidence of mercury elimination." When considering the amount of mercury the children might have been exposed to, though, and the expected volume of their stool, this rate of mercury elimination from the body would seem far too low to support a claim of "rapid excretion." Blaxill and Haley considered the 187.5 micrograms of ethylmercury a child could have received by six months of age during the 1990s, and infant stool volumes ranging from 6 to 18 grams (dry weight) per day covering the newborn to six-month age period. Assuming the excretion rate reported by Pichichero, Blaxill and Haley demonstrated that it could take children with low excretion rates of mercury in their stool almost four years to eliminate a 187.5 microgram mercury burden from their bodies.[376]

That finding followed from a study by Amy Holmes coauthored by Blaxill and Haley in 2003. It analyzed hair samples, collected by parents, from fully immunized babies' first haircuts. Compared to hair collected from older children in other studies, which failed to replicate Holmes' results, this first haircut hair was reasoned to be a better indicator by Holmes and coauthors of early childhood mercury exposure. Overall, the study revealed that children with autism between the ages of two and fifteen who had received Thimerosal-preserved vaccines excreted lower levels of mercury into their hair as infants compared with normal, same-aged children also receiving these vaccines. The Holmes study suggested therefore that mercury could be lodging in the brain and hindering neurological development.[377 378 379 380]

In 2006, Luis Maya and Flora Luna expanded the critique of Pichichero's study. The authors pointed out that while Pichichero's team had found ethylmercury to be excreted in appreciable quantities in the feces, the researchers did not study other body parts beyond the blood, such as the central nervous system. In agreement with Halsey and Goldman, Maya and Luna criticized Pichichero for neglecting to measure the peak serum levels of ethylmercury after the first hours of inoculation, though other investigations had documented substantially elevated blood concentrations in the first forty-eight to seventy-two hours after administration in pediatric vaccines. Maya and Luna also pointed out that the study was small and measured variables of pharmacokinetics (the actions of a drug within the body over time), so it was not designed to measure the biological effect of Thimerosal as a preservative.[381]

After such attacks on their methodology and conclusions, Pichichero and his colleagues conducted a similar analysis on a larger group of infants at two and six months as well as new-borns. This second paper in 2008 concluded that the half-life of ethylmercury in the blood was about four days. Pichichero and his colleagues wrote that "our measurements are unable to determine the fate of the mercury after it leaves the blood"; they also pointed out that "exposure guidelines based on oral methylmercury in adults may not be accurate for risk assessments in children who receive thimerosal-containing vaccines [because] of the differing pharmacokinetics of ethyl and methylmercury."[382]

By then, other research had clarified that while ethylmercury disperses quickly from the bloodstream, this is not evidence of safety. For example, a 2004 study by G. Jean Harry of the National Institute of Environmental Health Sciences noted that mice injected with Thimerosal accumulated mercury in both the brain and kidneys.[383] "By seven days" post-treatment, the study authors wrote, "mercury levels decreased in the blood but were unchanged in the brain" compared to levels measured just twenty-four hours after treatment, indicating slow clearance.[384]

A particularly significant study in this regard was conducted by the University of Washington's Thomas Burbacher and was published in 2005.[385] The researchers compared mercury levels in the blood and brains of infant macaques injected with Thimerosal-containing vaccines with monkeys who ingested equal amounts of methylmercury hydroxide via a feeding tube. The former group of primates were exposed to 20 micrograms of ethylmercury per kilogram of body weight on the day they were born and when they were seven, fourteen, and twenty-one days old, which was estimated to be within the range of doses that children at different developmental stages were receiving in the United States. The dosing methods were selected to mimic the routes of exposure in humans who eat mercury-containing foods and receive mercury-containing vaccines.

Subsequent tests showed a faster disappearance of mercury from the bloodstream of Thimerosal-injected monkeys than from the methylmercury group. Total mercury amounts in the brain were also threefold less for the Thimerosal-treated monkeys. However, the Thimerosal-injected monkeys had a higher ratio of brain-to-blood levels of mercury than the methylmercury group. In general, the primates injected with Thimerosal in the Burbacher study retained twice the level of inorganic mercury—a breakdown product of Thimerosal that has been suggested to be responsible for the brain damage associated with methylmercury—in their brains as the methylmercury-exposed primates. While all seventeen monkeys given Thimerosal had "readily" detectable levels of inorganic mercury in their brains, only nine of the seventeen exposed to methylmercury had detectable levels. Burbacher cited previous research ranging the half-life of inorganic mercury in various brain regions of primates from 227 to 540 days. In either case, that is a long time period for the toxic element to remain, especially if at higher levels from ethylmercury deposition versus methylmercury.

Burbacher and his colleagues wrote in summary that "[methylmercury] is not a suitable reference for risk assessment from exposure to thimerosal-derived [mercury]" and that:

Data from the present study support the prediction that, although little accumulation of [mercury] in the blood occurs over time with repeated vaccinations, accumulation of [mercury] in the brain of infants will occur. Thus, conclusion [sic] regarding the safety of thimerosal drawn from blood [mercury] clearance data in human infants receiving vaccines may not be valid, given the significantly slower half-life of [mercury] in the brain as observed in the infant macaques.[386]

A more recent 2012 study by Croatian researchers took a similar approach as Burbacher's study, but in suckling rats, and further evidences that the claims of ethylmercury's comparative safety to other forms of mercury is unwarranted. Maja Blanusa and colleagues gave rat pups either Thimerosal or inorganic mercury three times in their first 11 days of life, mimicking human infant vaccination schedules. The scientists then assessed the total retention of mercury and excretion over six days. The Thimerosal-exposed rats showed higher mercury retention rates in their brains, in line with some other results described in this chapter. Furthermore, these Thimerosal-exposed rats exhibited similar fecal excretion and much lower urinary excretion compared to the inorganic mercury-exposed rats. That second group also demonstrated higher retention rates of mercury in organs other than the brain.[387]

Two additional studies in the last few years by researchers in Brazil and Germany show, again, that methylmercury in particular should not be considered summarily more dangerous than ethylmercury. The studies found that cells similarly take up both forms of mercury. The former, by Luciana Zimmermann and colleagues, showed in 2013 that the methyl- and ethylmercury entered cultured rat cells in roughly equal measure and display similar toxicities.[388] The 2014 German study led by Christoph Wehe used novel laboratory techniques in concluding that methylmercury and ethylmercury in the form of Thimerosal accumulated in equal measure in a type of cultured human neural cell.[389]

Research on human beings that might firmly answer questions about methylmercury and ethylmercury toxicity is not ethical, of course. Many of the best insights that are available, however, into the toxicology of both ethylmercury and methylmercury in humans come from poisoning events several decades ago.

In addition to the major Minamata and Iraq methylmercury-poisoning outbreaks mentioned earlier in the book, many other large-scale food poisonings occurred involving ethylmercury fungicides, again in Iraq in 1956 and 1960, in Pakistan in 1961, and in Russia in the 1960s as well.[390 391 392 393] The episodes resulted in maladies ranging from basic tissue injury to heart and brain injury and even death.[394 395 396 397 398 399] Derban reported in 1974 on yet another instance—144 cases of mercury poisoning from the use of ethylmercury fungicide on a southern Ghana state farm.[400] Multiple other studies based on these poisoning events showed, as stated in a 1977 study by David Fagan, that the long-term neurological consequences produced by the "ingestion of either methyl or ethyl mercury-based fungicides are indistinguishable."[401 402 403]

Other human poisoning cases of note support some of the ethylmercury toxicity findings in animals. Ethylmercury compounds

THIMEROSAL'S DANGERS TO HUMAN HEALTH AND THE BRAIN

easily cross the placental barrier into human fetuses and into breast-feeding children for three to four years after maternal exposure, according to a 1968 study.[404] In 1977, Mukhtarova examined Russian adults who ate meat and dairy over a course of two to three months that had been exposed to ethylmercury-contaminated grain, containing mercury in micrograms or tenths of a microgram per kilogram. Many of the Russian patients still had clinical evidence of neurological injury, including vertigo, decreased vision and hearing, decreased memory, and pain and numbness in hands and feet, at least three years after exposure.[405] A 1979 case report concerned a fifteen-year-old boy who had eaten the meat of a pig that had fed on ethylmercury fungicide–treated seed. Documented effects on the boy included debilitating brain damage and loss of coordination, with high toxicity for the brain as well as the spinal motor neurons, peripheral nerves, skeletal muscles, and heart muscle. The boy died about one month after becoming ill.[406]

Ethylmercury's use as pesticide was eventually banned in many countries, including the United States and those in the European Union, and for good reason: A 1977 study gauged ethylmercury chloride's relative toxicity as a pesticide as the fifth most toxic of thirty substances tested, with a score of 12.7. That grade score almost matched that of DDT, at 14.2, an infamous pesticide banned in 1972.[407 408 409]

Many studies, as we have seen, present substantial evidence that ethylmercury could well be more invasive, more persistent in the brain, and ultimately more toxic than methylmercury, in direct contrast with the CDC's position. The next chapters will look a bit deeper into some of the relevant medical literature.

Notes

[330] Baker JP. Mercury, vaccines, and autism: one controversy, three histories. *Am J. Public Health*. 2008; 98:244–253.

[331] http://www.fda.gov/Food/FoodSafety/Product-SpecificInformation/Seafood/FoodbornePathogensContaminants/Methylmercury/ucm115662.htm.

[332] http://water.epa.gov/scitech/swguidance/fishshellfish/outreach/advice_index.cfm.

[333] http://toxics.usgs.gov/definitions/methylmercury.html.

[334] http://www.cdc.gov/vaccinesafety/Concerns/thimerosal/thimerosal_faqs.html.

[335] http://www.who.int/vaccine_safety/topics/thiomersal/statement_jul2006/en/.

[336] Al-Tikriti K, Al-Mufti AW. An outbreak of organomercury poisoning among Iraqi farmers. *Bull World Health Organ*. 1976;53 Suppl:15-21.

[337] Eyl TB. Organic-mercury food poisoning. *N Engl J Med*. 1971 Apr 1;284(13):706-9.

[338] http://www.nimd.go.jp/archives/english/tenji/e_corner/qa1/q6.html.

[339] http://www.fda.gov/BiologicsBloodVaccines/SafetyAvailability/VaccineSafety/UCM096228.

[340] Bakir F, Damluji SF, Amin-Zaki L, Murtadha M, Khalidi A, al-Rawi NY, Tikriti S, Dahahir HI, Clarkson TW, Smith JC, Doherty RA. Methylmercury poisoning in Iraq. *Science*. 1973 Jul 20;181(4096):230-41.

[341] http://www.epa.gov/mercury/exposure.htm.

[342] www.epa.gov/ncea/pdfs/methmerc.pdf.

[343] http://www.epa.gov/iris/subst/0073.htm.

[344] Mahaffey KR. Methylmercury: a new look at the risks. *Public Health Rep*. 1999 Sep-Oct;114(5):396-9, 402-13.

[345] http://www.inchem.org/documents/ehc/ehc/ehc101.htm.

[346] Committee on the Toxicological Effects of Methylmercury, Board on Environmental Studies and Toxicology, National Research Council. *Toxicological Effects of Methylmercury*. National Academy Press, Washington, DC. 2000.

[347] Gilbert SG, Grant-Webster KS. Neurobehavioral effects of developmental methylmercury exposure. *Environ Health Perspect*. 1995 Sep;103 Suppl 6:135-42.

[348] http://www.babycenter.com/average-fetal-length-weight-chart.

[349] Committee on Infectious Diseases and Committee on Environmental Health, American Academy of Pediatrics. Thimerosal in vaccines—an interim report to clinicians. *Pediatrics.* 1999 Sep;104(3 Pt 1):570-4.

[350] Haley BE. Mercury toxicity: genetic susceptibility and synergistic effects. *Med Veritas.* 2005; 2: 535-542.

[351] Guzzi G, Pigatto PD, Spadari F, La Porta CA. Effect of thimerosal, methylmercury, and mercuric chloride in Jurkat T Cell Line. *Interdiscip Toxicol.* 2012 Sep;5(3):159-61. doi: 10.2478/v10102-012-0026-1.

[352] Takeda Y, Kunugi T, Hoshino O, Ukita T. Distribution of inorganic, aryl, and alkyl mercury compounds in rats. *Toxicol Appl Pharmacol.* 1968 Sep;13(2):156-64.

[353] http://www.lu.se/lucat/user/ymed-ssk.

[354] http://www.epa.gov/oecaagct/ag101/pestlethal.html.

[355] Skerfving S. Organic mercury compounds—relation between exposure and effect. *Mercury in the Environment.* Friberg L, Vostal J, eds. CRC Press, Cleveland. 1972; 141-68.

[356] Tryphonas L, Nielsen N. Pathology of chronic alkymercurial poisoning in swine. *Am J Vet Research* 1973; 34: 379-392.

[357] Suzuki T, Takemoto TL, Kashiwazaki H, Miyama T. Metabolic fate of ethylmercury salts in man and animals. *Mercury, Mercurials, Mercaptans.* Miller, MW and Clarkson, TW, eds. Springfield, Illinois. 1973; 209-240 *as described* in Geier DA, Sykes LK, Geier MR 2007.

[358] Blair AMJN, Clark B, Clark AJ, Wood P. Tissue concentrations of mercury after chronic dosing of squirrel monkeys with thimerosal. *Toxicology.* 1975;3(2):171-6.

[359] Magos L, Brown AW, Sparrow S, Bailey E, Snowden RT, Skipp WR. The comparative toxicology of ethyl- and methylmercury. *Arch Toxicol* 1985 Sep; 57(4):260-7. PMID: 4091651.

[360] Aschner M1, Walker SJ. The neuropathogenesis of mercury toxicity. *Mol Psychiatry.* 2002;7 Suppl 2:S40-1.

[361] Léonard A, Jacquet P, Lauwerys RR. Mutagenicity and teratogenicity of mercury compounds. *Mutat Res.* 1983 Jan; 114(1):1-18

[362] Hempel M, Chau YK, Dutka BJ, McInnis R, Kwan KK, Liu D. Toxicity of organomercury compounds: bioassay results as a basis for risk assessment. *Analyst.* 1995 Mar;120(3):721-4.

[363] https://www.urmc.rochester.edu/people/20996550-michael-e-pichichero.

[364] Pichichero ME, Cernichiari E, Lopreiato J, Treanor J. Mercury concentrations and metabolism in infants receiving vaccines containing thiomersal: a descriptive study. *Lancet.* 2002 Nov 30; 360(9347):1737-1741.

[365] http://www.ewire.com/news-releases/safe-minds-and-mercury-policy-project-statement-on-mercury-concentrations-and-metabolism-in-infants-receiving-vaccines-containing-mercury-a-descriptive-study/.

[366] Westphal GA, Schnuch A, Schulz TG, Reich K, Aberer W, Brasch J, Koch P, Wessbecher R, Szliska C, Bauer A, Hallier E. Homozygous gene deletions of the glutathione S-transferases M1 and T1 are associated with thimerosal sensitization. *Int Arch Occup Environ Health.* 2000 Aug;73(6):384-8.

[367] Westphal GA, Asgari S, Schulz TG, Bünger J, Müller M, Hallier E. Thimerosal induces micronuclei in the cytochalasin B-block micronucleus test with human lymphocytes. *Arch Toxicol*. 2003; 77: 50–55.

[368] Westphal G, Hallier E. Mercury in infants given vaccines containing thiomersal. *Lancet*. 2003 Feb 22;361(9358):699; author reply 699.

[369] Geier DA, Geier MR. A case series of children with apparent mercury toxic encephalopathies manifesting with clinical symptoms of regressive autistic disorders. *J Toxicol Environ Health A*. 2007 May 15;70(10):837-51.

[370] http://www.urmc.rochester.edu/people/20996550-michael-e-pichichero/researchers.

[371] http://westernnyphysician.com/PDF/August-2011.pdf.

[372] http://www.aafp.org/afp/2000/0401/p2051.html.

[373] http://www.thelancet.com/journals/lancet/article/PIIS0140-6736%2804%2917133-X/fulltext.

[374] http://download.thelancet.com/flatcontentassets/authors/lancet-information-for-authors.pdf.

[375] Halsey NA, Goldman LR. Mercury in infants given vaccines containing thiomersal. *Lancet*. 2003 Feb 22;361(9358):698-9; author reply 699.

[376] http://adventuresinautism.blogspot.com/2008/03/mark-blaxill-and-boyd-haley-respond-to.html.

[377] Holmes AS, Blaxill MF, Haley BE. Reduced levels of mercury in first baby haircuts of autistic children. *Int J Toxic*. 2003;111(4):277-285.

[378] Ip P, Wong V, Ho M, Lee J, Wong W. Mercury exposure in children with autistic spectrum disorder: case-control study. *J Child Neurol*. 2004 Jun; 19(6): 431-4.

[379] DeSoto MC, Hitlan RT. Blood levels of mercury are related to diagnosis of autism: a reanalysis of an important data set. *J Child Neurol*. 2007 Nov; 22(11): 1308-1311.

[380] Olmsted D., Blaxill M. *The Age of Autism: Mercury, Medicine, and a Man-Made Epidemic*. St. Martin's Griffin. New York, New York. 2011.

[381] Maya L, Luna F. Thimerosal and children's neurodevelopmental disorders. *Ann Fac Med (Lima)* 2006; 67(3); 243-262 [Spanish], 32-page English translation *available at* http://www.safeminds.org/research/AnFacMedLima2006-67(3).pdf.

[382] Pichichero ME, Gentile A, Giglio N, Umido V, Clarkson T, Cernichiari E, Zareba G, Gotelli C, Gotelli M, Yan L, Treanor J. Mercury levels in newborns and infants after receipt of thimerosal-containing vaccines. *Pediatrics*. 2008 Feb;121(2):e208-14.

[383] http://www.niehs.nih.gov/research/atniehs/labs/ntp/nt/index.cfm.

[384] Harry GJ, Harris MW, Burka LT. Mercury concentrations in brain and kidney following ethylmercury, methylmercury and Thimerosal administration to neonatal mice. *Toxicol Lett*. 2004 Dec 30;154(3):183-9.

[385] http://depts.washington.edu/chdd/iddrc/res_aff/burbacher.html.

[386] Burbacher T, Shen D, Liberato N, Grant K, Cernichiari E, Clarkson T. Comparison of blood and brain mercury levels in infant monkeys exposed to methylmercury or vaccines containing thimerosal. *Environ Health Perspect*. 2005; 113(8):1015-1021.

387 Blanuša M1, Orct T, Vihnanek Lazarus M, Sekovanić A, Piasek M. Mercury disposition in suckling rats: comparative assessment following parenteral exposure to thiomersal and mercuric chloride. *J Biomed Biotechnol*. 2012;2012:256965. doi: 10.1155/2012/256965. Epub 2012 Jul 26.

388 Zimmermann LT, Santos DB, Naime AA, Leal RB, Dórea JG, Barbosa F Jr, Aschner M, Rocha JB, Farina M. Comparative study on methyl- and ethylmercury-induced toxicity in C6 glioma cells and the potential role of LAT-1 in mediating mercurial-thiol complexes uptake. *Neurotoxicology*. 2013 Sep;38:1-8. doi: 10.1016/j.neuro.2013.05.015. Epub 2013 May 30.

389 Wehe CA, Pieper I, Holtkamp M, Thyssen GM, Sperling M, Schwerdtle T, Karst U. On-line species-unspecific isotope dilution analysis in the picomolar range reveals the time- and species-depending mercury uptake in human astrocytes. *Anal Bioanal Chem*. 2014 Mar;406(7):1909-16. doi: 10.1007/s00216-013-7608-4. Epub 2014 Jan 18.

390 Jalili MA, Abbasi AH. Poisoning by ethyl mercury toluene sulphonanilide. *Br J Ind Med*. 1961; 18:303-308.

391 Al-Tikriti K, Al-Mufti AW. An outbreak of organomercury poisoning among Iraqi farmers. *Bull World Health Organ*. 1976;53 Suppl:15-21.

392 Eyl TB. Organic-mercury food poisoning. *N Engl J Med*. 1971 Apr 1;284(13):706-9.

393 Shustov VIA, Tsyganova SI. Clinical aspects of subacute intoxication with Granosan. *Kazansk Med Zh*. 1970; 2:78-79.

394 Al-Kasab S and Saigh N. Mercury and calcium excretion in chronic poisoning with organic mercury compounds. *J Fac Med Baghdad*. 1962; 4(3):118-123.

395 Samluji S. Granosan M. Mercurial poisoning with fungicide. *J Fac Med Baghdad*. 1962;4:83-103.

396 Dahhan SS, Orfaly H. Electrocardiographic changes in mercury poisoning. *Am J Cardiol*. 1964 Aug; 14:178-183.

397 Dahhan SS, Orfaly H. Mercury poisoning and electrocardiographic changes. *J Fac Med Baghdad*. 1962; 4(3): 104-111.

398 Nizov AA, Shestakov HM. Contribution to the clinical aspects of granosan poisoning. *Sov Med*. 1971; 11:150-152.

399 Zhang MD. Clinical observations in ethyl mercury chloride poisoning. *Am J Industr Med*. 1984; 5:251-258.

400 Derban LK. Outbreak of food poisoning due to alkyl-mercury fungicide on southern Ghana state farm. *Arch Environ Health*. 1974;28:49-52.

401 Mal'tsev PV. Granosan poisoning in children. *Feldsher Akush*. 1972; 37:14-16.

402 Ramanauskayte MB, Baublis PP. Clinical picture and treatment of organomercurial pesticide poisoning in children. *Pediatriya Moscow*. 1973; 35(2): 56-60.

403 Fagan DG, Pritchard JS, Clarkson TW, Greenwood MR. Organ mercury levels in infants with omphaloceles treated with organic mercurial antiseptic. *Arch Dis Child*. 1977 Dec; 52(12):962-964.

404 Bakulina AV. The effect of subacute Granosan poisoning on the progeny. *Soviet Med*. 1968; 31:60–63. [Russian] *as described in* Geier DA, Sykes LK, Geier MR 2007.

[405] Mukhtarova ND. Late sequelae of nervous system pathology caused by the action of low concentrations of ethyl mercury chloride. *Gig Tr Prof Zabol.* 1977 Mar; (3):4-7.

[406] Cinca I, Dumitrescu I, Onaca I, Serbänescu A, Nestorescu B. Accidental ethyl mercury poisoning with nervous system, skeletal muscle, and myocardium injury. *J Neurol Neurosurg Psychiatry.* 1980 Feb; 43(2): 143-149.

[407] http://www.chem.unep.ch/mercury/Report/Chapter7.htm#7.3.

[408] Weber, Jerome B. The pesticide scorecard. *Environ Sci Technol.* 1977: 11 (8); 56-761.

[409] http://www.epa.gov/pbt/pubs/ddt.htm.

Chapter 5:
A Wide Range of Animal Studies Show Thimerosal's Toxicity

In addition to studies involving animals and humans cited in previous chapters, many other lines of research have shown that even at very low doses, Thimerosal and ethylmercury-containing compounds can kill or cause severe brain and organ damage in a host of species.

Studies have indicated that mercury from Thimerosal crosses the blood-brain barrier and becomes highly incorporated in the brains of rabbits, as well as their fetuses.[410] As shown in other animals such as pigs and monkeys, mercury can persist in the brain for many months.[411 412] Experiments looking at cells from the brains of mice indicate that Thimerosal causes cell damage and cell death, in line with findings in human cells cited elsewhere in this document, and could increase rates of death in mice that received Thimerosal-containing vaccines.[413 414 415 416]

Overall, research has demonstrated Thimerosal- or ethylmercury-
-related damage in many animals exposed to the substances,
including guinea pigs, poultry, pheasants, cattle, sheep, and
cats.[417 418 419 420 421 422 423] Numerous other studies of animals previously mentioned, including mice and pigs, have further bolstered
the case for the dangers of Thimerosal.[424 425 426 427]

In particular, peer-reviewed animal studies have shown Thimerosal
can do harm to animal fetuses. A 1987 study found that nearly half of
chicken embryos died when 0.1 mg of Thimerosal was injected into
their eggs for six days during their incubation. Furthermore, more
than a third of the exposed embryos suffered serious defects, including syndactyly (joining of digits), visceroptosis (drooping of internal
organs), thinning of the abdominal wall, and abnormalities in the
growth of the wings and the body. In contrast, the control group's
eggs all appeared viable with no evidence of malformations.[428]

A prior study in 1972 involving rabbit fetuses indicated that
Thimerosal injections to the connective tissue of pregnant rabbits
caused a significant increase in fetal death.[429] Other studies have
similarly shown damage to embryonic eggs and fetal mice, and that
Thimerosal is toxic to proteins important for cell structure using
extracts from pig brains.[430 431 432 433] A 1993 study found Thimerosal to
be a "strong inhibitor" in bovine cells of microtubule assembly, which,
among other functions, is essential for proper cellular division.[434] In
some of the earliest work with Thimerosal, a 1935 study determined
that Thimerosal was more than thirty-five times as toxic to living
animal tissue—in this case embryonic chicken heart tissue—as to the
bacteria that causes staph infections, *Staphylococcus aureus*.[435]

Thimerosal and mercury have likewise been implicated in
impairing fertility. A 1990 study showed that Thimerosal inhibited

the beating function of cilia, the tiny hairs found on many creatures' cells, including human cells that, among other functions, remove debris in the windpipe and are thought to be important for moving women's eggs to the uterus through the fallopian tubes and in sperm motility.[436][437] Hints of this kind of effect have appeared in humans. Scientists have proposed such a hypothesis to justify the high rates of infertility among men who in their infancy suffered acrodynia, or "pink disease." Acrodynia is caused by exposure to tooth powders containing a mercury compound called Calomel, the trade name for mercurous chloride (about 85 percent mercury by weight). These Calomel-containing powders were commonly used from the late 1800s into the 1930s in the United States and until the mid-1950s in the United Kingdom.[438]

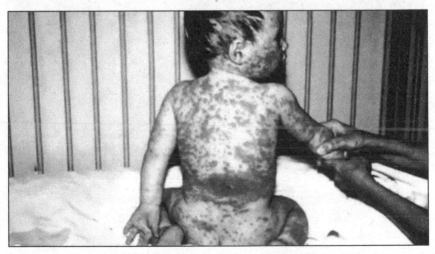

A baby suffering from pink disease. Credit: "Repeating History"/SafeMinds, http://www.youtube.com/watch?v=4d4j8GGbQ5g

A number of animal studies have also demonstrated that organic mercury diminishes reproductive capacity in laboratory animals, including rats, guinea pigs, and monkeys.[439] Inorganic mercury, one of the derivatives of Thimerosal, has been demonstrated to hamper fertility as well.[440] FDA toxicologist Abu Kahn showed in a 2004 study that mice exposed to mercuric chloride suffered reduced fertility and survival of their offspring. Reproductive health changes, such as reduced ovary size, occurred in mice that showed no outward signs of mercury toxicity.[441] Furthermore, a 1971 study on rats showed that female rats exposed to ethylmercury compounds suffered impaired fertility and that the impairment persisted in their progeny for two generations.[442] J. W. Spann and colleagues, meanwhile, reported that pheasants exposed to ethylmercury died or suffered reproductive problems, including reduced egg production and survival.[443]

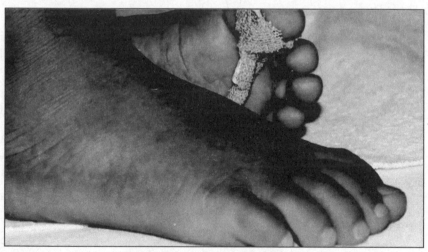

A close-up of the foot of a victim of pink disease. Credit: "Repeating History"/ SafeMinds, http://www.youtube.com/watch?v=4d4j8GGbQ5g

We now move from the extensive animal literature to how Thimerosal's prescribed use in people has changed since the chemical's introduction to medicine.

Notes

[410] Gasset AR, Itoi M, Ishii Y, Ramer RM. Teratogenicities of ophthalmic drugs. II. *Arch Ophthalmol.* 1975; 93: 52-55 *as described in* Geier DA, Sykes LK, Geier MR 2007.

[411] Saley PL. Evaluation of slaughter products from Granosan-poisoned animals. *Veterinariya.* 1970; 46: 102-103 *as described in* Geier DA, Sykes LK, Geier MR 2007.

[412] Burbacher T, Shen D, Liberato N, Grant K, Cernichiari E, Clarkson T. Comparison of blood and brain mercury levels in infant monkeys exposed to methylmercury or vaccines containing Thimerosal. *Environ Health Perspect.* 2005; 113(8): 1015-1021.

[413] Nelson EA, Gottshall RY. Enhanced toxicity for mice of pertussis vaccines when preserved with merthiolate. *Appl Microbiol.* 1967; 15: 590-593.

[414] Mukai N. An experimental study of alkylmercurial encephalopathy. *Acta Neuropathol.* 1972;22(2):102-9.

[415] Yonaha M, Ishikura S, Uchiyama M. Toxicity of organic mercury compounds. III. Uptake and retention of mercury in several organs by mice by long term exposure of alkoxyethylmercury compounds. *Chem Pharm Bull.* 1975;23(8): 1718-1725.

[416] Ueha-Ishibashi T, Oyama Y, Nakao H, Umebayashi C, Nishizaki Y, Tatsuishi T, Iwase K, Murao K, Seo H. Effect of thimerosal, a preservative in vaccines, on intracellular Ca2+ concentration of rat cerebellar neurons. *Toxicology.* 2004 Jan 15;195(1):77-84.

[417] Cummins SL. Merthiolate in the treatment of tuberculosis. *Lancet.* 1937; 230: 962-963.

[418] Besredka A. *Ann Inst Pasteur.* 1921; 55: 291.

[419] Tishkov AL, Saley P, Vitkalov VP. Poultry poisoning with Granosan. *Veterinariya.* 1968; 45: 58 *as described in* Geier DA, Sykes LK, Geier MR 2007.

[420] Spann JW, Heath RG, Kreitzer JF, Locke LN. Ethyl-mercury-p-toluene-sulfonanilde: Lethal and Reproductive Effects on Pheasants. *Science.* 1972; 175(4019): 328-331.

[421] Oliver WT, Platonow N. Studies on the Pharmacology of n-(ethylmercuri)-p-toluenesulfonanilide. *Am J Vet Res.* 1960 Sep; 21: 906-916 *as described in* Geier DA, Sykes LK, Geier MR 2007.

[422] Palmer JS, Wright FC, Haufler M. Toxicologic and residual aspects of an alkyl mercury fungicide to cattle, sheep, and turkeys. *Clin Toxicol.* 1973;6(3):425-37.

[423] Morikawa N. Pathological studies in organic mercury poisoning, II. Experimental production of congenital cerebellar atrophy by bis-ethyl-mercuric sulfide in cats. *Kumamoto Med J.* 1961; 14, 87-93 *as described in* http://oehha.ca.gov/prop65/CRNR_notices/pdf_zip/hgbayer1.pdf.

[424] Trakhtenberg IM. The toxicity of organic mercury compounds (ethlmercuric phosphate and ethylmercuric chloride) in acute and chronic intoxication (experimental data). *Gig Sanit.* 1950; 6: 13-17 *as described in* Geier DA, Sykes LK, Geier MR 2007.

425 Ukita T, Takeda Y, Sato Y, Takahashi T. Distribution of 203Hg labeled mercury compounds in adult and pregnant mice determined by whole-body autoradiography. *Radioisotopes.* 1967; 16: 439-448 as described in Maya and Luna 2006.

426 Nelson EA, Gottshall RY. Enhanced toxicity for mice of pertussis vaccines when preserved with merthiolate. *Appl Microbiol.* 1967; 15(3): 590-593.

427 Birbin SS, Alekseeva AA, Bulatov AA. Poisoning of swine by grain treated with Granosan. *Veterinariia.* 1968; 45(8): 60-61 as described in Geier DA, Sykes LK, Geier MR 2007.

428 Digar A, Sensharma GC, Samal SN. Lethality and teratogenecity of organic mercury (Thimerosal) on the chick embryo. *J Anat Soc India.* 1987; 36: 153–156.

429 Itoi M, Ishii Y, Kaneko N. Teratogenicities of antiviral ophthalmics on experimental animals. *Jpn J Clin Ophthal.* 1972; 26:631–640 as described in Geier DA, Sykes LK, Geier MR 2007.

430 Witlin 1942 as described in Geier DA, Sykes LK, Geier MR 2007 [full reference not available].

431 Green and Berkeland 1944 as described in Geier DA, Sykes LK, Geier MR 2007 [full reference not available].

432 Oharazawa, H. 1968. Effect of ethylmercuric phosphate in the pregnant mouse on chromosome abnormalities and fetal malformation. *J Jpn Obstet Gynecol.* 20:1479–1487 as described in Geier DA, Sykes LK, Geier MR 2007.

433 Brunner M, Albertini S, Wurgler FE. Effects of 10 known or suspected spindle poisons in the in vitro porcine brain tubulin assembly assay. *Mutagenesis.* 1991; 6:65–70.

434 Wallin M, Hartley-Asp B. Effects of potential aneuploidy inducing agents on microtubule assembly in vitro. *Mutat Res.* 1993 May;287(1):17-22.

435 Salle AJ, Lazarus AS. A comparison of the resistance of bacteria and embryonic tissue to germicidal substances. *Proc Soc Exp Biol Med.* 1935; 32:665-667.

436 Batts AH, Marriotti C, Martini GP, Wood CF, Bond SW. The effect of some preservatives used in nasal preparations on mucus and ciliary components of mucociliary clearance. *J Pharm Pharmacol.* 1990 Mar; 42: 145-151.

437 Lyons RA, Saridogan E, Djahanbakhch O. The reproductive significance of human fallopian tube cilia. *Hum Reprod Update.* 2006 Jul-Aug;12(4):363-72.

438 Dally A. The rise and fall of pink disease. *Soc Hist Med.* 1997; 10: 291-304.

439 Clement Associates. *Toxicological Profile for Mercury.* Atlanta, Ga.: Department of Health and Human Services, Agency for Toxic Substances and Disease Registry, US Public Health Services; 1989.

440 Maya L, Luna F. Thimerosal and children's neurodevelopmental disorders. *Ann Fac Med (Lima).* 2006; 67(3): 243-262 [Spanish].

441 Kahn A, Atkinson A, Graham TC, Thompson SJ, Ali S, Shireen KF. Effects of inorganic mercury in reproductive performance of mice. *Food Chem Toxicol.* 2004 Apr;42(4):571-7.

442 Goncharuk G. Experimental investigation of the effect of organomercury pesticides on generative function and on progeny. *Hyg Sanit.* 1971; 36: 40-44 as described in Geier DA, Sykes LK, Geier MR 2007.

443 Spann JW, Heath RG, Kreitzer JF, Locke LN. Ethyl mercury p-toluene sulfonanilide: Lethal and reproductive effects on pheasants. *Science.* 1972; 175: 328-331.

Chapter 6:
Mounting Evidence of Thimerosal's Danger in Human Studies

Other studies and events dating back decades have lent credence to the idea that the ethylmercury in Thimerosal is as damaging to humans as it is to animals.

In cases of accidental high dosages, Thimerosal has caused human deaths. Clinicians in the 1940s used Thimerosal in an attempt to treat heart disease and noted its toxicity; at least one patient in a case series of thirteen patients died from documented mercury poisoning.[444] In 1969, five of six human patients (four children and two adults) died after being injected with an antimicrobial called chloramphenicol, which contained abnormally high levels of Thimerosal.[445] A 1983 report from the Ohio Board of Health Division of Epidemiology strongly implicated Thimerosal in the death of a twenty-one-month-old child.[446] A 1996 study even reported on a forty-four-year-old man in Germany who attempted suicide by consuming a large quantity of Thimerosal.[447][448]

Of course, many substances routinely ingested, injected, or otherwise placed into the human body for medical reasons can prove harmful or fatal if administered in excess. Yet the low levels long considered generally "safe" for Thimerosal in various products aroused suspicion in the medical community during the 1970s, and in some cases as soon as Thimerosal began appearing in many commercial products during the 1930s and 1940s.[449][450]

As described in Chapter 1, Thimerosal saw widespread use in topical medications, such as antiseptics and eyewashes. Accordingly, many studies in humans have focused on this mode of exposure. Even as early as 1943, scientists expressed concern that Thimerosal was toxic to some people who used it for eye care. Francis Ellis, an Army doctor in Baltimore, stated, "Since a patient may become sensitized to merthiolate while using the ophthalmic ointment, it may be advisable to withdraw this product from the market before a case of permanent ocular damage occurs."[451][452]

Several years later, anecdotal cases of reactions to Thimerosal began to mount. H. D. Cogswell and Alex Shoun noted: "Many severe reactions have been reported following the use of mercurial ointments and a lesser number due to antiseptics containing mercurials."[453] Skepticism about Thimerosal's effectiveness and its potential damage to humans continued, especially in light of the numerous animal studies and human exposure cases mentioned previously in this document.

Starting in 1975, the FDA undertook a comprehensive review of safety and effectiveness of over-the-counter (OTC) medicines containing Thimerosal.[454] A series of alarming studies that followed persuaded the agency to ban Thimerosal in topical medications. These studies included one funded by the US Veterans Administration (VA) and the US National Institutes of Health (NIH) showing that Thimerosal at the concentration used in ophthalmic products caused toxic effects on human cornea cells that were grown outside the body in a lab.[455] That study stated, "It is therefore concluded that ophthalmic solutions containing Thimerosal should not be used."

As part of the review, in 1977, the Boston University Medical Center published a large-scale human epidemiological study of birth defects among more than 50,000 pregnancies. The authors found that fifty-six of these mothers were exposed to topical Thimerosal during their pregnancy and that their offspring had an increased risk of birth defects.[456] Also, in the early 1970s, a study showed that ten infants with exomphalos (umbilical hernias) who had Thimerosal applied to them topically died and had blood and organ levels of mercury well beyond minimum toxic levels in adults and fetuses.[457]

After years of consistent findings from studies like these, in 1980, an FDA Advisory Review Panel on Over-the-Counter Miscellaneous External Drug Products concluded that Thimerosal is not safe for OTC topical drugs because of its potential for cell damage and allergic reactions. The FDA scientific panel's conclusions were clear and unequivocal that Thimerosal was deadly to human cells in vitro. In 1982, the FDA proposed to ban Thimerosal from nonprescription topical medications. However, that proposed ban from the list of permitted ingredients in OTC topical drug products was not implemented until 1998.[458] (One of the better known topical products containing organic mercury removed from the US market as a result of this FDA rule was the red, skin-staining topical antiseptic merbromin, marketed as mercurochrome, among other names.)[459][460]

It might seem surprising that the FDA would ban the OTC topical application of Thimerosal and mercury for being too dangerous, while allowing the same chemical to be injected into newborn babies. A possible explanation for the inconsistency is suggested by Sarah Bridges, whose son with autism revceived compensation for his injury from the federal "Vaccine Court." Bridges developed close relations with several FDA officials during the litigation process. According to Bridges, a scientist at the FDA told her, on condition of anonymity, that there was little communication between the FDA group charged with establishing safety for OTC medications and the group that regulates vaccines for human use.[461] (Over-the-counter medications are regulated by the Office of Drug Evaluation IV [ODE IV] in the FDA's Center for Drug Evaluation and Research [CDER].[462] Vaccines are regulated by the Office of Vaccines Research and Review [OVRR] in the FDA's Center for Biologics Evaluation and Research [CBER].[463])

Whether or not Bridges's source is correct, the FDA allowed Thimerosal to remain in vaccines, despite joint statements by the Public Health Service, including the FDA, NIH, and CDC, urging manufacturers to remove the ingredient.[464] Clearly, a substance that causes allergic reactions and toxicity to human cells in vitro when applied externally could be expected to do more harm when injected, as more of the chemical is likely to enter the blood and spread throughout the body via injection than through topical exposure.[465]

In the interim period between FDA's proposed banning of Thimerosal in OTCs to the ban's implementation, other studies indicated that the chemical could harm human tissues. There was a case of an eighteen-month-old girl who developed serious neurological injury, including loss of coordination and unprovoked screaming behavior, following ear irrigation with Thimerosal-containing solution.[466] A 1977 study published in a Sweden-based journal portrayed Thimerosal allergy as a sensitization brought on by unnecessary medical exposure, and thus preventable.[467] [468] A 1984 study showed that in the range of 5 to 8 percent of patients "using lens care solution with thimerosal exhibited solution intolerance (toxic to human cell tissue)."[469]

Other studies over this period described a specific molecular mechanism by which Thimerosal exposure results in toxicity in liver cells from rats.[470] An important 2003 report from Baskin bolstered the finding of Thimerosal-associated cellular toxicity in studies of both human nerve and skin cells. The study examined exposure to mercury concentrations around four times those once received by American children during their first six months of life.[471]

Meanwhile, in 1990, the California EPA's Office of Environmental Health Hazard Assessment (OEHHA) took the step of designating Thimerosal as a human reproductive toxin. The OEHHA's decision was informed by a review of federal EPA documents and many of the studies presented in this document. The report stated:

> The scientific evidence that demonstrates that Thimerosal causes reproductive toxicity is clear and voluminous. Thimerosal [breaks down] in the body into ethylmercury. The evidence for its reproductive toxicity includes severe mental retardation or malformations in human offspring who were poisoned when their mothers were exposed to ethylmercury or

thimerosal while pregnant, studies in animals demonstrating developmental toxicity after exposure to either ethylmercury or thimerosal, and data show interconversion to other forms of mercury that also clearly cause reproductive toxicity.[472]

During the last decade, numerous new studies have painted a grim picture of Thimerosal's destructive effect on neuronal cells in humans in addition to the animal-study proxies. As reviewed in a 2011 article by Jose Dórea, studies involving cultured human cells have shown that at vaccine-level concentrations, or even lower, Thimerosal exposure can trigger cell death.[473]

Amid these research efforts and findings, both published and behind-the-scenes, the CDC commissioned an epidemiological study that does not dispel suspicions about a link between Thimerosal and human injury.

Notes

[444] Kinsella RA. Chemotherapy of bacterial endocarditis. *Ann Intern Med.* 1941; 15: 982–986.

[445] Axton, JH. Six cases of poisoning after a parenteral organic mercurial compound (Merthiolate). *Postgrad Med J.* 1972 Jul;48(561):417-21.

[446] Anonymous. 1983. Mercury poisoning in child treated with aqueous Merthiolate. *MD State Med. J.* 32:523 *as described in* Geier DA, Sykes LK, Geier MR 2007.

[447] Pfab R, Mückter H, Roider G, Zilker T. Clinical course of severe poisoning with thiomersal. *J Toxicol Clin Toxicol.* 1996;34(4):453-60.

[448] http://www.fda.gov/BiologicsBloodVaccines/SafetyAvailability/VaccineSafety/UCM096228.

[449] Baker JP. Mercury, vaccines, and autism: one controversy, three histories. *Am J. Public Health.* 2008; 98:244–253.

[450] Geier DA, Sykes LK, Geier MR. A review of Thimerosal (Merthiolate) and its ethylmercury breakdown product: specific historical considerations regarding safety and effectiveness. *J Toxicol Environ Health, Part B,* 2007; 10: 575-596.

[451] Ellis FA. Possible danger in use of Merthiolate ophthalmic ointment. *Arch Ophthalmol.* 1943; 30: 265–266.

[452] Ellis FA. The sensitizing factor in Merthiolate. *J Allergy.* 1947; 18: 212–213.

[453] Cogswell, H.D., Shoun, A. 1948. Reaction following the use of tincture of Merthiolate. *Ariz Med.* 5:42–43.

[454] Department of Health and Human Services, Proposed Rules, CFR Part 333 Docket No. 75N-0183, Mercury-Containing Drug Products for Topical Antimicrobial Over-the-Counter Human Use; Establishment of a Monograph, Jan. 5, 1982.

[455] Van Horn DL, Edlehauser HF, Prodanovich G, Eiferman R, Pederson HJ. Effect of ophthalmic preservative Thimerosal on rabbit and human corneal endothelium. *Invest. Ophthalmol. Visual Sci.* 1977; 16: 273–280.

[456] Heinonen OP, Slone D, Shapiro S. *Birth Defects and Drugs in Pregnancy.* Littleton, Mass.: Publishing Sciences Group; 1977: 313.

[457] Fagan DG, Pritchard JS, Clarkson TW, Greenwood MR. Organ mercury levels in infants with omphaloceles treated with organic mercurial antiseptic. *Arch Dis Child.* 1977 Dec; 52(12): 962-964.

⁴⁵⁸ United States. Mercury in medicine report. *Congressional Record*. Washington: GPO, May 21, 2003: 1011-1030.

⁴⁵⁹ http://www.fda.gov/RegulatoryInformation/Legislation/FederalFoodDrugand-CosmeticActFDCAct/SignificantAmendmentstotheFDCAct/FDAMA/ucm100219.htm.

⁴⁶⁰ http://www.nlm.nih.gov/medlineplus/ency/article/002897.htm.

⁴⁶¹ Robert F. Kennedy Jr., telephone interview with Sarah Bridges, May 20, 2005.

⁴⁶² http://www.fda.gov/AboutFDA/CentersOffices/OfficeofMedicalProductsandTobacco/CDER/ucm093452.htm; http://www.fda.gov/AboutFDA/CentersOffices/OfficeofMedicalProductsandTobacco/CDER/ucm106342.htm.

⁴⁶³ http://www.fda.gov/NewsEvents/Testimony/ucm113267.htm?utm_campaign=-Google2&utm_source=fdaSearch&utm_medium=website&utm_term=Office%20of%20Vaccine%20Research%20and%20Review&utm_content=4.

⁴⁶⁴ http://www.fda.gov/BiologicsBloodVaccines/SafetyAvailability/VaccineSafety/UCM096228.

⁴⁶⁵ http://www.nursingtimes.net/nursing-practice/clinical-specialisms/prescribing/the-administration-of-medicines/288560.article.

⁴⁶⁶ Rohyans JA, Walson PD, Wood GA, MacDonald WA. Mercury toxicity following merthiolate ear irrigations. *Pediatrics*. 1984; 104(2): 311-313.

⁴⁶⁷ Möller H. Merthiolate allergy: a nationwide iatrogenic sensitization. *Acta Derm Venereol*. 1977;57(6):509-17.

⁴⁶⁸ http://www.medicaljournals.se/acta/index.php/contact-the-editorial-office.html.

⁴⁶⁹ Coward BD, Neumann R, Callender M. Solution intolerance among users of four chemical soft lens care regimens. *Am J Optom Physiol Opt*. 1984 Aug; 61(8): 523-527.

⁴⁷⁰ Anundi I, Högberg J, Stead AH. Glutathione depletion in isolated hepatocytes: its relation to lipid peroxidation and cell damage. *Acta Pharmacol Toxicol (Copenh)*. 1979 Jul;45(1):45-51.

⁴⁷¹ Baskin DS, Ngo H, Didenko VV. Thimerosal induces DNA breaks, caspase-3 activation, membrane damage, and cell death in cultured human neurons and fibroblasts. *Toxicol Sci*. 2003 Aug;74(2):361-8. Epub 2003 May 28.

⁴⁷² http://oehha.ca.gov/prop65/CRNR_notices/pdf_zip/hgbayer1.pdf.

⁴⁷³ Dórea JG. Integrating experimental (in vitro and in vivo) neurotoxicity studies of low dose thimerosal relevant to vaccines. *Neurochem Res*. 2011 Jun;36(6):927-38. Epub 2011 Feb 25.

Chapter 7: Findings of Epidemiological Studies: Links between Thimerosal and Neurological Damage

Multiple epidemiological studies have aimed to assess the impact of Thimerosal, if any, on neurodevelopmental health. The CDC has conducted, funded, or assisted in studies in this regard, which in their final, published form have not found statistically significant evidence of harm. However, studies conducted by scientists not connected to the CDC have found evidence, and in some cases very strong signals, correlating Thimerosal-containing vaccines with higher risks of neurodevelopmental disease.

The most controversial CDC-sponsored epidemiological study on the matter was published in *Pediatrics* in November 2003, with Thomas Verstraeten as the lead author. The study evaluated children in the Vaccine Safety Datalink (VSD) project, created in 1990 by the CDC to integrate medical event information, specific vaccine history, and selected demographic information from the computerized databases of several health maintenance organizations (better known by their acronym, HMOs).[474 475] Phase I of the Verstraeten analysis indicated increased risk of speech/language disorders and tics for children who received Thimerosal-containing vaccines between 1991 and 1997, but Phase II found no such associations. Ultimately, the study showed no significant associations between Thimerosal-containing vaccines and various neurodevelopmental disorders, including autism and attention disorders.[476]

The full story, however, was far more complex. As revealed through a Freedom of Information Act (FOIA) request by SafeMinds, a nonprofit organization advocating for the removal of mercury from medical products, the Verstraeten research had begun in late 1999. The initial analyses bore very different results from the published figures.[477] (In epidemiological studies, it should be noted, it is not unusual for early, crude analyses to show more striking associations with an exposure than later, more refined analyses that examine fully covariate-adjusted models. The evidence suggesting a massaging of the results rather than a normal course of data analysis will be explored thoroughly in Part Four of this book.)

Verstraeten shared an early data analysis with two of his paper's coauthors via email on December 17, 1999. This analysis indicated a strong dose-related connection between Thimerosal and a wide range of neurodevelopmental disorders. For those receiving the highest mercury dose, greater than 25 micrograms by one month of age, the initial Verstraeten results showed that these children were twice as likely to have speech/language delays, five-and-a-half times as likely to develop tics, more than six times as likely to have attention-deficit disorder (ADD), seven-and-a-half times as likely to have autism, and eight times as likely to have attention-deficit hyperactivity disorder (ADHD).[478][479]

The as-yet-unpublished study went through another analysis in February 2000. The study's figures had been reanalyzed and now represented far smaller risks; the relative risk for autism, for example, at three months of age in the highest Thimerosal-exposure category went down to 2.48 and then to 1.69.[480][481] This still represented a 69 to 148 percent increase in risk. Further analysis took place prior to publication. With each revision of the unpublished Verstraeten data, the relative risks for various neurodevelopmental disorders went down, and in the cases of autism and attention disorders, steeply so.[482]

The Verstraeten paper, along with four other epidemiological studies primarily done with the United Kingdom, Danish, and Swedish populations, became the cornerstone of the CDC's and the Institute of Medicine's (IOM) declaration in 2004 that there is no link between Thimerosal and autism.[483] (Part Four of this book will provide details on the methodological flaws of the five studies, as well as conflicts of interest concerning their authors.)

In 2004, Verstraeten himself, in a letter to *Pediatrics*, disavowed the CDC's efforts to present the published study as proof of Thimerosal's safety. The study, he said, had a "neutral" result, meaning that consistent associations between Thimerosal and neurodevelopmental delays were not found and that further research was required.[484] The CDC ignored Verstraeten's recommendation and in the opinion of this book has never seriously or properly reviewed the VSD data to explore the possible harm from Thimerosal-containing vaccines.

After the Verstraeten study, the CDC went on to publish two subsequent VSD studies, by William Thompson in 2007 and by Cristofer Price in 2010, in which Thompson served as second author. Thompson 2007's conclusions did "not support a causal association between early exposure to mercury from thimerosal-containing vaccines and immune globulins and deficits in neuropsychological functioning at the age of 7 to 10 years." The study reported some beneficial as well as detrimental associations, the latter of which included motor and phonic tics as well as poorer performance on a measure of speech articulation.[485]

Price's 2010 study explicitly evaluated the risk of autism associated with the receipt of Thimerosal-containing vaccines prenatally and through the first twenty months of life. Price concluded that there was no increased risk from Thimerosal exposure.[486] However, a review of the source report for this study, which was prepared by a public policy and business research and consulting firm, Abt Associates, indicates otherwise.[487][488] Two out of the six results obtained by Abt Associates showed a highly statistically significant increase in the risk for regressive autism spectrum disorder (ASD), which sets in after a child has developed normally. The highly significant increases for regressive ASD occurred with prenatal exposure of 16 micrograms of Thimerosal derived from maternal flu shots and anti-rho antibody formulations, such as Rhogam, given to some pregnant women to prevent Rh disease, which at the time contained Thimerosal. Using a more conservative statistical approach, all six results showed a significant increase in the risk for regressive ASD for children exposed prenatally to 16 micrograms of Thimerosal—as high as 8.73 times compared to a low-exposure group. That comprises a 773 percent increase in the risk of regressive autism in children who are exposed prenatally to a Thimerosal level lower than that of the seasonal flu shot currently recommended by the CDC for pregnant women.[489]

An additional critique of the Price study is that the study "overmatched" its autism case subjects with controls. Studies match cases and controls by age and gender, for example, to try to avoid potentially confounding variables. In Price's study, children with autism were matched by age, gender, and managed care organization, as well as by immunization schedule and vaccine manufacturer. As a result of this analytical approach, the cases and the controls had nearly identical Thimerosal exposures, in effect "matching out" any difference that might exist between them. Conclusions cannot be drawn because of this overmatching.[490] Also, notably, the top-tier journals *JAMA* and the *New England Journal of Medicine* rejected the Price study before *Pediatrics* eventually published it, according to documents obtained from the CDC by Representative Bill Posey (R-Florida) on December 18, 2012.[491 492 493 494] (Part Four of this book will review the conflicts of interest at *Pediatrics*, the journal that has published much of the literature avowing no link between Thimerosal and neurodevelopmental disorders.)

A final, recent study also in this vein and with CDC employees as authors, including Thompson, is John Barile's, published in 2012 in the *Journal of Pediatric Psychology*. The study used the same dataset as Thompson 2007. And like Thompson's 2007 study, this study did not support a causal association between early exposure to mercury from Thimerosal-containing vaccines and neuropsychological functioning at the age of seven to ten years, with the exception of tics, which could still indicate neurologic injury.[495]

The results of all three of these post-Verstraeten CDC-led studies have further come into question, and not by independent critics, but by Thompson himself. In a series of phone calls in 2014 with Simpson University associate professor of biology Brian S. Hooker, Thompson described how he was pressured by his superiors at the CDC to "water down" the Barile 2012 study's initial findings, as just one example.[496] [497] The analytical manipulation downplayed in the published study the significance of the association between Thimerosal exposure and the development of tics. Thompson also describes the "hostility" within the CDC with regard to objective study of potential injuries from vaccines.[498 498 499 500 501 502]

Hooker recorded four of the phone conversations with Thompson and released portions of the calls later in 2014. Thompson requested and was granted whistleblower protection in August 2014 as he cooperates with a Congressional inquiry into the described study data manipulation, which according to Thompson has occurred in other vaccine safety-related studies conducted by the CDC.[503 504] (Part Four of this book will go into further detail.)

Beyond VSD work, the CDC also funded a study by Alberto Eugenio Tozzi that assessed a population of Italian children exposed to Thimerosal through vaccinations in the early 1990s. This 2009 paper reported essentially no deficits.[505] However, in a July 28, 2014 conversation with Hooker, Thompson discusses how the paper's original analyses had found an association with tics and lower scores in a language test, in keeping with previously reported associations.[506]

None of these studies were of course available back in 2004, when the Verstraeten study was the only epidemiological study of US populations then considered credible by the IOM panel, and which it based its far-reaching conclusions on.[507] Several other studies, however, published and unpublished, that we will review existed at the time that showed significant correlations between Thimerosal exposure and neurodevelopmental disorders. These studies mostly used a separate resource from the VSD, called the Vaccine Adverse Event Reporting System (VAERS), an epidemiological database that has been maintained by the CDC since 1990 as a surveillance tool to evaluate vaccine safety. VAERS consists of physician- and parent-reported side effects associated with vaccines, whereas the VSD contains complete medical records.[508]

The research was conducted by Mark Geier and David Geier, a father-and-son team of independent medical researchers based in Maryland.[509] Since the early 2000s, the Geiers have published extensively on the topic of Thimerosal and its potential link to neurodevelopmental disorders, particularly autism.[510] Over the course of their careers, the Geiers have become lightning rods of controversy in the vaccine safety debate, and their credibility has been widely questioned.[511] [512] Yet it is worth noting that much of the Geiers' work has been subject to peer review and published accordingly in peer-reviewed publications.[513] [514] [515] [516] [517] The Geiers have published no fewer than thirteen epidemiological studies of the associations between Thimerosal and health effects in US populations, employing accepted statistical practices.[518] In addition, some studies were reviewed by renowned epidemiologist Walter

Spitzer.[519 520] Studies by the Geiers were also cited following publication in the Hazardous Substances Data Bank (HSDB) of the US National Library of Medicine.[521]

Altogether, the Geier epidemiological studies have shown a statistically significant correlation between Thimerosal exposure level and the risk of neurological damage. Using techniques developed and published by the CDC, the Geiers found significantly increased adjusted risk ratio in the VAERS database for various neurodevelopmental disorders, including autism, speech disorders, mental retardation, personality disorders, and thinking abnormalities in the group of children exposed to Thimerosal-preserved vaccines in the late 1980s through the 1990s.[522 523 524 525 526]

A few of these studies are presented here in further detail. A 2003 study in *Experimental Biology and Medicine* compared the medical records of children who had received a non-Thimerosal-preserved DTaP vaccine between 1997 and 2000 to those children who had received an additional 75 to 100 micrograms of mercury from Thimerosal-containing DTaP vaccines between 1992 and 2000. The study found a twofold to sixfold increase in neurodevelopmental disorders among children who had received the additional Thimerosal.[527] In a 2004 follow-up analysis, the Geiers concluded their results "demonstrate a connection between mercury exposure via infant vaccinations and the dramatic increase in autism and other neurodevelopmental disorders in the United States."[528]

A 2005 *Medical Science Monitor* study assessed Thimerosal exposure in about 110,000 children and found a statistically significant association between cumulative exposure to Thimerosal and neurodevelopmental disorders, including tics, ADD/ADHD, and speech and language delays.[529]

The Geiers conducted a more recent VAERS analysis, published in 2014 and based on VAERS data as updated through September 2013. The purpose of this study was to compare populations exposed to Thimerosal-containing DTaP vaccines administered between 1997 and 1999 and unexposed populations administered DTaP vaccines with trace amounts of Thimerosal between 2004 and 2006. The researchers reviewed a total of 5,591 adverse events reported to VAERS containing the mention of at least one of the following outcomes: autism, speech disorder, mental retardation or neurodevelopmental disorder, broadly. A control set of reports without these outcomes was considered as well. Overall, a comparison of the two groups revealed increased risks in the exposed group of 7.67 for autism, 3.49 for speech disorders, 8.73 for mental retardation and 4.84 for neurodevelopmental disorders.[530]

In addition to these papers, the Geiers have also published three studies, two of which published in 2008, using the CDC's VSD. Starting in 2002, the Geiers sought to use the VSD to investigate the associations originally found between Thimerosal-containing vaccines and neurodevelopmental disorders in the VAERS. Although a taxpayer-funded agency, the CDC was extremely uncooperative in granting the Geiers access to the database. The intervention of congressional representatives and staffers was necessary to obtain even limited access to the database.[531] [532] Initial runs of the VSD findings were presented to the IOM in 2004, but without acceptance, owing essentially to there not being enough information provided to evaluate the results, in the IOM's opinion.[533] (Part Four will go over some of the behind-the-scenes efforts by the CDC to discredit and stymie the Geiers in their research efforts.)

To date, the Geiers remain the only independent researchers who have queried the pre-2001 portion of the VSD with regards to Thimerosal. The Geiers had also wanted to review the Verstraeten VSD data sets, but the CDC claimed that these original data sets had not been maintained, and thus, in essence, were lost or destroyed.[534][535]

In the VSD, the Geiers found consistent, significantly increased rate ratios for autism, ASDs, tic disorders, developmental disorders/learning disorders, attention deficit disorder, and emotional disorders. The ratios were associated with a 100 microgram increase in the children's level of mercury exposure from Thimerosal-preserved childhood vaccines. Also, the rate ratios of medical conditions that the authors did not suspect would be linked to mercury exposure, such as pneumonia and congenital abnormalities, did not significantly change as mercury exposure from vaccines went up between 1990 and 1996.[536]

The second epidemiological study conducted by the Geiers in 2008 indicated that children exposed prenatally to Thimerosal-preserved Rho(D) immune globulins, which were routinely administered to Rh-negative mothers in the United States prior to 2002, were significantly more likely than their peers to suffer serious neurodevelopmental disorders.[537]

Finally, in 2013, the Geiers undertook a study with both VAERS and VSD data concerning an outcome of autism. The two-phased study first looked at the risk of autism spectrum disorder reported in VAERS between populations of children who were administered either Thimerosal-containing or Thimerosal-free

DTaP vaccines from 1998 through 2000. Phase I showed a two-fold increased risk of autism for the former, Thimerosal-exposed group compared to the latter, unexposed group. Phase II, using the VSD, considered the exposure levels to Thimerosal from HepB vaccines administered within the first, second and sixth month of life for children with autism born between 1991 through 1999, compared to controls who did not receive this vaccine at the same intervals as the autism cases. (The primary reason for this difference in exposure is the size of the windows for recommended vaccination at the time, with the first HepB shot between birth and two months of age, the second shot between one and four months of age, and a third shot between six and eighteen months of age.) For the first-month group, those exposed to 12.5 micrograms of ethylmercury from Thimerosal were about twice as likely as controls to eventually develop autism. The two-month group, comparing 25 microgram exposure to zero microgram exposure, had similar results. In the within-sixth-months-of-age group, children exposed to 37.5 micrograms were more than three times as likely to develop autism as those with no exposure.[538]

Other researchers beyond the Geiers and their coauthors have found further epidemiological evidence along these lines. In another 2008 study, Carolyn Gallagher and Melody Goodman examined the prevalence of receiving special education or intervention services in 1,824 children ages one to nine years who had received HepB vaccinations before 2000. In this group of children, the researchers observed that the odds of receiving special services were about nine times greater for boys receiving Thimerosal-containing HepB vaccinations than for those who did not receive the three-dose vaccine.[539] A study by the same authors in 2010 reported that vaccinated newborn boys had threefold greater odds of an autism diagnosis compared to unvaccinated boys or those who did not receive HepB vaccinations in their first month of life.[540]

Yet another 2008 study of eighty-two children in Brazil by Rejane Marques and his colleagues found a significant relationship between exposure to mercury from Thimerosal-preserved childhood vaccines and neurodevelopment deficits. The deficits were seen in the areas of motor development, language development, adaptive development, and general development.[541]

The suspicions raised about Thimerosal's safety by these epidemiological studies from medical researchers, through official CDC channels and otherwise, are joined by specific calls from scientists to eliminate the preservative from medicine entirely, as detailed in the next chapter.

Notes

[474] http://www.cdc.gov/vaccinesafety/Activities/VSD.html.

[475] http://www.nlm.nih.gov/medlineplus/managedcare.html.

[476] Verstraeten T, Davis RL, DeStefano F, Lieu TA, Rhodes PH, Black SB, Shinefield H, Chen RT. Safety of Thimerosal-Containing Vaccines: A Two-Phased Study of Computerized Health Maintenance Organization Databases. *Pediatrics.* 2003 Nov; 112(5): 1039-1048.

[477] SafeMinds. *What do epidemiological studies really tell us? available at* http://www.safeminds.org/news/documents/Vaccines%20and%20Autism.%20Epidemiology%20Rebuttal.pdf.

[478] Thomas Verstraeten, "It just won't go away," email to Robert Davis and Frank DeStefano, December 17, 1999.

[479] SafeMinds. *Generation Zero—Thomas Verstraeten's First Analyses of the Link Between Vaccine Mercury Exposure and the Risk of Diagnosis of Selected Neuro-Developmental Disorders Based on Data from the Vaccine Safety Datalink:* November-December 1999. September 2004.

[480] Verstraeten T, Davis R, DeStefano F. *Thimerosal VSD Study Phase I Update,* February 29, 2000.

[481] Verstraeten T, Davis R, and DeStefano F. *Risk of Neurologic and Renal Impairment Associated with Thimerosal-Containing Vaccines.* June 1, 2000.

[482] Verstraeten T. *Neurodevelopmental and Renal Toxicity of Thimerosal-Containing Vaccines: A Two-Phased Analysis of Computerized Databases.* PowerPoint presentation to the Institute of Medicine. July 2001.

[483] http://www8.nationalacademies.org/onpinews/newsitem.aspx?RecordID=10997.

[484] Verstraeten T. Letter to the editor: Thimerosal, the Centers for Disease Control and Prevention, and GlaxoSmithKline. *Pediatrics* 2004 Apr 1; 113(4): 932.

[485] Thompson WW, Price C, Goodson B, Shay DK, Benson P, Hinrichsen VL, Lewis E, Eriksen E, Ray P, Marcy SM, Dunn J, Jackson LA, Lieu TA, Black S, Stewart G, Weintraub ES, Davis RL, DeStefano F; Vaccine Safety Datalink Team. Early Thimerosal exposure and neuropsychological outcomes at 7 to 10 years. *N Engl J Med.* 2007; 357: 1281-1292.

[486] Price CS, Thompson WW, Goodson B, Weintraub ES, Croen LA, Hinrichsen VL, Marcy M, Robertson A, Eriksen E, Lewis E, Bernal P, Shay D, Davis RL, DeStefano F. Prenatal and infant exposure to thimerosal from vaccines and immunoglobulins and risk of autism. *Pediatrics.* 2010 Oct;126(4):656-64. doi: 10.1542/peds.2010-0309. Epub 2010 Sep 13.

[487] http://abtassociates.com/reports/Aut_Tech_Report_Vol1_090310.pdf.

[488] http://www.abtassociates.com/.

[489] Brian S. Hooker, correspondence with book researchers.

[490] DeSoto MC, Hitlan RT. *Vaccine Safety Study as an Interesting Case of "Over-Matching."* *Recent Advances in Autism Spectrum Disorders—Volume I.* Michael Fitzgerald, ed. March 6, 2013 under CC BY 3.0 license *available at* http://www.intechopen.com/books/recent-advances-in-autism-spectrum-disorders-volume-i/vaccine-safety-study-as-an-interesting-case-of-over-matching-.

[491] http://www.journal-ranking.com/ranking/listCommonRanking.html?citingStart-Year=1901&externalCitationWeight=1&journalListId=370&selfCitationWeight=1.

[492] http://posey.house.gov/.

[493] JAMA rejection letter of Price manuscript [date unavailable].

[494] onbehalfof@scholarone.com on behalf of editorial@nejm.org. "New England Journal of Medicine 09-07936," email to Frank DeStefano, August 31, 2009.

[495] https://www.linkedin.com/pub/brian-hooker-ph-d-p-e/8/834/891.

[496] http://simpsonu.edu/Pages/About/Connect/Faculty-Directory.htm.

[497] http://www.mothering.com/articles/thimerosal-vaccines-autism-let-science-speak/.

[498] https://vimeo.com/104141199.

[499] Transcript. Conversation between Brian Hooker and William Thompson. May 8, 2014. Not publicly available.

[500] Transcript. Conversation between Brian Hooker and William Thompson. May 24, 2014. Not publicly available.

[501] Transcript. Conversation between Brian Hooker and William Thompson. July 28, 2014. Not publicly available.

[502] http://www.morganverkamp.com/august-27-2014-press-release-statement-of-william-w-thompson-ph-d-regarding-the-2004-article-examining-the-possibility-of-a-relationship-between-mmr-vaccine-and-autism/.

[503] Tozzi AE, Bisiacchi P, Tarantino V, De Mei B, D'Elia L, Chiarotti F, Salmaso S. Neuropsychological performance 10 years after immunization in infancy with thimerosal-containing vaccines. *Pediatrics.* 2009 Feb;123(2):475-82."

[504] Tozzi AE, Bisiacchi P, Tarantino V, De Mei B, D'Elia L, Chiarotti F, Salmaso S. Neuropsychological performance 10 years after immunization in infancy with thimerosal-containing vaccines. Pediatrics. 2009 Feb;123(2):475-82.

[505] Transcript. Conversation between Brian Hooker and William Thompson. June 12, 2014. Not publicly available.

[506] Tozzi AE, Bisiacchi P, Tarantino V, De Mei B, D'Elia L, Chiarotti F, Salmaso S. Neuropsychological performance 10 years after immunization in infancy with thimerosal-containing vaccines. *Pediatrics.* 2009 Feb;123(2):475-82.

[507] Barile JP, Kuperminc GP, Weintraub ES, Mink JW, Thompson WW. Thimerosal exposure in early life and neuropsychological outcomes 7-10 years later. *J Pediatr Psychol.* 2012 Jan-Feb;37(1):106-18. doi: 10.1093/jpepsy/jsr048. Epub 2011 Jul 23.

508 Immunization Safety Review Committee Board on Health Promotion and Disease Prevention, IOM. *Final Report, Immunization Safety Review: Vaccines And Autism.* May 2004.

509 http://www.cdc.gov/vaccinesafety/vaccine_monitoring/history.html.

510 http://www.autismtreatmentclinics.com/Staff.html.

511 http://www.ncbi.nlm.nih.gov/pubmed?term=Mark%20Geier%20AND%20David%20 Geier%20AND%20thimerosal.

512 http://articles.baltimoresun.com/2011-05-06/health/bs-hs-doctor-suspen-sion-20110505_1_david-geier-mark-geier-autism-commission.

513 http://www.chicagotribune.com/health/ct-nw-autism-geiers-charged-20110519,0,5269435. story.

514 http://www.ncbi.nlm.nih.gov/pubmed?term=Mark%20Geier%20AND%20David%20 Geier.

515 http://www.ane.pl/.

516 http://onlinelibrary.wiley.com/journal/10.1111/(ISSN)1442-200X/homepage/ForAuthors. html.

517 http://icmr.nic.in/ijmr/aboutijmr.htm.

518 http://www.tandfonline.com/action/aboutThisJournal?show=readership&journal-Code=uteh20.

519 http://www.ncbi.nlm.nih.gov/pubmed?term=Mark%20Geier%20AND%20David%20 Geier%20AND%20thimerosal.

520 http://aje.oxfordjournals.org/content/164/6/607.full.pdf.

521 Book researcher interview with David Geier, September 14, 2012.

522 http://toxnet.nlm.nih.gov/cgi-bin/sis/htmlgen?HSDB; enter search term "Thimerosal," click on first returned query marked "1. THIMEROSAL 54-64-8".

523 Geier DA, Geier MR. An assessment of the impact of thimerosal on childhood neurodevel-opmental disorders. *Pediatr Rehabil.* 2003 Apr-Jun; 6(2):97-102.

524 Geier MR, Geier DA. Neurodevelopmental disorders after thimerosal-containing vaccines: a brief communication. *Exp Biol Med (Maywood).* 2003 Jun; 228(6):660-4.

525 Geier MR, Geier DA. Thimerosal in childhood vaccines, neurodevelopment disorders, and heart disease in the United States. *J Am Phys Surg.* 2003;8:6-11.

526 Geier DA, Geier MR. Neurodevelopmental disorders following thimerosal-containing childhood immunizations: a follow-up analysis. *Int J Toxicol.* 2004 Nov-Dec;23(6):369-76.

527 Geier DA, Kern JK, King PG, Sykes LK, Geier MR. The risk of neurodevelopmental dis-orders following a Thimerosal-preserved DTaP formulation in comparison to its Thimerosal-reduced formulation in the vaccine adverse event reporting system (VAERS). *J Biochem Pharmacol Res.* 2014 Jun 1;2(2):64-73.

528 Geier DA, Geier MR. An evaluation of the effects of thimerosal on neurodevelopmental disorders reported following DTP and Hib vaccines in comparison to DTPH vaccine in the United States. *J Toxicol Environ Health A.* 2006 Aug;69(15):1481-95.

[529] Geier MR, Geier DA. Neurodevelopmental disorders after Thimerosal-containing vaccines: a brief communication. *Exp Biol Med (Maywood)*. 2003 Oct; 228(9): 991-992; discussion 993-994.

[530] Geier DA, Geier MR. Neurodevelopmental disorders following Thimerosal-containing childhood immunizations: a follow-up analysis. *Int J Toxicol*. 2004 Nov-Dec; 23: 369-376.

[531] Geier DA, Geier MR. A two-phased population epidemiological study of the safety of thimerosal-containing vaccines: a follow-up analysis. *Med Sci Monit*. 2005 Mar; 24(4): CR160-CR170.

[532] Book researcher interview with David Geier, September 14, 2012.

[533] Kirby D. *Evidence of Harm: Mercury in Vaccines and the Autism Epidemic: A Medical Controversy*. New York: St. Martin's Press, 2005.

[534] Immunization Safety Review Committee Board on Health Promotion and Disease Prevention, IOM. *Final Report, Immunization Safety Review: Vaccines And Autism*. May 2004.

[535] Geier DA, Hooker BS, Kern JK, King PG, Sykes LK, Geier MR. A two-phase study evaluating the relationship between Thimerosal-containing vaccine administration and the risk for an autism spectrum disorder diagnosis in the United States. *Transl Neurodegener*. 2013 Dec 19;2(1):25. doi: 10.1186/2047-9158-2-25.

[536] Book researcher interview with David Geier, September 14, 2012.

[537] Kirby D. *Evidence of Harm: Mercury in Vaccines and the Autism Epidemic: A Medical Controversy*. New York: St. Martin's Press, 2005.

[538] Young HA, Geier DA, Geier MR. Thimerosal exposure in infants and neurodevelopmental disorders: an assessment of computerized medical records in the Vaccine Safety Datalink. *J Neurol Sci*. 2008 Aug 15;271(1-2):110-8. Epub 2008 May 15.

[539] Geier DA, Mumper E, Gladfelter B, Coleman L, Geier MR. Neurodevelopmental disorders, maternal Rh-negativity, and Rho(D) immune globulins: a multi-center assessment. *Neuro Endocrinol Lett*. 2008 Apr; 29(2): 272-280.

[540] Gallagher C, Goodman M. Hepatitis B triple series vaccine and developmental disability in US children aged 1-9 years. *Toxicol Environm Chem*. 2008; 90(5): 997-1008.

[541] Gallagher CM, Goodman MS. Hepatitis B vaccination of male neonates and autism diagnosis, NHIS 1997-2002. *J Toxicol Environ Health A*. 2010;73(24):1665-77.

[542] Marques RC, Bernardia JVE, Dórea JG, Bastos WR, Malm O. Principal component analysis and discrimination of variables associated with pre- and post-natal exposure to mercury. *Int J Hygiene Environ Health*. 2008 Oct; 211(5-6): 606-614.

Chapter 8:
Scientific Calls for a
Ban on Thimerosal

For more than seven decades, various European and American scientists have called for the removal of Thimerosal from vaccines in peer-reviewed studies and professional correspondences.

In 1947, Army doctor Francis Ellis warned, "It may be dangerous to inject a serum containing merthiolate into a patient sensitive to merthiolate."[543]

In 1948, H. D. Cogswell and Alex Shoun, doctors in Arizona, wrote, "Merthiolate is such a commonly used preservative for biologicals, plasma, cartilage, etc., that it would seem important to determine whether harm would result following its subcutaneous or intravenous injection in skin sensitive individuals."[544]

In 1977, David Fagan at The Hospital for Sick Children in Canada urged that topical organic mercurial antiseptics including Thimerosal be "heavily restricted or withdrawn from hospital use."[545]

David Matheson, also of The Hospital for Sick Children, and his team of research scientists wrote in 1980 that "merthiolate . . . represents a potential hazard to patients."[546]

In 1982, Martin Heyworth of the Department of Veterans Affairs Medical Center stated that "Thimerosal should no longer be added to [medications for preventing transplant rejection] or other materials which are intended for use in human subjects."[547]

Writing in 1983, the Russian scientist A. T. Kravchenko and his colleagues showed that Thimerosal not only killed human cells but also that mere contact with Thimerosal caused changes to cell properties. Kravchenko and his team marveled at the continued practice of putting Thimerosal in vaccines despite "numerous clinical studies confirming [Thimerosal's] damaging action on humans." The researchers concluded that Thimerosal should be banned from medicines, especially those used by children.[548]

Other studies, in particular those by Neil Cox and Angela Forsyth in 1988, Lars Förström in 1980, and JoAnn Royhans in 1984, pointed out the unsuitability of Thimerosal in vaccines because of its inherent toxicity, its capacity to induce allergic responses in upward of 29 percent of persons exposed to the preservative, and its poor antiseptic effectiveness.[549 550 551] In the Cox and Forsyth study, the authors wrote that "severe reactions to thiomersal [Thimerosal] demonstrate a need for vaccines with an alternative preservative." In the Förström study, the authors wrote, "Local reactions can be expected in such a high percentage of merthiolate-sensitive persons that merthiolate in vaccines should be replaced by another antibacterial agent."

In 1985, Harrison Stetler and his team from the CDC concluded that because Thimerosal was ineffective as a vaccine preservative and higher concentrations, which could be more effective, might "pose a health hazard to vaccine recipients . . . the only feasible and cost-effective preservative measure now available is careful attention to sterile technique when administering vaccines from multidose vials."[552]

A year later, K. A. Winship of the Department of Health and Social Security (now the Department of Health) in the United Kingdom wrote, "Multidose vaccines and allergy-testing extracts contain a mercurial preservative, usually 0.01% Thimerosal, and may present problems occasionally in practice. It is, therefore, now accepted that multidose injection preparations are undesirable and that preservatives should not be present in unit-dose preparations."[553]

In 1988, the head of Austria's Official Medicines Control Laboratory, Wolfgang Maurer, began calling for Thimerosal's removal from medicinal products. He had a Thimerosal-containing immunoglobulin pulled from that country's market, based on safety concerns he had from reading the literature on organo-mercurial use in medicines. That same year Maurer submitted a letter to two top-tier US journals entitled "Unconsidered Risk Due to Thiomersal in Anti-Lymphocytic Globulin Preparation." The article was not accepted. Maurer, however, continued urging a ban of Thimerosal in Europe in the 1990s and in a letter to US Congressman Dan Burton (R-Indiana) in 2002.[554][555]

Another particularly compelling call for the reduction or elimination of Thimerosal in vaccines was brought to light in lawsuits against the pharmaceutical industry in the United States. In a 1991 memo obtained by plaintiffs' lawyers, Maurice Hilleman, one of the fathers of Merck's vaccination programs, warned Gordon Douglas, then-president of the company's vaccine division, that six-month-old children administered the shots on schedule would have cumulative mercury exposures about eighty-seven times the daily Swedish safety standard. Hilleman calculated:

> For babies: The 25 μg [micrograms] of mercury in a single 0.5 ml dose and extrapolated to a 6 lb. baby would be 25X the adjusted Swedish daily allowance of 1.0 μg for a baby of that size. . . . If 8 doses of thimerosal-containing vaccine were given in the first six months of life (3 DPT, 2 HIB, and 3 Hepatitis B), the 200 μg of mercury given, say an average size of 12 lbs., would be about 87X the Swedish daily allowance of 2.3 μg of mercury for a baby of that size. When viewed in this way, the mercury load appears rather large.

(The 200 micrograms of mercury example that Hilleman used is about 350 times the US EPA RfD of 0.1 microgram of mercury per kilogram of body weight per day.)

Based on a perception in the public that Thimerosal might not be safe, which could in turn hurt vaccine sales, Hilleman recommended that Thimerosal use be discontinued, "especially where use in infants and young children is anticipated." He also noted that regulators in Sweden, elsewhere in Scandinavia, and in the United Kingdom, Japan, and Switzerland had expressed concern about the mercury-containing vaccine preservative, but that the US FDA "does not have this concern about thimerosal." Hilleman also recommended reducing the preservative level of Thimerosal used and that "it is worthy of consideration to find another acceptable preservative."[556][557]

The same year that the Hilleman memo was written, other scientists made their professional opinions known on the matter of Thimerosal. Writing in *The Lancet*, David Seal and his colleagues from the Moorsfield Eye Hospital in the United Kingdom observed, "Thimerosal is a weak antibacterial agent that is rapidly broken down to products, including ethylmercury residues, which are neurotoxic. Its role as a preservative in vaccines has been questioned, and the pharmaceutical industry itself considers its use as historical."[558]

Also in 1991, Werner Aberer of the University of Vienna, Austria, published an article titled "Topical Mercury Should Be Banned—Dangerous, Outmoded, but Still Popular" in the *Journal of the American Academy of Dermatology*. Aberer did not limit his criticism to just topical applications, however. He wrote:

> The presence of mercury in over-the-counter drugs for the eye, ear, nose, throat, and skin; in bleaching creams; as preservative in cosmetics, tooth pastes, lens solutions, vaccines, allergy test and immuno-therapy solutions, in antiseptics, disinfectants, and contraceptives; in fungicides and herbicides; in dental fillings and thermometers; and many other products, makes it a ubiquitous source of danger. . . . Despite calls for abandonment and a general prohibition in 1967, mercury is still listed in many pharmacopeias, including that of the United States . . . thus mercury is still much more frequently used than is generally believed. This seems incomprehensible because side effects are not only potentially disastrous but also numerous and well documented.

He listed among the well-known effects of Thimerosal "neurologic and psychiatric symptoms, renal toxicity, erythroderma and other signs of poisoning after percutaneous absorption." Furthermore, he stated that "knowledge of all these side effects has been available for some time." He concluded by arguing:

> Recommendations not to use mercury salts in children or only on prescription are insufficient. Removal from textbooks seems overdue. . . . However, calls for their abandonment (as early as 1960) or restricted use have not sufficed. Only a general ban and their removal from the pharmacopeias will be effective in stopping the use of these dangerous, outmoded substances.[559]

In 1992, Manfred Hause of the Paul-Ehrlich-Institut, a medical regulatory body in Germany, wrote a letter expressing official concern about Thimerosal to the European Medicine Agency's Commission of the European Communities, Committee for Proprietary Medicinal Products. Hause wrote:

> It is well known that even low amounts of organic mercury compounds may cause rare untoward reactions in man, mainly allergic reactions. Other undesired properties have also have [sic] been seen in experimental studies or were described in the scientific literature: mutagenicity, teratogenicity, embryo- and neurotoxicity. . . . Based upon the principle that whenever an additive which can be a matter of concern is not necessary to ensure some essential property of a medicinal product its use should be avoided[,] in June of 1991 the Paul-Ehrlich-Institut has encouraged manufacturers to discontinue the addition

of organic mercury compounds into immunoglobulins. This initiative has been generally appreciated and in the meantime nearly all manufacturers have informed our institute on the measures taken to implement the recommend change. It can be predicted that this will be achieved by the end of 1992.[560]

In a June 1999 memo, the Executive Director of the European Agency for the Evaluation of Medicinal Products (EMEA), Fernand Sauer, advised Elaine Esber of the FDA on limiting exposure to Thimerosal among vulnerable populations.[561] [562] Sauer wrote: "For vaccination in infants and toddlers, the use of vaccine without thiomersal and other mercurial-containing products should be encouraged." He also stated: "The main concern with thiomersal are the induction of allergic reactions and due to the presence of ethylmercury, the potential risks of neurotoxicity."[563]

In 2001, Leslie Ball and her colleagues with the FDA warned in a risk assessment published in *Pediatrics* that "inadvertent high dose exposure to thimerosal includes acute neurotoxicity and nephrotoxicity [toxicity in the kidneys]." The authors wrote, "Limited data on toxicity from low-dose exposures to ethylmercury are available, but toxicity may be similar to that of methylmercury. . . . Exposure of infants to mercury in vaccines can be reduced or eliminated by using products formulated without thimerosal as a preservative."[564] For at least a few years prior, Ball had debated with colleagues about the possible danger stemming from Thimerosal. In a 1998 memo, Ball wrote:

On a strictly scientific basis, yes, there are no data that have looked at the specific issue of thimerosal in vaccines. However, there are factors/data that would argue for the removal of thimerosal, including data on methylmercury exposure in infants and the knowledge that thimerosal is not an essential component to vaccines.[565]

Following a comprehensive literature review of the well-documented neurodevelopmental damage from Thimerosal, in 2006, two doctors in Lima, Peru, requested to establish the legal framework to remove Thimerosal from the remaining vaccines in Peru as quickly as possible.[566]

In a 2011 Brazilian paper in *Neurochemical Research*, representing perhaps the most comprehensive review ever undertaken of existing peer-reviewed literature studying Thimerosal's toxic effects in vitro and in vivo, in both animals and humans at doses comparable to those of vaccines, Jose Dórea of the University of Brasilia concluded that Thimerosal is highly toxic and has the potential to have neurodevelopmental effects. This review calls for banning the use of Thimerosal in the vaccines used in the developing nations.[567]

Notes

[543] Ellis FA. The sensitizing factor in Merthiolate. *J Allergy.* 1947; 18: 212-213.

[544] Cogswell HD, Shoun A. Reaction following the use of tincture of Merthiolate. *Ariz Med.* 1948; 5: 42–43.

[545] Fagan DG, Pritchard JS, Clarkson TW, Greenwood MR. Organ mercury levels in infants with omphaloceles treated with organic mercurial antiseptic. *Arch Dis Child.* 1977 Dec; 52(12): 962-964.

[546] Matheson DS, Clarkson TW, Gelfand EW. Mercury toxicity (acrodynia) induced by long-term injection of gammaglobulin. *J Pediatr.* 1980 Jul;97(1):153-5.

[547] Heyworth MF. Clinical experience with antilymphocyte serum. *Immunol Rev.* 1982; 65: 79–97.

[548] Kravchenko AT, Dzagurov SG, Chervonskaia GP. Evaluation of the toxic action of prophylactic and therapeutic preparations on cell cultures. Communication III. Revealing the toxic properties of medical biological preparations from the degree of cell damage in continuous cell line L132. *Zh Mikrobiol Epidemiol Immunobiol.* 1983; 3: 87-92 *as described in* Geier DA, Sykes LK, Geier MR 2007.

[549] Cox NH, Forsyth A. Thimerosal allergy and vaccination reactions. *Contact Dermatitis.* 1988 April;18(4):229-33.

[550] Forstrom L, Hannuksela M, Kousa M, Lehmuskallio E. Merthiolate hypersensitivity and vaccination. *Contact Dermatitis.* 1980 Jun;6(4): 241-5.

[551] Rohyans J, Walson PD, Wood GA, MacDonald WA. Mercury toxicity following Merthiolate ear irrigations. *J Pediatr.* 1984 Feb;104(2):311-3.

[552] Stetler HC, Garbe PL, Dwyer DM, Facklam RR, Orenstein WA, West GR, Dudley KJ, Bloch AB. Outbreaks of group A streptococcal abscesses following diphtheria-tetanus toxoid-pertussis vaccination. *Pediatrics.* 1985 Feb;75(2):299-303.

[553] Winship KA. Organic mercury compounds and their toxicity. *Adverse Drug React Acute Poisoning Rev.* 1986 Autumn;5(3).141-80 *as described in* Geier DA, Sykes LK, Geier MR 2007.

[554] Wolfgang Maurer, "Thiomersal," memo to Dan Burton, December 4, 2002 *available at* http://www.putchildrenfirst.org/media/1.11.pdf.

[555] Elizabeth Birt and James Moody, "timeline," memo to Lauren Fuller, July 15, 2005 *portions available at* http://www.putchildrenfirst.org/media/e.19.pdf.

111

[556] Maurice Hilleman, "Vaccine Task Force Assignment Thimerosal (Merthiolate) Preservative—Problems, Analysis, Suggestions for Resolution," memo to Gordon Douglas, March 27, 1991.

[557] http://articles.latimes.com/print/2005/feb/08/business/fi-vaccine8.

[558] Seal D, Ficker L, Wright P, Andrews V. The case against Thimerosal. *Lancet*. 1991 Aug 3;338(8762): 315-6.

[559] Aberer W. Topical mercury should be banned—dangerous, outmoded, but still popular. *J Am Acad Dermatol*. 1991 Jan;24(1):150-1 *as described in* Geier DA, Sykes LK, Geier MR 2007.

[560] Elizabeth Birt and James Moody, "timeline," memo to Lauren Fuller, July 15, 2005 *portions available at* http://www.putchildrenfirst.org/media/e.19.pdf.

[561] http://www.ema.europa.eu/docs/en_GB/document_library/Press_release/2009/11/WC500015019.pdf.

[562] http://www.fda.gov/OHRMS/DOCKETS/98fr/cd006.pdf.

[563] Elizabeth Birt and James Moody, "timeline," memo to Lauren Fuller, July 15, 2005 *portions available at* http://www.putchildrenfirst.org/media/e.19.pdf.

[564] Ball LK, Ball R, Pratt RD. An assessment of thimerosal use in childhood vaccines. *Pediatrics*. 2001 May;107(5):1147-1154.

[565] Elizabeth Birt and James Moody, "timeline," memo to Lauren Fuller, July 15, 2005 *portions available at* http://www.putchildrenfirst.org/media/e.19.pdf.

[566] Maya L, Luna F. Thimerosal and children's neurodevelopmental disorders. *Ann Fac Med (Lima)*. 2006; 67(3); 243-262 [Spanish].

[567] Dórea JG. Integrating experimental (in vitro and in vivo) neurotoxicity studies of low dose thimerosal relevant to vaccines. *Neurochem Res*. 2011 Jun; 36(6): 927-938.

Chapter 9:
Official Reports against Thimerosal by Public Health and Other Agencies

In addition to individual physicians and researchers calling for bans on Thimerosal, more pointedly, many of America's and Europe's public health organizations and government agencies have also stated concerns over use of the preservative.

Food and Drug Administration (FDA): In 1982, the FDA recommended that Thimerosal be banned from topical over-the-counter products.[568] [569] In August of 1998, an FDA internal Point Paper was prepared by the Maternal Immunization Working Group. That document officially recommended that for "investigational

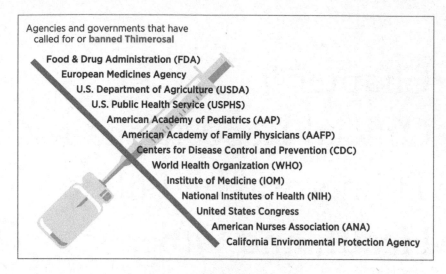

Agencies and governments that have
called for or **banned Thimerosal**

Food & Drug Administration (FDA)
European Medicines Agency
U.S. Department of Agriculture (USDA)
U.S. Public Health Service (USPHS)
American Academy of Pediatrics (AAP)
American Academy of Family Physicians (AAFP)
Centers for Disease Control and Prevention (CDC)
World Health Organization (WHO)
Institute of Medicine (IOM)
National Institutes of Health (NIH)
United States Congress
American Nurses Association (ANA)
California Environmental Protection Agency

FIGURE 10

vaccines indicated for maternal immunization, the use of single-dose vials should be required to avoid the need of preservative in multidose vials. Of concern here is the potential neurotoxic effect of mercury especially when considering cumulative doses of this component in early infancy."[570][571]

European Medicines Agency: The European Medicines Agency—previously known as the European Agency for the Evaluation of Medicinal Products (EMEA)—is responsible for the scientific evaluation of medicines developed by pharmaceutical companies for use within the European Union.[572][573] The agency issued a report in June 1999 recommending that "for vaccination in infants and toddlers . . . although there is no evidence of harm caused by the level of exposure from vaccines, it would be prudent to promote the general use of vaccines without thiomersal. . . . This should be done within the shortest possible time-frame."[574] The then-EMEA made their assessment of risk associated with thiomersal in vaccines based on toxicity data of methylmercury.[575] In 2007, the EMEA reiterated that "the development of vaccines without thiomersal or with the lowest possible levels of thiomersal and other mercury-containing preservatives should continue to be promoted."[576]

US Department of Agriculture (USDA): In a July 2, 1999, email, Ruth Etzel of the USDA noted, "We must follow the three basic rules: (1) act quickly to inform pediatricians that the products have more mercury than we realized; (2) be open with consumers about why we didn't catch this earlier; (3) show contrition. . . . If the public loses faith in the Public Health Services recommendations, then the immunization battle will falter. To keep faith, we must be open and honest now and move forward quickly to replace these products."[577]

US Public Health Service (USPHS): In July 1999, the USPHS called for Thimerosal's removal from all vaccines.[578]

American Academy of Pediatrics (AAP): The AAP joined the USPHS in calling for Thimerosal's removal from all vaccines in July 1999. The AAP requested that vaccine manufacturers reduce or eliminate the mercury in their vaccines as soon as possible and that the FDA expedite review of licenses for vaccines with eliminated or reduced mercury.[579] [580] In 2001, the AAP Committee on Environmental Health concluded that "the developing fetus and young children are thought to be disproportionately affected by the exposure to mercury, because many aspects of development, particularly brain maturation, can be disturbed by the presence of mercury. Minimizing mercury exposure is, therefore, essential to optimal child health."[581] The AAP has since affirmed that Thimerosal does not pose a risk to vaccine recipients.[582]

American Academy of Family Physicians (AAFP): In 1999, the AAFP joined the AAP and the USPHS in recommending the removal of Thimerosal from routine infant vaccines as soon as possible, and in 2000, the AAFP together with the AAP, the USPHS, and the CDC's Advisory Committee on Immunization Practices (ACIP) recommended that the policy to rapidly move away from Thimerosal-preserved vaccines continue.[583]

Centers for Disease Control and Prevention (CDC): In 1999, the CDC, as part of the USPHS, was also a signatory of the joint statement urging vaccine makers to eliminate or reduce Thimerosal in vaccines as soon as possible.[584] On behalf of CDC's official position that Thimerosal should be banned, Roger Bernier, chief science advisor to the CDC, testified to the Government Reform Committee of the United States Congress on July 18, 2000: "We agree that we do not need to have thimerosal in vaccines. If it doesn't need to be there, we should take it out. And we should take it out as rapidly as possible. We have agreed to that. The Public Health Service, the vaccine makers, and the academies are all in agreement."[585][586] The CDC has since maintained that Thimerosal, however, is safe. On a frequently asked questions webpage concerning Thimerosal, the CDC states: "Thimerosal has a proven

THIMEROSAL'S DANGERS TO HUMAN HEALTH AND THE BRAIN

track record of being very safe. Data from many studies show no convincing evidence of harm caused by the low doses of thimerosal in vaccines."[587]

World Health Organization (WHO): Although the WHO remains a strong defender of Thimerosal use, in January 2000 the organization issued a qualified endorsement of the USPHS and AAP position.[588] In its *Weekly Epidemiological Record*, the WHO stated that it "supports a statement made on 7 July 1999 by the American Academy of Pediatrics and the United States Public Health Service regarding prospective phasing out of thiomersal. . . . However, the Organization underlines the importance of continuing to use currently available children's vaccines containing thiomersal." The statement's summary further read:

> [W]ith the weight of public opinion against the use of mercury of any sort, WHO and other agencies have begun the process of reducing and removing thiomersal from vaccines. In the short term (the next 3 years), modifications to existing strategies will result in a reduction in exposure to thiomersal. Over the long term (beyond 3 years), efforts will be focused on new vaccine-delivery technologies, alternative preservatives and combination vaccines, further reducing and eventually, perhaps, eliminating thiomersal from vaccines.[589]

Institute of Medicine (IOM): A 2001 report by the Institute of Medicine (IOM), an "independent" agency founded in 1970 by the National Academy of Sciences, a society that Congress mandated in 1863 to "advise the federal government on scientific and technical matters," could not rule out a biologically plausible link between Thimerosal and neurological disorders. The IOM advised accordingly that "full consideration be given to removing thimerosal from any biological or pharmaceutical product to which infants, children, and pregnant women are exposed."[590]

A follow-up report published by the IOM in 2004 backed away from this language, however. That report deliberately limited its scope to examining the hypothesis that Thimerosal-containing vaccines cause autism, and concluded that "the evidence favors rejection of a causal relationship between thimerosal-containing vaccines and autism."[591] The controversy surrounding these reports will be covered in Part Four of this book.

National Institutes of Health (NIH): In 2001, NIH nominated Thimerosal to the US National Toxicology Program for further study. The NIH report stated that there is some evidence from animal studies that Thimerosal is a carcinogen and can be deadly to fetuses.[592]

United States Congress: In May 2003, the Committee on Government Reform of the US Congress found that "the committee, upon a thorough review of the scientific literature and internal documents from government and industry did find evidence that Thimerosal did pose a risk" and "our public health agencies' failure to act is indicative of institutional malfeasance for self-protection and misplaced protectionism of the pharmaceutical industry." The report also stated, "The continued response from agency officials that 'there is no proof of harm' is a disingenuous response. The lack of conclusive proof does not mean that there is no connection between thimerosal and vaccine-induced autism. What the lack of conclusive proof indicates is that the agency has failed in its duties to assure that adequate safety studies were conducted prior to marketing. Furthermore, in the last two decades, after determining that thimerosal was no longer 'generally recognized as safe' for topical ointments, the agency did not extend their evaluation to other applications of thimerosal, in particular as a vaccine preservative."[593]

American Nurses Association (ANA): In 2006, the ANA issued a position statement on mercury in vaccines. ANA, it states, "insists that pharmaceutical companies develop technology to produce seasonal influenza vaccine without using thimerosal as a preservative and cease using thimerosal as a preservative in vaccines immediately." The statement also called for "pharmaceutical companies [to] increase the availability of single-dose vials and pre-filled syringes to meet the subsequent increased demand with discontinuation of the use of thimerosal as a preservative in multidose vials of seasonal influenza vaccine."[594]

California Environmental Protection Agency (Cal/EPA): In 2004, the Cal/EPA stated, "The scientific evidence that . . . thimerosal causes reproductive toxicity is clear and voluminous . . . [and] includes severe mental retardation or malformations in human offspring who were poisoned when their mothers were exposed to ethyl mercury or thimerosal while pregnant."[595] In addition, effective July 1, 2006, the state of California has banned administration of Thimerosal-preserved vaccines to children under three and to pregnant women, with the exception of the influenza vaccine, for which the level of mercury cannot exceed one microgram per 0.5 mL dose, except in an emergency.[596]

Besides California, several other US states have passed laws aimed at reducing Thimerosal exposure to pregnant women and young children. The laws, passed in states including Delaware, Illinois, Iowa, Missouri, New York, and Washington, require that vaccines contain no Thimerosal or only trace amounts when administered to infants, children, and pregnant women.[597] [598] [599] Efforts to ban Thimerosal on the state level have come up in many other jurisdictions, including Maryland, Massachusetts, and Rhode Island.[600] [601]

On an international level, numerous countries have phased out Thimerosal from their childhood vaccine armamentaria, including Denmark (in 1992), Sweden (in 1989), and the United Kingdom (as of September 27, 2004).[602] [603] [604] [605] Other countries have announced intended phaseouts and have expressed a preference for Thimerosal-free formulations for children, including Australia (starting as early as 2000), Canada (as of March 1, 2003), and France (July 4, 2000).[606] [607] [608] Meanwhile, efforts are under way in Chile and elsewhere to limit childhood exposure to Thimerosal.[609]

Having thus presented the case for the health hazards of Thimerosal, as well as the calls by scientists and medical organizations based on these hazards to ban the chemical, we will review the evidence suggesting that Thimerosal is actually ineffective and is a poor choice as a vaccine preservative.

Notes

[568] United States. Mercury in medicine report. *Congressional Record*. Washington: GPO, May 21, 2003: 1011-1030.

[569] U.S. National Archives and Records Administration, Office of the Federal Register. Status of certain additional over-the-counter drug category II and III active ingredients. *Federal Register*. 1998 Apr; 63(77): 19799-19802.

[570] United States. Mercury in medicine report. *Congressional Record*. Washington: GPO, May 21, 2003: 1011-1030.

[571] Geier DA, Sykes LK, Geier MR. A review of Thimerosal (Merthiolate) and its ethylmercury breakdown product: specific historical considerations regarding safety and effectiveness. *J Toxicol Environ Health B Crit Rev*. 2007 Dec;10(8):575-96.

[572] http://www.ema.europa.eu/ema/index.jsp?curl=pages/about_us/general/general_content_000235.jsp&mid=WC0b01ac058001ce7d.

[573] http://www.epha.org/IMG/pdf/EMEA_Communication_NewVisualIdentity_en.pdf.

[574] http://www.ema.europa.eu/docs/en_GB/document_library/Scientific_guideline/2009/09/WC500003902.pdf.

[575] http://www.ema.europa.eu/docs/en_GB/document_library/Scientific_guideline/2009/09/WC500003904.pdf.

[576] http://www.ema.europa.eu/docs/en_GB/document_library/Scientific_guideline/2009/09/WC500003905.pdf.

[577] Ruth Etzel, "Message from Ruth Etzel, M.D.," email to Lauri Hall, Ray Koteras, Hope Hurley, Roger Suchyta, July 2, 1999.

[578] Joint statement of the American Academy of Pediatrics (AAP) and the United States Public Health Service (USPHS). *Pediatrics*. 1999 Sep;104(3 Pt 1):568-9.

[579] Committee on Infectious Diseases and Committee on Environmental Health, American Academy of Pediatrics. Thimerosal in vaccines—an interim report to clinicians. *Pediatrics*. 1999 Sep;104(3 Pt 1):570-4.

[580] http://www.fda.gov/BiologicsBloodVaccines/SafetyAvailability/VaccineSafety/UCM096228.

[581] Goldman LR, Shannon MW; American Academy of Pediatrics: Committee on Environmental Health. Technical report: mercury in the environment: implications for pediatricians. *Pediatrics*. 2001 Jul;108(1):197-205.

582 http://www2.aap.org/immunization/families/ingredients.html.

583 http://www.cdc.gov/mmwr/preview/mmwrhtml/mm4927a5.htm.

584 http://www.cdc.gov/mmwr/preview/mmwrhtml/mm4927a5.htm.

585 http://www.gpo.gov/fdsys/pkg/CHRG-106hhrg72722/html/CHRG-106hhrg72722.htm.

586 http://www.publichealth.uga.edu/epibio/about/directory/adjunct%20/roger_bernier.

587 http://www.cdc.gov/vaccinesafety/concerns/thimerosal/thimerosal_faqs.html.

588 http://www.who.int/vaccine_safety/committee/topics/thiomersal/statement_jul2006/en/.

589 http://www.who.int/docstore/wer/pdf/2000/wer7502.pdf.

590 Kathleen Stratton, Alicia Gable, and Marie C. McCormick, eds.; Immunization Safety Review Committee, Board on Health Promotion and Disease Prevention, Institute of Medicine. *Immunization Safety Review: Thimerosal-Containing Vaccines and Neurodevelopmental Disorders.* The National Academies Press. Washington, DC. October 1, 2001.

591 Immunization Safety Review Committee, Board on Health Promotion and Disease Prevention, Institute of Medicine. *Immunization Safety Review: Vaccines and Autism.* National Academies Press. Washington, DC. May 2004.

592 http://www.ntp.niehs.nih.gov/ntp/htdocs/Chem_Background/ExSumPDF/Thimerosal.pdf.

593 United States. Mercury in medicine report. *Congressional Record.* Washington: GPO, May 21, 2003: 1011-1030.

594 http://nursingworld.org/MainMenuCategories/Policy-Advocacy/Positions-and-Resolutions/ANAPositionStatements/Position-Statements-Alphabetically/Mercury-in-Vaccines.html.

595 http://oehha.ca.gov/prop65/CRNR_notices/pdf_zip/hgbayer1.pdf.

596 http://www.leginfo.ca.gov/pub/03-04/bill/asm/ab_2901-2950/ab_2943_bill_20040928_chaptered.html.

597 http://www.cga.ct.gov/2010/rpt/2010-R-0352.htm.

598 http://www.ama-assn.org/amednews/2006/04/24/hll20424.htm.

599 http://www.gpo.gov/fdsys/pkg/CREC-2005-02-09/html/CREC-2005-02-09-pt1-PgH481-4.htm.

600 http://www.whale.to/vaccine/ayoub.html.

601 http://www.petitiononline.com/HgBill/petition.html.

602 Madsen KM, Lauritsen MB, Pedersen CB, Thorsen P, Plesner A-M, Andersen PH, Mortensen PB. Thimerosal and the occurrence of autism: negative ecological evidence from Danish population-based data. *Pediatrics.* 2003 Sep; 112(3): 604-606.

603 Marta Granstrom, "Re: vaccine preservatives," email to Diane Simpson, June 22, 2001.

604 Bedford H, Elliman D. Misconceptions about the new combination vaccine. *BMJ.* 2004 Aug 21;329(7463):411-2.

605 http://web.archive.org/web/20070609114311/http://www.advisorybodies.doh.gov.uk/jcvi/mins011004.htm.

[606] Brown I, Austin D. Maternal transfer of mercury to the developing embryo/fetus: is there a safe level? *Toxicological & Environmental Chemistry.* 2012 94:8, 1610-1627.

[607] http://www.collectionscanada.gc.ca/webarchives/20071125012841/http://www.phac-aspc.gc.ca/publicat/ccdr-rmtc/03pdf/acs-dcc-29-1.pdf.

[608] http://web.archive.org/web/20081210134413/http://agmed.sante.gouv.fr/htm/10/filcoprs/excom.htm.

[609] http://www.prnewswire.com/news-releases/chile-stops-use-of-mercury-in-vaccines-145939975.html.

PART TWO:

THE UNNECESSARY USE OF THIMEROSAL

Chapter 10: The Ineffectiveness of Thimerosal as a Germicide

Given the safety issues regarding Thimerosal known since its invention and further revealed in the following decades, one might assume that the compound had "earned its keep" as a potent germicide. Perhaps some of the threats to health that Thimerosal could pose have been offset by its effectiveness at preventing microbial contamination in vaccines and other medicinal products. Yet numerous studies and accounts from over the years have shown Thimerosal to be poorly suited to the task it is intended to serve.

A disinfectant that ends up in the human body, as Thimerosal does, must be more effective at killing pathogens than destroying human cells. Thimerosal does not meet this criterion, according to several studies.[610] For example, a 1935 study found that Thimerosal was 35.3 times as toxic to embryonic chick cells as to the bacteria

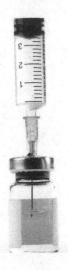

Staphylococcus aureus.[611] Studies in 1939 and 1940 showed Thimerosal to be among the most toxic to animal tissue of ten germicides tested.[612] [613]

Many other studies in this early era of Thimerosal's evaluation similarly suggested that the chemical may be more toxic to human tissue than to bacterial cells, as reviewed in a 1950 study by Frank Engley.[614] A 1956 study by the same author also concluded that "mercurial antiseptics proved to be more toxic than the antibiotics in common usage."[615] Engley also questioned Thimerosal's effectiveness, noting that myriad other studies dating back to the late 1800s had "shown that the antibacterial activity of mercurials is only slowly bactericidal [bacteria-killing] and mainly bacteriostatic [bacteria growth–inhibiting]." A 1948 study had found, for example, that Thimerosal is not "highly germicidal," as advertised, especially in the presence of the portion of blood known as serum.[616]

More recent studies have likewise graded Thimerosal's performance as a preservative as poor. A 1974 FDA panel that performed a comprehensive review of Thimerosal in over-the-counter products found it to be a weak antimicrobial that could cause cell damage when applied to broken skin or trigger an allergic response.[617] As a result of the panel's report, the FDA issued a proposed rule in 1982 to ban Thimerosal from over-the-counter topical products because they were not "generally recognized as safe and effective."[618]

A 1985 investigation provides an example of Thimerosal failing to preserve vaccine product. A streptococcus outbreak occurred in children after they received DTP vaccines, and the study reported that the bacteria survived fourteen days after inoculation in a multidose DTP vaccine vial. The study authors wrote that the "thimerosal preservative present in DTP vaccine requires substantial time to kill organisms and cannot be relied upon to prevent transmission of bacteria under conditions of practice when a vial is used over a short period."[619] A 1991 study used harsher language to describe Thimerosal, noting:

> Thimerosal is a weak antibacterial agent that is rapidly broken down to products, including ethylmercury residues, which are neurotoxic. Its role as a preservative in vaccines has been questioned, and the pharmaceutical industry itself considers its use as "historical."[620]

As previously discussed elsewhere in this document, although Thimerosal has been phased out of childhood vaccines, it is still used in flu vaccines.[621] A 2004 incident involving flu vaccine prepared with Thimerosal highlights the compound's ineffectiveness as a preservative. Chiron—a biotechnology company acquired by Novartis in 2006—produced forty-eight million doses, about half of the United States' flu vaccine for the 2004 to 2005 flu season.[622 623] In August 2004, Chiron announced that some vaccine lots made at a plant in Liverpool, United Kingdom, might not be sterile.[624] Regulatory authorities in Britain prohibited the use of vaccines from the plant, and a flu vaccine shortage ensued, in which thirty million fewer doses were available than were offered for the previous season. The bacteriological contamination of the vaccine stock by an organism known as *Serratia marcescens* should not have been possible if Thimerosal functioned as advertised, argued David Kirby, journalist and author of *Evidence of Harm: Mercury in Vaccines and the Autism Epidemic.*[625] [626] [627] [628]

We will now examine the issue of aluminum's use in Thimerosal-containing vaccines.

Notes

[610] Geier DA, Sykes LK, Geier MR. A review of Thimerosal (Merthiolate) and its ethylmercury breakdown product: specific historical considerations regarding safety and effectiveness. *J Toxicol Environ Health B Crit Rev.* 2007 Dec;10(8):575–96.

[611] Salle AJ, Lazarus AS. A comparison of the resistance of bacteria and embryonic tissue to germicidal substances. *Proc Soc Exp Biol Med.* 1935;32:665–667.

[612] Welch H. Mechanism of the toxic action of germicides on whole blood measured by the loss of phagocytic activity of leucocytes. *J. Immunol.* 1939; 37:525–533.

[613] Welch H, Hunter AC. Method for determining the effect of chemical antisepsis on phagocytosis. *Am J Public Health.* 1940; 30: 129-137.

[614] Engley FB. Evaluation of mercurial compounds as antiseptics. *Annal New York Acad Sci.* 1950, 53: 197–206.

[615] Engley FB. *Mercurials as Disinfectants: Evaluation of Mercurial Antimicrobic Action and Comparative Toxicity for Skin Tissue Cells.* Chicago: 42nd Mid-Year Meeting of the Chemical Specialties Manufacturer's Association. 1956 *as described in* Geier DA, Sykes LK, Geier MR 2007.

[616] Morton HE, North LL, Engley FB. Council of Pharmacy and Chemistry, the American Medical Association 1948 report: the bacteriostatic and bactericidal actions of some mercury compounds on hemolytic streptococci in vivo and in vitro studies. *JAMA.* 1948; 136(1): 36-41.

[617] United States. Mercury in medicine report. *Congressional Record.* Washington: GPO, May 21, 2003: 1011-1030.

[618] http://www.fda.gov/ohrms/dockets/98fr/042298a.pdf.

[619] Stetler HC, Garbe PL, Dwyer DM, Facklam RR, Orenstein WA, West GR, Dudley KJ, Bloch AB. Outbreaks of group A streptococcal abscesses following diphtheria-tetanus toxoid-pertussis vaccination. *Pediatrics.* 1985 Feb; 75(2): 299-303.

[620] Seal D, Ficker L, Wright P, Andrews V. The case against Thimerosal. *Lancet.* 1991; 338: 315-316.

[621] http://answers.flu.gov/questions/7082.

[622] http://www.hhs.gov/asl/testify/t041118c.html.

[623] Offit PA. Why are pharmaceutical companies gradually abandoning vaccines? *Health Aff (Millwood).* 2005 May-Jun;24(3):622-30.

[624] Danzon PM, Pereira NS, Tejwani SS. Vaccine supply: a cross-national perspective. *Health Aff (Millwood).* 2005 May-Jun;24(3):706-17.

[625] http://www.washingtonpost.com/wp-dyn/articles/A18795-2004Oct8.html.

[626] http://www.upi.com/Business_News/Security-Industry/2004/10/13/Commentary-Facing-the-flu-all-alone/UPI-97701097716817/.

[627] St. Martin's Press. *Flu Vaccination Shortage—Is Thimerosal to Blame?* Press release. October 7, 2004.

[628] http://www.nature.com/news/2004/041004/full/news041004-8.html.

Chapter 11:
Amplification of Thimerosal Toxicity by Aluminum in Vaccines

In addition to its questionable effectiveness, Thimerosal is also a very poor choice for vaccine preservation because its toxicity is thought to be compounded when used with aluminum, a common component of vaccines.

Aluminum has been added to vaccines as an "adjuvant" for more than seventy years. Adjuvants enhance the immune response to a vaccine, thus helping to generate stronger and longer-lasting immunity. In the United States, children typically receive aluminum-containing vaccines as part of their regular schedule in DTaP, Tdap, Hib, HepA, HepB, human papillomavirus (HPV), and pneumococcus vaccines.[629][630] Other vaccines using aluminum adjuvants include those for anthrax and rabies.[631]

Despite their widespread use, significant gaps exist in the basic knowledge of how aluminum adjuvants interact with the immune system. Although there is general acceptance that aluminum adjuvant is safe and effective in vaccines, more studies are needed to explicate its toxicology and pharmacology, particularly in infants and children.[632]

This relatively poor understanding is surprising given that aluminum is a known neurotoxin.[633] Mercury and aluminum share some common poisonous properties: Both elements have been shown to affect neurotransmitters, interfere with neuronal membranes, inhibit the formation of microtubules in nerve cells, increase oxidative stress in cells, damage mitochondria, possibly promote DNA damage by binding DNA, and serve as endocrine disruptors.[634 635 636 637 638 639 640 641 642 643 644 645]

Research has demonstrated links between several diseases involving the immune system and aluminum-adjuvanted vaccines. These diseases include Gulf War syndrome, chronic fatigue syndrome, macrophagic myofasciitis, and autism spectrum disorders.[646] In the case of Gulf War syndrome, Petrik 2007 demonstrated brain damage in mice given comparable injection levels of aluminum adjuvants to those of humans with the condition.[647] Macrophagic myofasciitis, meanwhile, is a condition that produces diffuse muscle weakness and pain. Patients with the condition show evidence of chronic overstimulation of their immune systems associated with the injection of aluminum adjuvants.[648] Immune cells called macrophages enter the muscle tissue in these patients at the site of the vaccine injection, as revealed by diagnostic biopsy.[649] Interestingly, aluminum adjuvant has been found in mouse studies to activate a type of macrophage cell in the brain called microglia.[650 651] Microglial activation is identified as a possible major cause of damage in numerous neurodegenerative illnesses, including Alzheimer's and Parkinson's, as well as neurodevelopmental disorders, including autism.[652 653 654 655 656 657]

Given a possible aluminum-autism connection, a 2011 study by Lucija Tomljenovic and Christopher Shaw took the crucial step of comparing the prevalence rates of autism to the levels of aluminum adjuvants administered to children in select countries. The study came to three important conclusions: One, children from countries that have the highest prevalence of autism spectrum disorders seem to have the highest exposure to aluminum via vaccines; two, the increase in exposure to aluminum in vaccines correlates significantly with the rise over the last two decades in the United States in autism spectrum disorders; and, three, there is a significant correlation between the amounts of aluminum administered to infants and young children and the current prevalence of autism spectrum disorders in seven Western countries.[658]

Tomljenovic and Shaw summarized research regarding aluminum toxicity to the central nervous system in 2013, and then later that year built on their epidemiological work with an animal model.[659] In a study, male and female mice were injected with high and low aluminum adjuvant levels, selected to correlate with the US and Scandinavian pediatric vaccine schedules, respectively. A control group received saline injections. In the high-aluminum-adjuvant, US group, male and female mice exhibited more anxiety-like behaviors than controls in a particular test; females in even the low-adjuvant, Scandinavian group also showed higher anxiety. In a separate test, high-adjuvant males demonstrated reduced exploratory tendencies, although females did not. The results suggested that aluminum exposure can produce changes in at least the murine central nervous system. The authors concluded about their preliminary study:

> Our current results are consistent with the existing evidence on the toxicology and pharmacokinetics of [aluminum] adjuvants which altogether strongly implicate these compounds as contributors to the rising prevalence of neurobehavioural disorders in children. Given that autism has devastating consequences in a life of a child, and that currently in the developed world over 1% of children suffer from some form of ASD, it would seem wise to make efforts towards reducing infant exposure to [aluminum] from vaccines.[660]

More evidence that the aluminum in some vaccines is working synergistically with Thimerosal in causing harm comes from a 2005 study by Haley. The research demonstrated that aluminum and Thimerosal together quickly ramp up the cell death of neurons in culture. After five hours, aluminum and Thimerosal separately led to the death of about 5 percent of neuronal cells. Aluminum and Thimerosal combined, however, killed about half the available cells in the same time period. Over twenty-four hours, aluminum by itself killed about 10 percent of the neurons in culture; Thimerosal, meanwhile, killed about 65 percent. When the two substances were again placed together, around 90 percent of the neuronal cells died.[661] In terms of basic chemical interactions, a 1972 case report indicated that aluminum and Thimerosal can also cause burns when placed together on skin.[662] And in a final item of interest for this chapter, a small study presented in 2012 showed that autistic children have higher-than-normal aluminum levels in their hair, blood, and/or urine.[663]

Clearly, more research would appear to be warranted on the possible neurotoxic effects of aluminum in vaccines, especially in the presence of Thimerosal.

Notes

[629] http://www.cdc.gov/vaccinesafety/Concerns/adjuvants.html.

[630] Lindblad, EB. Aluminium compounds for use in vaccines. *Immunology and Cell Biology.* 2004 Oct; 82(5): 497–505.

[631] Shingde M, Hughes J, Boadle R, Wills EJ, Pamphlett R. Macrophagic myofasciitis associated with vaccine-derived aluminium. *Med J Aust.* 2005 Aug 1;183(3):145-6.

[632] Eickhoff TC, Myers M. Workshop summary. Aluminum in vaccines. *Vaccine.* 2002 May 31;20 Suppl 3:S1-4.

[633] Keith LS, Jones DE, Chou CH. Aluminum toxicokinetics regarding infant diet and vaccinations. *Vaccine.* 2002 May 31;20 Suppl 3:S13-7.

[634] Sanfeliu C, Sebastià J, Cristòfol R, Rodríguez-Farré E. Neurotoxicity of organomercurial compounds. *Neurotox Res.* 2003;5(4):283-305.

[635] Verstraeten SV, Aimo L, Oteiza PI. Aluminium and lead: molecular mechanisms of brain toxicity. *Arch Toxicol.* 2008 Nov;82(11):789-802. Epub 2008 Jul 31.

[636] Walum E, Marchner H. Effects of mercuric chloride on the membrane integrity of cultured cell lines. *Toxicol Lett.* 1983 Aug;18(1-2):89-95.

[637] Keith LS, Jones DE, Chou CH. Aluminum toxicokinetics regarding infant diet and vaccinations. *Vaccine.* 2002 May 31;20 Suppl 3:S13-7.

[638] Kumar V, Gill KD. Aluminium neurotoxicity: neurobehavioural and oxidative aspects. *Arch Toxicol.* 2009 Nov;83(11):965-78. Epub 2009 Jul 1.

[639] Sharpe MA, Livingston AD, Baskin DS. Thimerosal-derived ethylmercury is a mitochondrial toxin in human astrocytes: possible role of Fenton chemistry in the oxidation and breakage of mtDNA. *J Toxicol.* 2012;2012:373678. doi: 10.1155/2012/373678. Epub 2012 Jun 28.

[640] Crespo-López ME, Macêdo GL, Pereira SI, Arrifano GP, Picanço-Diniz DL, do Nascimento JL, Herculano AM. Mercury and human genotoxicity: critical considerations and possible molecular mechanisms. *Pharmacol Res.* 2009 Oct;60(4):212-20. Epub 2009 Mar 9.

[641] Tan SW, Meiller JC, Mahaffey KR. The endocrine effects of mercury in humans and wildlife. *Crit Rev Toxicol.* 2009;39(3):228-69. doi: 10.1080/10408440802233259.

[642] Hamza H, Cao J, Li X, Li C, Zhu M, Zhao S. Hepatitis B vaccine induces apoptotic death in Hepa1-6 cells. *Apoptosis.* 2012 May;17(5):516-27. doi: 10.1007/s10495-011-0690-1.

[643] Gump BB, MacKenzie JA, Dumas AK, Palmer CD, Parsons PJ, Segu ZM, Mechref YS, Bendinskas KG. Fish consumption, low-level mercury, lipids, and inflammatory markers

in children. *Environ Res.* 2012 Jan;112:204-11. doi: 10.1016/j.envres.2011.10.002. Epub 2011 Oct 24.

[644] Guo C, Huang C, Chen S, Wang Hsu G. Serum and testicular testosterone and nitric oxide products in aluminum-treated mice. *Environ Toxicol Pharmacol.* 2001 Jun;10(1-2):53-60.

[645] http://www.pca.state.mn.us/index.php/view-document.html?gid=3892.

[646] Tomljenovic L, Shaw CA. Do aluminum vaccine adjuvants contribute to the rising prevalence of autism? *J Inorg Biochem.* 2011 Nov;105(11):1489-99.

[647] Petrik MS, Wong MC, Tabata RC, Garry RF, Shaw CA. Aluminum adjuvant linked to Gulf War illness induces motor neuron death in mice. *Neuromolecular Med.* 2007;9(1):83-100.

[648] Gherardi R. Lessons from macrophagic myofasciitis: towards definition of a vaccine adjuvant-related syndrome. *Rev Neurol (Paris).* 2003; 159: 162-164.

[649] Shoenfeld Y, Agmon-Levin N. "ASIA"—autoimmune/inflammatory syndrome induced by adjuvants. *J Autoimmun.* 2011 Feb;36(1):4-8.

[650] Tomljenovic L, Shaw CA. Do aluminum vaccine adjuvants contribute to the rising prevalence of autism? *J Inorg Biochem.* 2011 Nov;105(11):1489-99.

[651] Rock RB, Gekker G, Hu S, Sheng WS, Cheeran M, Lokensgard JR, Peterson PK. Role of microglia in central nervous system infections. *Clin Microbiol Rev.* 2004 Oct;17(4):942-64, table of contents.

[652] Blaylock R. Interactions of cytokines, excitotoxins, and reactive nitrogen and oxygen species in autism spectrum disorders. *J Amer Nutr Assoc.* 2003; 6: 21-35.

[653] Blaylock R. The central role of excitotoxins in autism spectrum disorders. *J Amer Nutr Assoc.* 2003; 6: 7-19.

[654] Blaylock R. Chronic microglial activation and excitotoxicity secondary to excessive immune stimulation: possible factors in Gulf War Syndrome and autism. *J Amer Phys Surg.* 2004; 9: 46-51.

[655] Morgan JT, Chana G, Pardo CA, Achim C, Semendeferi K, Buckwalter J, Courchesne E, Everall IP. Microglial activation and increased microglial density observed in the dorsolateral prefrontal cortex in autism. *Biol Psychiatry.* 2010 Aug 15;68(4):368-76.

[656] Badoer E. Microglia: activation in acute and chronic inflammatory states and in response to cardiovascular dysfunction. *Int J Biochem Cell Biol.* 2010 Oct;42(10):1580-5. Epub 2010 Jul 16.

[657] Vargas DL, Nascimbene C, Krishnan C, Zimmerman AW, Pardo CA. Neuroglial activation and neuroinflammation in the brain of patients with autism. *Ann Neurol.* 2005 Jan;57(1):67-81.

[658] Tomljenovic L, Shaw CA. Do aluminum vaccine adjuvants contribute to the rising prevalence of autism? *J Inorg Biochem.* 2011 Nov;105(11):1489-99.

[659] Shaw CA, Tomljenovic L. Aluminum in the central nervous system (CNS): toxicity in humans and animals, vaccine adjuvants, and autoimmunity. *Immunol Res.* 2013 Jul;56(2-3):304-16. doi: 10.1007/s12026-013-8403-1.

[660] Shaw CA, Li Y, Tomljenovic L. Administration of aluminium to neonatal mice in vaccine-relevant amounts is associated with adverse long term neurological outcomes. *J Inorg Biochem.* 2013 Nov;128:237-44. doi: 10.1016/j.jinorgbio.2013.07.022. Epub 2013 Jul 19.

661 M.M. Lopes, L.Q.A. Caldas. Young children with autism spectrum disorders: Can aluminium body-burden cause metabolism disruption? *Toxicology Letters Volume 205, Supplement.* 28 August 2011, Pages S92.

662 Haley BE. Mercury toxicity: Genetic susceptibility and synergistic effects. *Med Veritas.* 2005; 2: 535-542.

663 Jones HT. Danger of skin burns from thimerosal. *BMJ.* 1972; 2: 504-505.

Chapter 12: Safer and Cost-Effective Alternatives to Thimerosal

On top of its questionable effectiveness and possibly dangerous interactions with aluminum, Thimerosal can also be replaced in vaccines with safer, better alternatives. Vaccines should not contain toxic additives as preservatives at all. Nevertheless, it is worth noting that vaccine manufacturers have developed preservatives with far fewer toxicity concerns than Thimerosal.

One of these, 2-phenoxyethanol (2-PE), is already being used as a preservative in the polio vaccine Ipol.[664] It is also present at nonpreservative levels in the DTaP vaccine Daptacel, the DTaP-IPV/Hib vaccine Pentacel, and the Tdap vaccine Adacel.[665 666 667 668]

A 2010 study showed that 2-PE is about seventy times less toxic than Thimerosal to human cells, compared to bacterial cells, when tested at levels similar to vaccine-preservative levels.[669] A joint report issued that same year by a group of researchers at Pfizer found that "Thimerosal is not an effective preservative compared to 2-PE." The report, later published in *Vaccine*, further commented that "the data support the use of 2-PE as a more effective preservative with the potential to replace thimerosal, the most commonly used preservative in multidose vaccine formulations."[670]

The chief reason for preservatives in vaccines is to protect against the growth of microbes that could get into multidose vaccine vials when a needle is inserted into the vial to withdraw a vaccine dose.[671][672] Making vaccines single-dose rather than multidose would eliminate the need for a preservative, such as 2-PE or Thimerosal.[673]

Manufacturing multidose vaccine vials, however, is less expensive than manufacturing single-use vaccine vials. Further cost-effectiveness of multidose vials arises because they use less packaging and take up less cold-storage space than do single dose vials.[674] Neal Halsey of the Johns Hopkins Bloomberg School of Public Health and Institute for Vaccine Safety, and Paul Offit of the Children's Hospital of Philadelphia, said that single-dose vaccines cost five to ten times the price of the multidose inoculations.[675][676][677][678]

Advocates for the continued use of Thimerosal point to this cost argument. The World Health Organization (WHO), for example, has long held that switching to single-dose vials could raise the costs of immunization programs in developing countries, thus jeopardizing the organization's international vaccine efforts.[679][680][681][682] Ahead of the January 2013 negotiations over a multilateral environmental treaty backed by the United Nations Environment Programme (UNEP) aiming to restrict human and environmental mercury exposure, the WHO prepared a new impact assessment of Thimerosal removal from vaccines. The analysis was based on a survey of manufacturers, data from selected countries, and modeling based on procurement patterns by the United Nations Children's Fund (UNICEF) and the Pan American Health Organization (PAHO). The assessment claimed that switching to single-dose from multidose vials would raise annual costs to UNICEF or PAHO by $300 million, per increased costs in manufacturing, shipping, cold-chain storage, administration, and waste-handling infrastructure.[683 684]

While those costs are inarguably high, the societal costs of potentially poisoning generations of children in developing countries with mercury could be far greater. In March 2012, a study by Autism Speaks—with guidance and technical assistance from WHO—estimated the annual economic costs in just the United States, and from autism alone, to be a staggering $137 billion. The study, presented at an international conference in Hong Kong in collaboration with Goldman Sachs and the Child Development Centre of Hong Kong, took into account such factors as lost family income and productivity as well as the direct costs of autism-associated care.[685 686 687]

Furthermore, single-dose vaccines might ultimately be more cost-effective than multidose vials in some cases. A comprehensive analysis in 2003 of the pricing issue by a team of researchers at the Program for Appropriate Technology in Health (PATH), a nonprofit organization based in Seattle, bears this out. The per-dose production cost of the most common size multidose vial, the ten-dose vial, is around $0.10, compared to $0.25 for a single-dose vial, according to figures compiled by PATH at the time. The study posits that single-dose vials may make more economic sense, particularly for expensive vaccines, because they lead to less vaccine wastage; historically, the rate of wastage of ten-dose vials has been as high as 60 percent. To avoid having to waste leftover vaccine solution, health care workers have also shown reluctance in opening a multidose vial for vaccinating only one or two children, the PATH report noted. Single-dose vials would prevent this gap in coverage. The single-dose format offers the other important benefit of reducing contamination risk.[688] Other studies have since further explored the cost-benefit analysis of single-dose versus multidose vaccines, similarly supporting an approach that gauges the optimal number of doses per vial based on the type of vaccine, geographical considerations, and patient demand.[689]

In conclusion, better preservatives and wiser deployment of single-use vaccine vials over multidose vials could significantly reduce exposure to the mercury in Thimerosal worldwide.

Notes

[664] http://www.fda.gov/downloads/BiologicsBloodVaccines/Vaccines/ApprovedProducts/UCM133479.pdf.

[665] http://www.cdc.gov/vaccines/pubs/pinkbook/downloads/appendices/b/excipient-table-2.pdf.

[666] http://www.drugs.com/pro/daptacel.html.

[667] http://dailymed.nlm.nih.gov/dailymed/about.cfm.

[668] http://www.fda.gov/BiologicsBloodVaccines/SafetyAvailability/VaccineSafety/UCM096228.

[669] Geier DA, Jordan SK, Geier MR. The relative toxicity of compounds used as preservatives in vaccines and biologics. *Med Sci Monit.* 2010 May;16(5):SR21-7.

[670] Khandke L, Yang C, Fan J, Han H, Rashidbaigi KKA, Green BA, Jansen KU. *Development of a Multidose for Prevnar 13™. Vaccine Technology III.* John G. Auniņš, Barry C. Buckland, Kathrin U. Jansen, Paula Marques Alves, eds., ECI Symposium Series, Volume P13. 2010.

[671] Khandke L, Yang C, Krylova K, Jansen KU, Rashidbaigi A. Preservative of choice for Prev(e)nar 13™ in a multidose formulation. *Vaccine.* 2011 Sep 22;29(41):7144-53. doi: 10.1016/j.vaccine.2011.05.074. Epub 2011 Jun 7.

[672] http://www.cdc.gov/injectionsafety/providers/provider_faqs_multivials.html.

[673] Lee BY, Norman BA, Assi TM, Chen SI, Bailey RR, Rajgopal J, Brown ST, Wiringa AE, Burke DS. Single versus multidose vaccine vials: an economic computational model. *Vaccine.* 2010 Jul 19;28(32):5292-300. Epub 2010 Jun 3.

[674] http://www.fda.gov/BiologicsBloodVaccines/Vaccines/QuestionsaboutVaccines/ucm070430.htm.

[675] Drain PK, Nelson CM, Lloyd JS. Single dose versus multidose vaccine vials for immunization programmes in developing countries. *Bull World Health Organ.* 2003;81(10):726-31. Epub 2003 Nov 25.

[676] http://www.jhsph.edu/faculty/directory/profile/934/Halsey/Neal.

[677] http://www.chop.edu/doctors/offit-paul-a.html.

[678] Robert F. Kennedy, Jr., telephone interview with Neal Halsey, May 2005.

[679] Robert F. Kennedy, Jr., telephone interview with Paul Offit, May 4, 2005.

[680] http://www.who.int/vaccines-documents/DocsPDF03/www720.pdf.

[681] Bigham M, Copes R. Thiomersal in vaccines: balancing the risk of adverse effects with the risk of vaccine-preventable disease. *Drug Saf.* 2005;28(2):89-101.

[682] http://www.who.int/vaccine_safety/topics/thiomersal/Jun_2012/en/index.html.

[683] King K, Paterson M, Green SK. Global justice and the proposed ban on thimerosal-containing vaccines. *Pediatrics.* 2013 Jan;131(1):154-6. doi: 10.1542/peds.2012-2976. Epub 2012 Dec 17.

[684] http://www.who.int/immunization_delivery/systems_policy/IPAC_2012_April_report.pdf.

[685] http://www.autismspeaks.org/science/science-news/%E2%80%98costs-autism%-E2%80%99-summit.

[686] http://www.autismspeaks.org/science/science-news/autism%E2%80%99s-costs-nation-reach-137-billion-year.

[687] http://www.cdc.gov/media/releases/2012/t0329_Autism_Telebriefing.html.

[688] Drain PK., Nelson CM, Lloyd JS. Single dose versus multidose vaccine vials for immunization programmes in developing countries. *Bull World Health Organ.* 2003;81(10):726-31. Epub 2003 Nov 25.

[689] Lee BY, Norman BA, Assi TM, Chen SI, Bailey RR, Rajgopal J, Brown ST, Wiringa AE, Burke DS. Single versus multidose vaccine vials: an economic computational model. *Vaccine.* 2010 Jul 19;28(32):5292-300. doi: 10.1016/j.vaccine.2010.05.048. Epub 2010 Jun 3.

PART THREE:

THIMEROSAL AND AUTISM

Author's Note: Part One of this book addressed the scientific evidence supporting the link between Thimerosal exposure and neurological damage. Part Two then indicated Thimerosal's questionable efficacy and how it could be replaced or completely phased out of the vaccine supply. I believe that this information alone is sufficient to warrant an immediate removal of Thimerosal from vaccines. Because it is a thorny and controversial issue that provokes fierce reactions on both sides, I initially considered leaving any discussion of the Thimerosal-autism debate out of the book altogether. In the end, however, it became clear that, given the weight of scientific evidence suggesting a link between Thimerosal exposure and autism, no discussion of Thimerosal could be considered complete without including a review of this material. I elected to isolate the review of this research under a separate heading, Part Three, in order to avoid the conflations between these two separate but interlinked topics of neurological damage in general, and autism in particular. This sort of conflation has been a hallmark of a hitherto confusing debate.

Chapter 13:
Is the Autism
Epidemic Real?

Autism is a "new" disorder, having only been definitively described and named in the 20th century. In 1943, the first known cases of autism were documented by Leo Kanner in children born in the very years, as it happens, after Eli Lilly began marketing Thimerosal for vaccines and other products in the 1930s.[690][691][692] Kanner, who was one of the fathers of American childhood psychiatry, remarked

---

The Three Main Types of Autism Spectrum Disorder
according to the *Diagnostic and Statistical Manual of Mental Disorders,* Fourth Edition (DSM-IV).

Autistic Disorder	Asperger Syndrome	Pervasive Developmental Disorder—Not Otherwise Specified (PDD-NOS)
Also known as "classic autism" or simply "autism," this is the most common and severe form of the spectrum disorder. People with Autistic Disorder usually have significant language delays, social and communication challenges, unusual repetitive behaviors, and restricted interests. Many people with autistic disorder also have intellectual disability.	Also known as "high-functioning autism," Asperger Syndrome is a milder form of Autistic Disorder. Symptoms include social interaction difficulties and unusual behaviors and interests. People with Asperger Syndrome typically do not have problems with language or intellectual disability.	Also called "atypical autism," PDD-NOS is a diagnosis for people who meet some but not all of the criteria for Autistic Disorder or Asperger Syndrome. As with Asperger Syndrome, those with PDD-NOS usually have fewer and milder symptoms than those with Autistic Disorder. The symptoms might cause only social and communication challenges. Note that the term "Pervasive Developmental Disorder" can be used interchangeably with "Autism Spectrum Disorder."

FIGURE 11

some years later on the disorder as "a behavior pattern not known to me or anyone else theretofore."[693] [694]

Since the coining of the term "autism" seventy years ago, cases of the condition have surged worldwide, and markedly so in about the last twenty-five years. When researchers conducted the first surveys of autism prevalence in the mid-1960s through the 1980s, results indicated that around 1 in 2,500 children had autism. That figure rose dramatically from 1 in 333 to 1 in 166 in studies conducted in the late 1990s and early 2000s.[695] [696] [697] [698] [699] [700] A 2012 review study of worldwide prevalence rates for autism spectrum disorders (ASDs) found an estimated median global prevalence in remarkable agreement with the higher figure.[701] A report in California documented the rapid increase in that state alone since the 1980s, noting as of 2003 that "autism, once a rare disorder, is now more prevalent than childhood cancer, diabetes and Down Syndrome."[702] In reports issued over the last several years, the rate of the late 1990s and early 2000s had soared still higher, with a CDC survey of parents published in 2013 estimating the US ASD rate (assessed in 2011 to 2012) at 1 in every 50 children (and 1 in 31 boys), and in 2014 the agency reported a more reliable, though still alarming ASD prevalence of 1 in 68 children aged eight years as of 2010.[703] [704] [705]

To date, doctors can tie only around 15 to 20 percent of autism cases to a metabolic disease, a genetic syndrome, specific mutations, or an environmental agent.[706] [707] Isolated genetic mutations over one or two human generations—and across multiple countries—are considered extremely unlikely as the source of autism's rise.[708]

A major debate has centered, then, on whether the skyrocketing prevalence of autism is a possible artifact of expanded diagnostic criteria coupled with increased parental and clinical awareness of the malady.[709] On its face, this contention seems unlikely, as it assumes doctors and parents several decades ago did not notice the sheer number of people with autism in the population as is apparent nowadays. In a 2000 journal editorial, the late Bernard Rimland, founder of the Autism Research Institute and a pioneer in the field, recalled the infrequency of the disorder earlier in his career:[710][711]

> I saw the word autism for the first time in the spring of 1958, five years after I had earned my PhD in psychology. My wife and I had taken our implacable, screaming newborn son to our pediatrician two years earlier. Dr. Black had been in practice for 35 years and had never seen a child like Mark. Nor had any other physician we consulted. When Mark was two years old, his strange, aloof, ritualistic behavior reminded my wife of a child she had read about in an old college textbook. There, in that textbook, I first saw the word "autism."
>
> William Crook of Tennessee, a pediatrician who had received his medical training in the 1940s at Johns Hopkins, where Leo Kanner taught, became intrigued by autism and actively sought such cases by letting his pediatric colleagues throughout the South know of his special interest. It was not until 1973, 24 years after starting his practice, that he had his first autistic patient. Then came more. "I am absolutely certain that there is a huge increase in autism," Dr. Crook told me. I have heard similar tales from many physicians as well as special education teachers and school administrators whose experience dates back to the early 1970s and before. Autism was truly rare in those days.[712]

Boyd Haley, the retired chairman of the chemistry department at the University of Kentucky, of whom we first learned in Part One, put it more simply to us in an interview. Haley said, "Missing autism is like missing a train wreck."[713]

Diagnostic criteria for autism spectrum disorders did become more expansive, both in 1987 and then again in 1994 with the publication of the third (revised) and fourth editions of the *Diagnostic and Statistical Manual of Mental Disorders* (DSM), the American Psychiatric Association's (APA) widely used guide for diagnosing mental illness.[714][715]

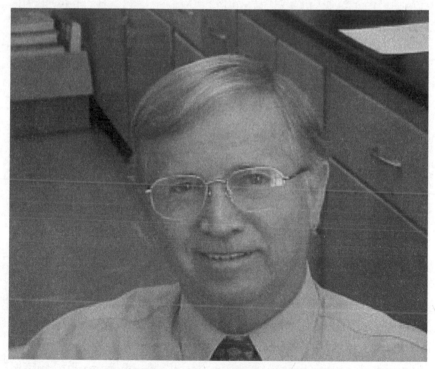

Boyd Haley. Credit: University of Kentucky,
http://www.chem.uky.edu/research/haley/

(A fifth DSM edition, with further changes to how autism spectrum disorders are diagnosed, published in May 2013.[716] Significantly, the four-category system of DSM-IV [also including the rarely diagnosed childhood disintegrative disorder] was condensed to an umbrella diagnostic categorical term of "autism spectrum disorder." As most of the research cited in this book dates from the DSM-IV era, the three main categories of autism spectrum disorder recognized then will appear often. It is not yet clear if autism prevalence will rise or fall as a result of the DSM-5 changes [which also extend to dispensing with Roman numerals in the edition numbering]. But a 2012 study by Marisela Huerta suggests the changes will not be significant, according to the APA.)[717] [718]

A recent study from researchers at Columbia University has shown that the shift in diagnostic criteria in 1987 and 1994 can account for only about a quarter of the increased caseload seen over time. The study's authors looked at a population of children in California diagnosed with an autism spectrum disorder between 1992 and 2005 and found that a substantial number of cases previously classified as mental retardation now fell under the definition of autism.[719] Even so, a wide gap in the expected number of autism cases over time remains. As Haley asked, "If the change is just diagnostic, then where are all the 30-year-old people with autism?"[720]

Social factors can help explain some of the remaining disparity. In a 2010 study, the same research team from Columbia demonstrated that 16 percent of the rise in the autism caseload in California between 2000 and 2005 could be chalked up to parents' increased awareness of the disorder. The study found that children living in close proximity to those already diagnosed with autism had significantly greater odds of being diagnosed with the illness themselves. The researchers offered that communication between parents about autism in neighborhoods is a possible explanation for this prevalence clustering.[721]

A third factor often cited for why autism rates might have gone up is an increase in the average age of parents compared to decades past.[722] Various childhood developmental disorders are associated with advanced parental age, and studies have noted a similar link for autism.[723 724 725 726]

Altogether, the ongoing Columbia research suggests that around half of the rise in autism's prevalence can be attributed to diagnostic, social, and demographic changes and influences.[727] That leaves an additional half for which an environmental trigger of some sort stands as a highly plausible causative agent.

Other studies support that an epidemic of autism in recent decades is in fact real. For example, in California, the Department of Developmental Services experienced an increase of 273 percent in reported cases of autism between 1987 and 1998.[728] The California state legislature responded by commissioning the University of California's Medical Investigation of Neurodevelopmental Disorders (MIND) Institute to conduct a comprehensive study to determine the reason for this increase. That study did not find evidence that the observed increase could be explained by changing diagnostic criteria, misclassification, or migration of children with autism into California.[729]

A 2009 study expanded on the California work and looked at autism cases per year (incidence) from 1990 to 2006. Incidence shot up 700 to 800 percent over this period. The authors concluded that changes in diagnostic criteria (as described a few paragraphs prior), the inclusion of milder cases, and an earlier age at diagnosis could explain only 120, 56, and 24 percent, respectively, of the caseload spike.[730] "These are fairly small percentages compared to the size of the increase that we've seen in the state," lead author and UC Davis MIND researcher Irva Hertz-Picciotto said in a statement at the time. "It's time to start looking for the environmental culprits responsible for the remarkable increase in the rate of autism in California."[731]

As a further example, a study of children in Olmsted County, Minnesota, also offered no evidence of diagnostic substitution behind autism rates rising since the early 1980s.[732] In a 2004 review article citing more than fifty studies on estimates of the frequency of autism, Mark Blaxill also found that the large increases in prevalence cannot be chalked up merely to changes in diagnostic criteria or improvements in case ascertainment.[733]

A 2005 study by Craig Newschaffer also strongly discounted diagnostic substitution. The study looked at all US children six to seventeen years of age between 1992 and 2001 in various disability category classifications as documented by state departments of education and reported to the federal Department of Education. Newschaffer found:

> The [autism] increases were greatest for annual cohorts born from 1987 to 1992. For cohorts born after 1992, the prevalence increased with each successive year but the increases did not appear to be as great, although there were fewer data points available within cohorts. No concomitant decreases in categories of mental retardation or speech/language impairment were seen.[734]

The US Department of Education's Office of Special Education Programs (OSEP) statistics on which Newschaffer relied document a steep rise in autism cases. In 1992, OSEP first began collecting autism statistics from the states on the number of students identified as having autism and receiving special education and related services under the Individuals with Disabilities Education Act (IDEA). That year, there were 5,208 students ages six through twenty-one reported to have autism nationwide. As recorded in a recent 2009 report, by 2004, the number had jumped to 166,424.[735]

In a 2000 editorial, the late Bernard Rimland spoke bluntly about the debate over autism's rise, even before some of the findings described above were reached:

> While there are a few Flat-Earthers who insist that there is no real epidemic of autism, only an increased awareness, it is obvious to everyone else that the number of young children with autism spectrum disorders (ASD) has risen, and continues to rise, dramatically.[736]

Researchers for pharmaceutical giant Eli Lilly, the company that introduced Thimerosal in the 1930s, have additionally confirmed that the increase in prevalence of autism is genuine and cannot be attributed to diagnostic criteria or misclassification.[737][738] They suggest that some environmental cause is partly responsible for the epidemic.[739][740]

The coincidence in the rise of autism cases alongside an increase in the number of pediatric vaccines administered and total exposure to Thimerosal makes Thimerosal causation an attractive, if speculative, hypothesis. Moreover, as the number of administered vaccines rose after 1989 and on through the 1990s, so did a previously little-seen pattern of autism onset called regressive autism.[741] In regressive autism, children developing normally over their first year or two suddenly become autistic, losing language and social skills they had previously acquired.[742] A 2005 study objectively validated the phenomenon of regressive autism by reviewing home videotapes of children's birthdays, documenting greater attention and use of vocalizations at twelve months compared to typical children or early onset cases of autism.[743] Many published case reports of patients have described developmental regressions with autism symptoms following fetal or early childhood mercury exposure.[744 745 746]

Although studies have differed on the percentage of cases that can be categorized as regressive, owing largely to how regression is defined and reported, some researchers argue that the rise has been sharp. Data collected since 1965 by the Autism Research Institute indicate that the onset of autism at eighteen months, rather than closer to birth, is a recent development.[747] According to Rimland, writing in 2003, "Late onset autism, (starting in the 2nd year), was almost unheard of in the '50s, '60s, and '70s; today such cases outnumber early onset cases 5 to 1, the increase paralleling the increase in required vaccines."[748] This changeover, some have suggested, implies that regressive autism cannot be attributed to genetics, but rather is an acquired condition.[749 750]

In the next few chapters, this book will review the striking similarities between mercury poisoning and autism. This observation provides a basis in part for the epidemiological literature that has shown a correlation between the spike in autism cases and the increased use of vaccines preserved with mercury-containing

Thimerosal. As shown thereafter, several studies have indicated that children with an autism spectrum disorder diagnosis have higher levels of mercury body burden relative to other, healthy children. Furthermore, the neurological damage caused by mercury is consistent with the abnormalities found in the brains of children diagnosed with an autism spectrum disorder. Mercury, research suggests, not only directly kills brain cells but also disrupts the critical mechanisms and pathways needed to eliminate it from the brain, thus exacerbating its poisonous impact.

Notes

[690] Marshall MS. The Merthiolate—a new antiseptic. *Cal West Med*. 1931 Jul;35(1):43–44.

[691] Baker JP. Mercury, vaccines, and autism: one controversy, three histories. *Am J. Public Health*. 2008; 98:244–253.

[692] Kanner L. Autistic disturbances of affective contact. *Nerv Child*. 1943;2:217-250.

[693] Eisenberg L, Leo Kanner, 1894-1981. *Am J Psychiatry*. 1981 August;138(8):1122-5.

[694] Citations Classics, Kanner Letter written in 1978 and published 1979, http://garfield.library. upenn.edu/classics.html; http://garfield.library.upenn.edu/classics1979/A1979HZ31800001. pdf.

[695] Ritvo ER, Freeman BJ, Pingree C, Mason-Brothers A, Jorde L, Jenson WR, McMahon WM, Petersen PB, Mo A, Ritvo A. The UCLA-University of Utah epidemiologic survey of autism: prevalence. *Am J Psychiatry*. 1989 Feb;146(2):194-9.

[696] Fombonne E. The epidemiology of autism: a review. *Psychol Med*. 1999 Jul;29(4):769-86.

[697] Rimland B. The Autism epidemic, vaccinations, and mercury. *J Nut Environ Med*. 2000; 10: 261-6.

[698] Rutter M. Incidence of autism spectrum disorders: Changes over time and their meaning. *Acta Paediatr*. 2005 Jan;94(1):2-15.

[699] Newschaffer CJ, Falb MD, Gurney JG. National autism prevalence trends from United States Special Education Data. *Pediatrics*. 2005 Mar; 115(3): e277-e282.

[700] Fombonne, E. Epidemiology of pervasive developmental disorders. *Pediatr Res*. 2009 Jun; 65(6): 591-598.

[701] Elsabbagh M, Divan G, Koh YJ, Kim YS, Kauchali S, Marcín C, Montiel-Nava C, Patel V, Paula CS, Wang C, Yasamy MT, Fombonne E. Global prevalence of autism and other pervasive developmental disorders. *Autism Res*. 2012 Jun;5(3):160-79. doi: 10.1002/aur.239. Epub 2012 Apr 11.

[702] California Department of Developmental Services. *Autistic Spectrum Disorders—Changes in the California Caseload—An Update: 1999 through 2002*. Sacramento, CA: State of California; 2003.

[703] http://www.cdc.gov/media/releases/2013/a0320_autism_disorder.html.

[704] http://www.cdc.gov/nchs/data/nhsr/nhsr065.pdf.

[705] http://www.cdc.gov/mmwr/preview/mmwrhtml/ss6302a1.htm?s_cid=ss6302a1_w.

[706] http://www.genome.gov/25522099.

[707] Benvenuto A, Manzi B, Alessandrelli R, Galasso C, Curatolo P. Recent advances in the pathogenesis of syndromic autisms. *Int J Pediatr.* 2009;2009:198736. Epub 2009 Jun 21.

[708] Liu K, Zerubavel N, Bearman P. Social demographic change and autism. *Demography.* 2010 May;47(2):327-43.

[709] Fombonne E. Epidemiology of autism. Elsabbagh M, Clarke ME, topic eds. In: Tremblay RE, Boivin M, Peters RDeV, eds. *Encyclopedia on Early Childhood Development [online].* Montreal, Quebec: Centre of Excellence for Early Childhood Development and Strategic Knowledge Cluster on Early Child Development; 2012:1-5.

[710] http://www.autism.com/index.php/about_rimland.

[711] http://select.nytimes.com/gst/abstract.html?res=F4091EF93B5A0C7B8ED-DA80994DE404482.

[712] Rimland B. The Autism epidemic, vaccinations, and mercury. *J Nut Environ Med.* 2000; 10: 261-6.

[713] Robert F. Kennedy, Jr., telephone interview with Boyd Haley, May 5, 2005.

[714] Miller JS, Bilder D, Farley M, Coon H, Pinborough-Zimmerman J, Jenson W, Rice CE, Fombonne E, Pingree CB, Ritvo E, Ritvo RA, McMahon WM. Autism spectrum disorder reclassified: a second look at the 1980s Utah/UCLA autism epidemiologic study. *J Autism Dev Disord.* 2012 Jun 13. [Epub ahead of print].

[715] http://www.psychiatry.org/practice/dsm/dsm-history-of-the-manual.

[716] http://www.dsm5.org/Pages/Default.aspx.

[717] http://www.dsm5.org/Documents/Autism%20Spectrum%20Disorder%20Fact%20Sheet.pdf.

[718] Huerta M, Bishop SL, Duncan A, Hus V, Lord C. Application of DSM-5 criteria for autism spectrum disorder to three samples of children with DSM-IV diagnoses of pervasive developmental disorders. *Am J Psychiatry.* 2012 Oct;169(10):1056-64. doi: 10.1176/appi.ajp.2012.12020276.

[719] King M, Bearman P. Diagnostic change and increased prevalence of autism. *Int J Epidemiol.* 2009 Oct;38(5):1224-34. Epub 2009 Sep 7.

[720] Robert F. Kennedy, Jr., telephone interview with Boyd Haley, May 5, 2005.

[721] Liu KY, King M, Bearman P. Social influence and the autism epidemic. *AJS.* 2010 Mar;115(5):1387-434.

[722] Child Trends; Halle, Tamara. *Charting Parenthood: A Statistical Portrait of Fathers and Mothers in America,* 2002. http://fatherhood.hhs.gov/charting02/.

[723] Grether JK, Anderson MC, Croen LA, Smith D, Windham GC. Risk of autism and increasing maternal and paternal age in a large North American population. *Am J Epidemiol.* 2009 Nov 1;170(9):1118-26. Epub 2009 Sep 25.

[724] King MD, Fountain C, Dakhlallah D, Bearman PS. Estimated autism risk and older reproductive age. *Am J Public Health.* 2009 Sep;99(9):1673-9. Epub 2009 Jul 16.

[725] Kong A, Frigge ML, Masson G, Besenbacher S, Sulem P, Magnusson G, Gudjonsson SA, Sigurdsson A, Jonasdottir A, Jonasdottir A, Wong WS, Sigurdsson G, Walters GB, Steinberg S, Helgason H, Thorleifsson G, Gudbjartsson DF, Helgason A, Magnusson OT, Thorsteinsdottir U, Stefansson K. Rate of de novo mutations and the importance of father's age to disease risk. *Nature*. 2012 Aug 23;488(7412):471-5.

[726] Liu K, Zerubavel N, Bearman P. Social demographic change and autism. *Demography*. 2010 May;47(2):327-43.

[727] http://understandingautism.columbia.edu/about.html.

[728] California Department of Developmental Services. *Autistic Spectrum Disorders—Changes in the California Caseload—An Update: 1999 through 2002*. Sacramento, CA: State of California; 2003.

[729] Byrd RS, Sage AC, Keyzer J, Shefelbine R, Gee K, Enders K, Neufeld J, Do N, Heung K, Hughes T, Baron R, Moore A, Walbridge B, Samuels S, Tancredi D, He J, Calvert E, Elsdon A, Lee L, Wong D, Sigman M, Bono M, Beck C, Clavell S, Lizaola E, Meyerkova V. *Report to the Legislature on the Principal Findings from The Epidemiology of Autism in California: A Comprehensive Pilot Study*. 2002 Oct 17 http://www.feat.org/LinkClick.aspx?fileticket=R-RD%2FsTcWUmc%3D&tabid=78&mid=583.

[730] Hertz-Picciotto I, Delwiche L. The rise in autism and the role of age at diagnosis. *Epidemiology*. 2009 Jan;20(1):84-90.

[731] http://www.ucdmc.ucdavis.edu/welcome/features/20090218_autism_environment/index.html.

[732] Gurney JG, Fritz MS, Ness KK, Sievers P, Newschaffer CJ, Shapiro EG. Analysis of prevalence trends of autism spectrum disorder in Minnesota. *Arch Pediatr Adolesc Med*. 2003 Jul; 157: 622-7.

[733] Blaxill M. What's going on? The question of time trends in autism. *Public Health Rep*. 2004; 119: 536-51.

[734] Newschaffer CJ, Falb MD, Gurney JG. National autism prevalence trends from United States special education data. *Pediatrics*. 2005 Mar;115(3):e277-82.

[735] U.S. Department of Education, Office of Special Education and Rehabilitative Services, Office of Special Education Programs. *28th Annual Report to Congress on the Implementation of the Individuals with Disabilities Education Act, 2006, vol. 1*. Washington, D.C., 2009.

[736] Rimland B. The Autism epidemic, vaccinations, and mercury. *J Nut Environ Med*. 2000; 10: 261-266.

[737] http://www.lilly.com/about/Pages/default.aspx.

[738] http://www.hhs.gov/fda/faq/vaccines/1858.html.

[739] Gerlai J, Gerlai R. Autism: a large unmet medical need and a complex research problem. *Physiol Behav*. 2003 Aug;79(3):461-70.

[740] Gerlai R, Gerlai J. Autism: a target of pharmacotherapies? *Drug Discov Today*. 2004 Apr 15;9(8):366-74.

[741] http://www.cdc.gov/vaccines/pubs/vacc-timeline.htm.

[742] Ozonoff S, Heung K, Byrd R, Hansen R, Hertz-Picciotto I. The onset of autism: patterns of symptom emergence in the first years of life. *Autism Res*. 2008 Dec;1(6):320-8.

[743] Werner E, Dawson G. Validation of the phenomenon of autistic regression using home videotapes. *Arch Gen Psychiatry*. 2005; 62: 788-794.

[744] Geier DA, Geier MR. A prospective study of mercury toxicity biomarkers in autistic spectrum disorders. *J Toxicol and Environ Health, Part A*. 2007; 70(20): 1723-1730.

[745] Chrysochoou C, Rutishauser C, Rauber-Lüthy C, Neuhaus T, Boltshauser E, Superti-Furga A. An 11-month-old boy with psychomotor regression and auto-aggressive behavior. *European J Pediatrics*. 2003; 162(7-8): 559-561.

[746] Corbett SJ, Poon CCS. Letter: Toxic levels of mercury in Chinese infants eating fish congee. *Med J Australia*. 2008 Jan; 188(1): 59-60.

[747] Rimland B. The Autism epidemic, vaccinations, and mercury. *J Nut Environ Med*. 2000; 10: 261-266.

[748] http://www.autismautoimmunityproject.org/Rimland.htm.

[749] Ewing GE. What is regressive autism and why does it occur? Is it the consequence of multi-systemic dysfunction affecting the elimination of heavy metals and the ability to regulate neural temperature? *N Am J Med Sci*. 2009 Jul;1(2):28-47. http://www.ncbi.nlm.nih.gov/pmc/articles/PMC3364648/.

[750] Pangborn J, Baker S. Autism: effective biomedical treatments. Individuality in an epidemic. Autism Research Institute Publication, 2005, *as described by* Maya L, Luna F. Thimerosal and children's neurodevelopmental disorders. *Ann Fac Med (Lima)*. 2006; 67(3); 243-262 [Spanish].

Chapter 14:
Similar Symptoms in Autism and Mercury Poisoning

The similarities in symptomology between autism spectrum disorders and chronic low-dose mercury poisoning suggest a causal relationship between Thimerosal and the disorders.

As described in Part One, mercury occurs in the environment in three broad forms: elemental, inorganic, and organic. The last of those categories includes the methylmercury in fish and shellfish, for which the EPA has exposure limit guidelines, and ethylmercury found in Thimerosal.[751] Knowledge of the symptoms of mercury poisoning in humans comes from several areas of clinical and anecdotal study. These areas include studies of people with too rich a diet of fish and shellfish, who were exposed to grains treated with mercury-containing fungicides, or who used mercury-containing tooth powders.[752][753][754] Another source of information on mercury's effects is individual instances of poisoning in occupational settings. A classic example is Mad Hatter disease, which afflicted hatters in the 19th century with slurred speech, tremors, irritability, shyness, depression, and other neurological symptoms, owing to the use of mercury in hat manufacturing in poorly ventilated work spaces.[755]

A study published in 2001 in the journal *Medical Hypotheses* by Sallie Bernard, cofounder and president of SafeMinds, documented the high degree of overlap in the number and type of symptoms that can occur in autism and mercury poisoning.[756] Although each condition is highly variable in its presentation—that is, no two people with autism or victims of poisoning may be exactly alike in their constellation of symptoms—the conditions still share approximately one hundred universal or common traits, as shown in Figures 12 and 13.

Of these traits, shared examples of psychiatric disturbances include social deficits, shyness, stereotypic behaviors, mood swings, impaired facial recognition, lack of eye contact, anxiety, irritability, and aggression, among others. Victims of autism and mercury poisoning also experience speech and language deficits, including delayed or failure to develop speech, speech comprehension difficulties, verbalizing and word retrieval problems, and "echolalia" (repetition of words). Sensory abnormalities are also common, in the mouth and extremities, for example, as well as sound sensitivity, hearing loss, touch aversion, light sensitivity, and blurred vision. Still other similarities in symptomology occur with motor disorders, including unusual postures, circling, rocking, twitching, intentional movement problems, abnormal gait, clumsiness, and deficits in hand-eye coordination. Interestingly, the unusual motor

1. List of overlapping traits of autism and mercury poisoning

Psychiatric disturbances Social deficits, shyness, social withdrawal Repetitive, preseverative, stereotypic behaviors, obsessive-compulsive tendencies Depression/depressive traits, mood swings, flat affect, impaired face recognition Anxiety, schizoid tendencies, irrational fears Irritability, aggression, temper tantrums Lacking eye contact, impaired visual fixation, problems in joint attention	**Motor disorders** Flapping, myoclonal jerks, chloreiform movements, circling, rocking, toe walking, unusual postures Deficits in eye-hand coordination, limb apraxia, intention tremors, problems with intentional movement or imitation Abnormal gait and posture, clumsiness and incoordination, difficulties sitting, lying, crawling, walking, problem on one side of body	**Unusual behaviors** Self injurious behavior (e.g. head banging) ADHD traits Agitation, unprovoked crying, grimacing, staring spells Sleep difficulties **Physical disturbances** Hyper- or hypotonia, abnormal reflexes, decreased muscle strength (especially upper body), incontinence, problems chewing, swallowing Rashes, dermatitis, eczema, itching
Speech and language deficits Loss of speech, delayed language, failure to develop speech Dysarthria, articulation problems Speech comprehension deficits Verbalizing and word retrieval problems,echolalia, word use and pragmatic errors	**Cognitive impairments** Borderline intelligence, mental retardation—some cases reversable Poor concentration, attention, response inhibition, shifting attention Uneven performance on IQ subtests, verbal IQ higher than performance IQ Poor short term, verbal and auditory memory	Diarrhea, abdominal pain/discomfort, constipation, "colitis" Anorexia, nausea, vomiting, poor appetite, restricted diet Lesions of ileum and colon, increased gut permeability
Sensory abnormalities Abnormal sensation in mouth and extremities Sound sensitivity, mild to profound hearing loss Abnormal touch sensations, touch aversion Over-sensitivity to light, blurred vision	Poor visual and perceptual motor skills, impairment in simple reaction time, lower performance on timed tests Deficits in understanding abstract ideas and symbolism, degeneration of higher mental powers, sequencing, planning and organizing, difficulty carrying out complex commands	**Source:** *Autism: a novel form of mercury poisoning* S. Bernard, A. Enayati, L. Redwood, H. Roger, T. Binstock 2001

FIGURE 12

behavior of hand-flapping is common to those with a diagnosis in the autism spectrum and to victims of mercury poisoning.

People with autism and victims of mercury poisoning also suffer cognitive impairments. These include borderline intelligence, mental retardation, poor concentration, poor short-term memory, poor verbal and auditory memory, deficits in understanding abstract ideas and symbolism, and difficulty carrying out complex commands. In addition, both groups display unusual behaviors, including self-in-

2. Summary comparison of biological abnormalities in autism and mercury exposure

Mercury exposure	Autism
Biochemistry	
Binds-SH groups; blocks sulfate transporter in intestines, kidneys	Low sulfate levels
Reduces glutathione availability; inhibits enzymes of glutathione metabolism; glutathione needed in neurons, cells, and liver to detoxify heavy metals; reduces glutathione peroxidase and reductase	Low levels of glutathione; decreased ability of liver to detoxify xenobiotics; abnormal glutathione peroxidase activities in erythrocytes
Disrupts purine and pyrimidine metabolism	Purine and pyrimidine metabolism errors lead to autistic features
Disrupts mitochondrial activities, especially in brain	Mitochondrial dysfunction, especially in brain
Immune system	
Sensitive individuals more likely to have allergies, asthma, autoimmune-like symptoms, especially rheumatoid-like ones	More likely to have allergies, asthma, familial presence of auto-immune diseases, especially rheumatoid arthritis; IgA deficiencies
Can produce an immune response in CNS; causes brain/MBP autoantibodies	On-going immune response in CNS; brain/MBP autoantibodies present
Causes overproduction of the Th2 subset; kills/inhibits lymphocytes, T-cells, and monocytes, decreases NK T-cell activity; induces or suppresses IFNg & IL-2	Skewed immune-cell subset in the Th2 direction; decreased responses to T-cell mitogens; reduced NK T-cell function; increased IFNg & IL-2
CNS structure	
Selectively targets brain areas unable to detoxify or reduce Hg-induced oxidative stress	Specific areas of brain pathology; many functions spared
Accumulates in amygdala, hippocampus, basal ganglia, cerebral cortex; damages Purkinje and granule cells in cerebellum; brain stem defects in some cases	Pathology in amygdala, hippocampus, basal ganglia, cerebral cortex; damage to Purkinje and granule cells in cerebellum; brain stem defects in some cases
Causes abnormal neuronal cytoarchitecture; disrupts neuronal migration, microtubules, and cell division; reduces NCAMs	Neuronal disorganization, increased neuronal cell replication, increased glial cells; depressed expression of NCAMs
Progressive microcephaly	Progressive microcephaly and macrocephaly
Neuro-chemistry	
Prevents presynaptic serotonin release and inhibits serotonin transport; causes calcium disruptions	Decreased serotonin synthesis in children; abnormal calcium metabolism
Alters dopamine systems; peroxidine deficiency in rats resembles mercurialism in humans	Either high or low dopamine levels; positive response to peroxidine which lowers dopamine levels
Elevates epinephrine and norepinephrine levels by blocking enzyme that degrades epinephrine	Elevated norepinephrine and epinephrine
Elevates glutamate	Elevated glutamate and asparate
Leads to cortical acetylcholine deficiency; increases muscarinic receptor density in hippocampus and cerebellum	Cortical acetylcholine deficiency; reduced muscarinic receptor binding in hippocampus
Causes demyelinating neuropathy	Demyelination in brain
Neurophysiology	
Causes abnormal EEGs, epileptiform activity, variable pattern, e.g., subtle, low amplitude seizure activities	Abnormal EEGs, epileptiform activity, variable patterns, including subtle, low amplitude seizure activities
Causes abnormal vestibular nystagmus responses; loss of sense of position in space	Abnormal vestibular nystagmus responses; loss of sense of position in space
Results in autonomic disturbance; excessive sweating, poor circulation, elevated heart rate	Autonomic disturbance; unusual sweating, poor circulation, elevated heart rate

FIGURE 13

jurious behavior such as head banging, agitation, unprovoked crying, grimacing, and staring spells. Furthermore, physical disturbances, including abnormal reflexes, decreased muscle strength, problems chewing and swallowing, rashes, incontinence, diarrhea, constipation, abdominal pain, nausea, and vomiting all occur in the autism population and in mercury poisoning cases.[757]

Beyond this array of outward manifestations, the specific biological effects of mercury exposure on neuronal development are compatible with the brain pathology observed in autism. To quote the technical literature, in a review article published in the *Journal of Immunotoxicology* in 2011, Helen Ratajczak wrote of Sallie Bernard's work:

> Not only is every major symptom of autism documented in cases of mercury poisoning but also biological abnormalities in autism are very similar to the side effects of mercury poisoning itself (Bernard et al., 2001): these include psychiatric disturbances (e.g., impairments in sociality, stereotypic behaviors, depression, anxiety disorder, and neuroses), increased incidences of allergies and asthma, increases in the presence of IgG autoantibodies against brain and myelin basic proteins, reductions in natural killer cell function, and increases in neopterin levels (indicative of immune activation). Autistic brains show neurotransmitter irregularities that are virtually identical to those arising from mercury exposure, i.e., changes in serotonin and dopamine concentrations, elevated epinephrine and norepinephrine levels in the plasma and brain, elevated serum glutamate levels, and an acetylcholine deficiency in the hippocampus (Bernard et al., 2001). Due to the extensive parallels between autism and mercury poisoning, the likelihood of a causal relationship is great.[758]

Other researchers have also reported and commented on the remarkable similarities between mercury exposure and autism spectrum disorders. A review study by Austin in 2008 similarly pulled together multiple lines of evidence, noting that the "biochemical abnormalities found in autism are consistent with mercury poisoning."[759] In a case study of nine patients with regressive autism, published in 2007, Geier noted that "in the course of evaluating these patients, differential diagnosis generally revealed no apparent factors contributing to/causing the children's autistic disorders other than their mercury exposure" from Thimerosal-containing vaccines and Thimerosal-containing Rho(D)-immune globulin given during pregnancy.[760]

Some scientists have argued, however, that the brain abnormalities associated with autism differ from those associated with mercury poisoning. These views were expressed in a 2003 commentary by Karin Nelson and Margaret Bauman published in *Pediatrics*. (Part Four of this book will review conflicts of interest regarding the American Academy of Pediatrics [AAP], publisher of this journal, and its financial ties with the pharmaceutical industry.) Nelson and Bauman disagreed with Bernard's summary of similar autism and mercury poisoning symptoms, writing, "[Bernard's] table does not distinguish typical and characteristic manifestations of either disorder from the rare, unusual, and highly atypical" and that "at sufficient dose mercury is indeed a neurotoxin, but the typical clinical signs of mercurism are not similar to the typical clinical signs of autism." Nelson and Bauman also cited numerous studies indicating major differences in the brain pathologies and neuroanatomic findings of autism and mercury poisoning.[761]

The scientific literature, in short, is not in agreement on the matter (or meaning) of specific or even broad similarities between autism and mercury poisoning. Indeed, the ability for mercury to cause neurodevelopmental disorders in children is not in question, but whether this causation extends to autism remains unproven. "There is no doubt that mercury exposure causes learning and developmental disorders; the controversy regards the level of exposure," stated a scientific consensus statement on environmental agents associated with neurodevelopmental disorders, released by the international Collaborative on Health and the Environment's Learning Developmental Disabilities Initiative in 2008.[762]

Nevertheless, as this book will continue to contend, more than enough "circumstantial" evidence exists that should prompt the utter removal of Thimerosal from the worldwide vaccine supply. There are nearly four million children born every year in the United States and about 137 million children born annually around the world.[763][764] While Thimerosal has been removed from the routine pediatric vaccines in the United States and in some European countries, it remains in many of the childhood vaccines distributed in the developing world. Accordingly, a substantial number of those 137 million children may be at risk for neurodevelopmental disorders stemming from Thimerosal exposure. As we will show in the next chapter, many epidemiological studies have implied that the levels of mercury in Thimerosal-preserved vaccines have, in fact, been high enough to cross a threshold into causing neurological injury.

Notes

[751] http://www.cdc.gov/vaccinesafety/updates/thimerosal_faqs_mercury.htm.

[752] http://www.epa.gov/ttnatw01/112nmerc/volume1.pdf.

[753] http://www.fda.gov/BiologicsBloodVaccines/SafetyAvailability/VaccineSafety/UCM096228.

[754] Bernard S, Enayati A, Redwood L, Roger H, Binstock T. Autism: a novel form of mercury poisoning. *Med Hypotheses.* 2001 Apr; 56(4): 462-471.

[755] http://www.cdc.gov/niosh/updates/upd-03-04-10.html.

[756] http://www.safeminds.org/about/executive-board.html.

[757] Bernard S, Enayati A, Redwood L, Roger H, Binstock T. Autism: a novel form of mercury poisoning. *Med Hypotheses.* 2001 Apr; 56(4): 462-471.

[758] Ratajczak HV. Theoretical aspects of autism: causes—a review. *J Immunotoxicol.* 2011 Jan-Mar;8(1):68-79.

[759] Austin D. An epidemiological analysis of the "autism as mercury poisoning" hypothesis. *Int J Risk & Safety Med.* 2008; 20(3): 135-142.

[760] Geier DA, Geier MR. A case series of children with apparent mercury toxic encephalopathies manifesting with clinical symptoms of regressive autistic disorders. *J Toxicol Environ Health A.* 2007 May 15;70(10):837-51.

[761] Nelson KB, Bauman ML. Thimerosal and autism? *Pediatrics.* 2003 Mar;111(3):674-9.

[762] Collaborative on Health and the Environment's Learning Developmental Disabilities Initiative. *Scientific Consensus Statement on Environmental Agents Associated with Neurodevelopmental Disorders.* 2008.

[763] http://www.cdc.gov/nchs/fastats/births.htm.

[764] http://www.who.int/whr/2005/media_centre/facts_en.pdf.

Chapter 15:
Links between Mercury Exposure and Autism Spectrum Disorders

Many studies have found positive correlations between environmental mercury exposure and autism spectrum disorders. As first described in Chapter 7, some of these studies have found specific and statistically significant relationships between Thimerosal exposure in vaccines and neurodevelopmental disorders.

The first such study of this kind was published in a peer-reviewed journal in 2003, conducted by the Geiers.[765][766] The study compared records in the Vaccine Adverse Events Reporting System (VAERS) database for children who had received a Thimerosal-free DTaP vaccine to children who had received Thimerosal-containing DTaP vaccines. The results showed that the latter group, which received 75 to 100 micrograms of Thimerosal from Thimerosal-containing

DTaP vaccines, was six times as likely to develop autism as the former group. In the study, the Geiers wrote:

> We were initially highly skeptical that differences in the concentrations of thimerosal in vaccines would have any effect on the incidence rate of neurodevelopmental disorders after childhood immunization. This study presents the first epidemiologic evidence, based upon tens of millions of doses of vaccine administered in the United States, that associates increasing thimerosal from vaccines with neurodevelopmental disorders.[767]

Two other 2003 studies by the Geiers showed that the risk of autism increased along with the dosage of mercury via DTaP vaccines administered in the 1990s.[768 769]

The year of 2003 also saw the publication of the controversial Verstraeten study, described in Part One and explored thoroughly in the upcoming Part Four. The Verstraeten analyses initially reported a strong causal link between Thimerosal-containing vaccines and autism, but after additional rounds of research concluded that it could neither accept nor reject such a hypothesis.[770]

A further analysis of DTaP vaccines, published in 2004 by the Geiers, also concluded that children receiving the Thimerosal-containing versions were at a greater risk of autism.[771] An additional two-phased study, published in 2005, evaluated DTaP vaccine administration and adverse reports in VAERS. The study also used Vaccine Safety Datalink (VSD) information to assess cumulative, early-life exposures to mercury from Thimerosal-containing vaccines for infants born from 1992 through 1997

173

and neurodevelopmental disorder outcomes. Exposure to mercury turned out to be a consistent risk factor for neurodevelopmental disorder diagnoses.[772]

The Geiers continued their research and published more studies looking at Thimerosal-preserved vaccines. A 2006 study compared children who received DTP and Hib vaccines to those who received a combination DTP-Hib vaccine, called DTPH. The former group of children could have received 100 micrograms more mercury within their first eighteen months of life than those who received fewer injections (and thus less Thimerosal) by receiving DTPH. The VAERS data showed that the children who received more mercury had significantly greater odds of developing neurodevelopmental disorders, including autism.[773]

In 2008, the Geiers, along with lead author Heather Young, published one of their most important epidemiological studies in the *Journal of the Neurological Sciences*.[774] Through the VSD, the study assessed the HMO medical records of 278,624 children born in 1990 through 1996 with calculated exposure windows to Thimerosal from birth to seven months and birth to thirteen months. The results consistently showed elevated risks for various neurodevelopmental disorders, including autism associated with mercury exposure. For comparison's sake, three control conditions not expected to be associated with Thimerosal exposure—namely, pneumonia, congenital abnormalities, and failure to thrive—were assessed, and indeed the risks for these outcomes were not elevated.[775]

A more recent study by the Geiers and colleagues in the same vein published in 2013, using both VAERS and VSD data concerning an outcome of autism. It found that children administered Thimerosal-containing DTaP vaccines 1998 through 2000 had twice the risk of developing autism as children administered Thimerosal-free DTaP vaccines. The VSD data revealed that variances in the age of receipt of Thimerosal-containing HepB vaccines correlated with autism diagnoses variances. The highest autism risk found was about three-fold for children exposed to 37.5 micrograms (three shots' worth) in their first six months of life compared to children with no exposure.[776]

Other researchers have found positive correlations between Thimerosal exposure and autism. Gallagher and Goodman, as noted in Chapter 7, studied health survey records for boys who received HepB vaccinations as newborns prior to 1999, when the vaccines still contained Thimerosal. The study reported that vaccinated newborn boys had threefold greater odds of an autism diagnosis compared to unvaccinated boys or those who did not receive vaccinations in their first month of life.[777]

Aside from scheduled childhood vaccines with Thimerosal content, studies have also assessed Thimerosal-containing Rho(D) immune globulin vaccines. These injections are given to pregnant women with Rh-negative blood who have fetuses with Rh-positive blood in order to prevent injury to the developing baby.[778]

A 2001 study by Naya Juul-Dam published in *Pediatrics* reported a 12 percent and 10 percent incidence of Rh-factor disease in pregnancies for children with autism or PDD-NOS, respectively, versus a 3 percent incidence for controls.[779] It is very likely that women with Rh-factor disease received Rho(D) immune globulin injections, which could have contained Thimerosal.

A study by the Geiers in 2007 showed that children with ASDs were more likely to have mothers who received Rho(D) immune globulins.[780] A second Geier study in 2008 pivoted on the fact that Thimerosal was removed from Rho(D) immune globulin preparations in 2002. The hypothesis was as follows: If prenatal exposure to Thimerosal-containing Rho(D) immune globulins were a risk factor for neurodevelopmental disorders, more children with neurodevelopmental disorders would have Rh-negative mothers; but after 2002, children with neurodevelopmental issues would be born to both Rh-negative and Rh-positive mothers at about the same rate. That is indeed what the study found; children with neurodevelopmental disorders, including autism, had a maternal Rh-negativity frequency that closely matched the control group.[781]

Two other Rho(D) immune globulin studies were published around the same time as the last two referenced Geier studies, though both reported no correlation between a mother's Rh status or receipt of the injection with her child developing autism. We will take a few moments to review some of the issues with these studies.

The first, a 2007 study by Judith H. Miles and T. Nicole Takahashi, was sponsored by Johnson & Johnson, the manufacturer of the Thimerosal-containing Rho(D) immune globulin product Rhogam and thus posing an inherent conflict of interest.[782] Of additional concern, SafeMinds reviewed an earlier version of the study data that the authors presented at a 2005 conference. Contradicting the published study's findings, the earlier data showed an increased rate of Rho(D) immune globulin administration during the pregnancy of children who were eventually diagnosed with an ASD compared to siblings without an ASD. Several possible reasons for the discrepancy exist. About one-third of the original sample families were removed from the final data set, and nearly three out of five eligible families declined to participate or were lost during follow-up, potentially introducing selection bias. The control group in the journal version of the study had too few families—just 27—to confer statistical power.[783][784] In a chapter for the 2011 textbook *Autism Spectrum Disorders*, Hertz-Picciotto pointed out other shortcomings of the study, including that "no information was provided on race/ethnicity or other relevant demographic or medical factors. A larger and better-defined comparison series for the thimerosal analysis would have provided more convincing evidence. This study also did not adjust for any confounders."[785][786]

The second Rho(D) immune globulin study, published in 2008, is by Lisa Croen and colleagues.[787] While stronger in many respects compared to the Miles and Takahashi study, it, too, contained a significant flaw. Exposure risk calculations could have been compromised because the authors in both studies assumed that Rhogam constituted all the administered Rho(D) immune globulins. This is unlikely, however, as this Thimerosal-containing brand had only around half of the market share during the pregnancy period for most study participants. "Rhogam" had at that point emerged as a generic term, like "Kleenex," irrespective of brand.[788] Hertz-Picciotto noted that this flaw could have produced a "[p]ossible strong downward bias resulting from high misclassification, as many Rhogam manufacturers did not use thimerosal."

Beyond vaccines, other recent studies have found significant associations between environmental sources of mercury exposure and autism spectrum disorders. A study supported by the CDC implicated mercury, among other metals, as the air pollutant most associated with higher risks of autism spectrum disorder diagnoses among a sample of children born in the San Francisco Bay area in 1994.[789] A follow-up study extended the findings to other parts of California.[790] Meanwhile, a master's thesis completed at Louisiana State University in 2006 noted an association between mercury in fish and air emissions and developmental disorders, including autism.[791]

Also in 2006 and then in 2009, researchers demonstrated that increases in environmental mercury (from power plants, for instance) and distance from point sources of mercury exposure in Texas were significantly related to the risk of an individual being diagnosed with an ASD. The 2006 study found that "on average, for each 1000 lb of environmentally released mercury, there was a 43% increase in the rate of special education services and a 61% increase in the rate of autism."[792] The 2009 study reported that "for every additional 10 miles of distance from industrial or power plant sources, there was an associated decreased autism Incident Risk of 2.0% and 1.4%, respectively."[793] A 2013 study similarly looked at air pollution and ASD incidence and found that exposure to mercury, amongst other pollutants, in the perinatal period indeed upped the odds of ASD development later in life.[794]

In 2009, other scientists undertook an evaluation in the United States, on a state-by-state basis, of ASD prevalence among three-to five-year-old children from 2000 to 2006 and environmental mercury exposure levels from 1996 to 2006. These investigators observed that mercury concentration in the environment among children one year old or younger had a significant association with ASD prevalence three years later.[795]

A 2013 study, primarily from Harvard researchers, found that women exposed to air pollutants such as metals and diesel particles had an increased risk of autism in their children by an average of 30 to 50 percent compared to women exposed to the lowest levels. Of the contaminants, "multi-pollutant models suggested mercury and methylene chloride to be the most robustly associated with autism," the study said.[796 797]

Another important and illustrative example of a link between autism risk and mercury exposure involves dental amalgams, used for filling cavities.[798] Amalgams composed of about 50 percent mercury have been used in dentistry since the 19th century. The CDC and the FDA maintain that mercury-containing amalgams are safe, though studies have suggested leaching of the element and mercury vapor release do occur and contribute to mercury body burden.[799 800] A 2009 study revealed that mercury exposure from maternal dental amalgams during pregnancy may significantly impact the severity of ASD diagnoses. Subjects whose mothers had more than six amalgams during pregnancy were more than three times as likely to be diagnosed with severe autism, as opposed to milder forms of ASD, than subjects whose mothers had five or fewer amalgams during pregnancy.[801] Notably, the Minamata Convention on Mercury, an international treaty approved in January 2013 to restrict human mercury exposure, calls for a global phasedown of mercury amalgams but has an exemption for Thimerosal in vaccines.[802]

A final example of a link between mercury exposure and autism also involves an oral route of ingestion. In the first half of the 20th century, teething powders often contained an ingredient called calomel, which is mercurous chloride. Around 1 in 500 children exposed to calomel developed "pink disease," also known as infantile acrodynia. The disease was eventually linked to calomel, the removal of which from teething powders in 1954 essentially eliminated the disease. The fact that only 1 in 500 children developed pink disease was attributed to individual susceptibilities to mercury. A 2011 Australian study explored autism prevalence in the descendants of individuals with a mercury sensitivity who survived pink disease. Sure enough, the prevalence rate of autism in grandchildren of pink disease survivors turned out to be 1 in 25—far higher than the general population prevalence figure of 1 in 160 documented in Australia at the time.[803]

Notes

[765] http://ebm.rsmjournals.com/site/misc/authors.xhtml.

[766] http://www.autismtreatmentclinics.com/Staff.html.

[767] Geier MR, Geier DA. Neurodevelopmental disorders after thimerosal containing vaccines: a brief communication. *Exp Biolo Med.* 2003;228:660-4.

[768] Geier MR, Geier DA. Thimerosal in childhood vaccines, neurodevelopmental disorders, and heart disease in the United States. *J Am Phys Surg.* 2003;8:6-11.

[769] Geier DA, Geier MR. An assessment of the impact of thimerosal on neurodevelopmental disorders. *Pediatr Rehabil.* 2003;6:97-102.

[770] Verstraeten T, Davis RL, DeStefano F, Lieu TA, Rhodes PH, Black SB, Shinefield H, Chen RT. Safety of thimerosal-containing vaccines: a two-phased study of computerized health maintenance organization databases. *Pediatrics.* 2003 Nov;112:1039-1048.

[771] Geier DA, Geier MR. Neurodevelopmental disorders following thimerosal containing childhood immunizations: a follow-up analysis. *Int J Toxicol.* 2004;23:369-75.

[772] Geier DA, Geier MR. A two-phased population epidemiological study of the safety of thimerosal containing vaccines: a follow-up analysis. *Med Sci Monit.* 2005;11(4):CR160-CR170.

[773] Geier DA, Geier MR. An evaluation of the effects of thimerosal on neurodevelopmental disorders reported following DTP and Hib vaccines in comparison to DTPH vaccine in the United States. *J Toxicol Environ Health A.* 2006 Aug;69(15):1481-95.

[774] http://www.epa.gov/scipoly/sap/pubs/biographies/youngh.htm.

[775] Young HA, Geier DA, Geier MR. Thimerosal exposure in infants and neurodevelopmental disorders: An assessment of computerized medical records in the Vaccine Safety Datalink. *J Neurological Sci.* 2008 Aug 15; 271(1): 110-118.

[776] Geier DA, Hooker BS, Kern JK, King PG, Sykes LK, Geier MR. A two-phase study evaluating the relationship between Thimerosal-containing vaccine administration and the risk for an autism spectrum disorder diagnosis in the United States. *Transl Neurodegener.* 2013 Dec 19;2(1):25. doi: 10.1186/2047-9158-2-25.

[777] Gallagher CM, Goodman MS. Hepatitis B vaccination of male neonates and autism diagnosis, NHIS 1997-2002. *J Toxicol Environ Health A.* 2010;73(24):1665-77.

[778] http://www.mayoclinic.com/health/drug-information/DR601197.

779 Juul-Dam N, Townsend J, Courchesne E. Prenatal, perinatal, and neonatal factors in autism, pervasive developmental disorder-not otherwise specified, and the general population. Pediatrics. 2001 Apr;107(4):E63.

780 Geier DA, Geier MR. A prospective study of thimerosal-containing Rho(D)-immune globulin administration as a risk factor for autistic disorders. *J Matern Fetal Neonatal Med.* 2007 May;20(5):385-90.

781 Geier DA, Mumper E, Gladfelter B, Coleman L, Geier MR. Neurodevelopmental disorders, maternal Rh-negativity, and Rho(D) immune globulins: a multi-center assessment. *Neuro Endocrinol Lett.* 2008 Apr; 29(2): 272-280.

782 Miles JH, Takahashi TN. Lack of association between Rh status, Rh immune globulin in pregnancy and autism. *Am J Med Genet A.* 2007 Jul 1;143A(13):1397-407.

783 http://www.safeminds.org/news/2007/06-2007-1.html#article1.

784 http://www.fourteenstudies.org/HG_11_details.html.

785 Hertz-Picciotto I. Large Scale Epidemiologic Studies of Environmental Factors in Autism. *Autism Spectrum Disorders.* Amaral DG, Dawson G, Geschwind DH, eds. Oxford University Press, 2011.

786 http://www.ucdmc.ucdavis.edu/mindinstitute/ourteam/faculty_pdf/irva_hertzpicciotto.pdf.

787 Croen LA, Matevia M, Yoshida CK, Grether JK. Maternal Rh D status, anti-D immune globulin exposure during pregnancy, and risk of autism spectrum disorders. *Am J Obstet Gynecol.* 2008 Sep;199(3):234.e1-6. doi: 10. 1016/j.ajog.2008.04.044. Epub 2008 Jun 13.

788 Bernard S, Blaxill M, Redwood L. Re: Miles & Takahashi paper on RhIg and autism. *Am J Med Genet A.* 2008 Feb 1;146(3):405-6; author reply 407.

789 Windham GC, Zhang L, Gunier R, Croen LA, Grether JK. Autism spectrum disorders in relation to distribution of hazardous air pollutants in the San Francisco Bay area. *Environ Health Perspect.* 2006 Sep; 114(9): 1438–1444.

790 Windham G, King G, Roberts E, Croen L, Grether J. Autism and distribution of hazardous air pollutants at birth in California. *Epidemiology.* 2007 Sep; 18(5): S174. doi: 10.1097/01.ede.0000276871.78545.c6.

791 Rury J. *MS Thesis: Links Between Environmental Mercury, Special Education, and Autism in Louisiana.* Louisiana State University. 2006.

792 Palmer RF, Blanchard S, Stein Z, Mandell D, Miller C. Environmental mercury release, special education rates, and autism disorder: an ecological study of Texas. *Health Place.* 2006 Jun;12(2):203-9.

793 Palmer RF, Blanchard S, Wood R. Proximity to point sources of environmental mercury release as a predictor of autism prevalence. *Health Place.* 2009 Mar;15(1):18-24. doi: 10.1016/j.healthplace.2008.02.001. Epub 2008 Feb 12.

794 Roberts AL, Lyall K, Hart JE, Laden F, Just AC, Bobb JF, Koenen KC, Ascherio A, Weisskopf MG. Perinatal air pollutant exposures and autism spectrum disorder in the children of nurses' health study II participants. *Environ Health Perspect.* 2013 Aug;121(8):978-84. doi: 10.1289/ehp.1206187. Epub 2013 May 30.

795 Schweikert C, Li Y, Dayya D, Yens D, Torrents M, Hsu DF. *Analysis of Autism Prevalence and Neurotoxins Using Combinatorial Fusion and Association Rule Mining.* 9th IEEE international conference on bioinformatics and bioengineering. June 22–24, 2009, Taichung, China, 400-4.

796 https://imfar.confex.com/imfar/2013/webprogram/Paper14885.html.

797 http://online.wsj.com/article/SB10001424127887324766604578460533650317520.html#articleTabs%3Darticle.

798 http://www.fda.gov/medicaldevices/productsandmedicalprocedures/dentalproducts/dentalamalgam/default.htm.

799 http://www.epa.gov/hg/dentalamalgam.html.

800 Mutter J, Naumann J, Guethlin C. Comments on the article "the toxicology of mercury and its chemical compounds" by Clarkson and Magos (2006). *Crit Rev Toxicol.* 2007;37(6):537-49; discussion 551-2.

801 Geier DA, Kern JK, Geier MR. A prospective study of prenatal mercury exposure from maternal dental amalgams and autism severity. *Acta Neurobiol Exp (Wars).* 2009;69(2):189-97.

802 http://www.unep.org/newscentre/Default.aspx?DocumentID=2702&ArticleID=9373&l=en.

803 Shandley K, Austin DW. Ancestry of pink disease (infantile acrodynia) identified as a risk factor for autism spectrum disorders. *J Toxicol Environ Health A.* 2011;74(18):1185-94.

Chapter 16:
Autism Rates Decline when Thimerosal Exposure Levels Are Reduced

If the mercury in Thimerosal is indeed a major risk factor for autism spectrum disorders, reduced exposure to the toxin should result in reduced rates of the condition. Such a drop has not been officially declared or evidenced in the United States and other countries that have phased out Thimerosal in vaccines.[804] However, as Chapter 13 conveyed, considerable challenges have been posed in recent decades in arriving at consistent, "accurate" prevalence statistics for autism. Changing diagnostic definitions, greater public awareness, and social factors have complicated efforts in drawing clear comparisons between different time periods.[805] Younger ages of diagnosis and methods of reporting have also affected autism prevalence rate determinations, especially as these differ across geographical locations.[806] Nevertheless, as reviewed in this Chapter, multiple studies have indicated that autism rates did in fact decline when Thimerosal exposure levels were reduced. Some studies that have explicitly stated the contrary have suffered from methodological flaws and analytical limitations.

We will begin with the United States. In early 2003, the last childhood vaccines prepared for domestic use that contained Thimerosal expired, following a phaseout that began in 1999.[807] Since that time, reported ASD prevalence rates have continued their upward trajectory. However, as Part One explained, just as Thimerosal was being phased out of the standard pediatric vaccine schedule, the CDC began recommending Thimerosal-containing flu shots for healthy infants between six and twenty-three months of age.[808 809] That recommendation in 2002 came several years after pregnant women were advised by the Advisory Committee on Immunization Practices (ACIP) and CDC in 1997 to obtain flu shots in their second or third trimesters of pregnancy, or while breastfeeding.[810] Flu vaccine recommendations expanded further in the 2000s, and in 2010, to reduce the complexity of the recommendations and ensure that adults who might be at increased risk of flu complications received vaccinations, the CDC simply recommended that everyone ages six months or older obtain a flu shot.[811]

As a result—explained mathematically in Part One—a significant proportion of the mercury that children were exposed to during the 1990s, which was then removed from the vaccine schedule in 2003, has ultimately been replaced by the mercury in flu vaccines. Despite the lack of a clear before-and-after window for

THIMEROSAL: LET THE SCIENCE SPEAK

Thimerosal exposure in the United States in the last decade, four studies in particular have found evidence for autism prevalence declining when Thimerosal exposure has been reduced.

A 2004 study by the Geiers calculated an average mercury dose from vaccines for children in two birth cohorts, from 1981 to 1985 and from 1990 to 1996. The calculations were based on the CDC's Biological Surveillance Summaries and yearly live birth estimates. Figures for the number of autism cases came from US Department of Education data sets. The researchers compared this data and wrote:

> We have observed for birth cohorts from the mid-to-late 1980s through the early 1990s that as there was an increase in the average mercury dose from thimerosal-containing childhood vaccines a corresponding increase in the prevalence of autism occurred. A maximum in mercury from thimerosal-containing childhood vaccines and the prevalence of autism occurred for the birth cohort of 1993, and from 1993 through 1996, as the average mercury dose from thimerosal-containing vaccines decreased, a corresponding decrease in the prevalence of autism also ensued.[812]

A follow-up study in 2006 used two different sources of data from the CDC's VAERS database and the California Department of Developmental Services (DDS). In both registries, newly diagnosed autism and speech disorder cases rose from the year 1994 through mid-2002, closely tracking the rising content of Thimerosal in children's vaccines. (Given a lag time of about three to four years after birth for a neurodevelopmental disorder diagnosis, the 1994 reported cases were for children born predominantly in the late

1980s and early 1990s, when Thimerosal exposure levels began rising.) From mid-2002 through 2005, the number of newly diagnosed cases declined compared to an extrapolation of the trend line from previous years, consistent with Thimerosal's phaseout from pediatric vaccines starting in 1999.[813]

Another 2006 study assessed VAERS from the year 1991 to 2004. The peak of reports received in VAERS for autism, mental retardation, and speech disorders occurred in the period 2001 through 2002, which again with the lag time in diagnosis corresponds to vaccinations given in 1998. Report numbers declined in 2003 and 2004, consistent with reduced Thimerosal exposure.[814]

In 2014, the Geiers and their colleagues published perhaps the strongest epidemiological evidence of a decline in autism diagnoses following Thimerosal exposure reductions, owing to the growing span of time from when regulators phased out Thimerosal from the childhood vaccination schedule in the US As described first in Chapter 7, the Geiers used VAERS data, updated through September 2013, to compare populations exposed to Thimerosal-containing DTaP vaccines administered between 1997 and 1999 to unexposed populations administered DTaP vaccines with trace amounts of Thimerosal between 2004 and 2006. The researchers reviewed a total of 5,591 adverse events reported to VAERS containing the mention of at least one of the following outcomes: autism, speech disorder, mental retardation or neurodevelopmental disorder, broadly. A control set of reports without these outcomes was considered as well. Reports of these disorders declined in the second, unexposed group. An apples-to-apples comparison of the two groups revealed increased risks in the exposed group of 7.67 for autism, along with 3.49 for speech disorders, 8.73 for mental retardation and 4.84 for neurodevelopmental disorders.[815]

A 2008 study, based on California data, did not find the correlations in the Geier studies. It assessed children born from 1989 through 2003 who were reported to the DDS from 1995 to 2007. The study found that autism prevalence increased in children even after Thimerosal removal from vaccines from 1999 through 2002. Accordingly, the study said, the "data do not support the hypothesis that exposure to thimerosal during childhood is a primary cause of autism."[816]

SafeMinds, among others, critiqued the study's conclusion on several grounds. A trend toward autism ascertainment at earlier ages could bias the youngest birth cohorts in the study, increasing the post-Thimerosal prevalence figures to an extent. Infant flu vaccines containing Thimerosal administered per new federal recommendations in 2002 could have diluted any otherwise noticeable autism prevalence decreases in the last birth cohorts in 2002 and 2003. The study could not account for the leftover, not-yet-expired Thimerosal-containing vaccines administered by pediatricians through 2003. The California database also underwent administrative changes, with higher caseload numbers after 2002 because of improvements in the reporting system. The study only had young children four years and younger to assess for the most relevant years after 2002 when Thimerosal was largely reduced, compared to children as old as twelve years for 1990s birth cohorts, offering an incomplete and premature picture.[817]

Clearer examples of study limitations and flaws with the issue of Thimerosal reduction and autism prevalence come from Denmark.

The country removed Thimerosal from its childhood vaccines in 1992. Officially, Denmark did not immediately experience a decline in its rates of autism spectrum disorders.[818] But some of the key studies from this country relied on by health authorities in the United States as evidence against a link between Thimerosal and neurodevelopmental disorders do not cleanly show such a nonassociation.[819] (Part Four will discuss other issues with these Danish studies and conflicts of interest regarding their authors.)

A study lead-authored by Anders Hviid in 2003 reported that the risk of autism spectrum disorders did not differ significantly between populations of children who received Thimerosal-containing and Thimerosal-free vaccines. The study assessed all children born in Denmark from January 1990 to December 1996.[820] SafeMinds obtained a copy of the data set used from the Danish Psychiatric Central Research Register, covering the years 1980 to 2002.[821] The set is broken down into five-year age bands—zero- to four-year-olds, five- to nine-year-olds, and ten- to fourteen-year-olds. SafeMinds showed that case numbers declined for children transitioning from the five- to nine-year-old to ten- to fourteen-year-old category, most likely reflecting administrative error. Overall, in the ten years preceding 2000, 815 cases were lost as they moved through the registry, a number that exceeds the 710 logged in the system as of 2000. Missing records for older children, therefore, could bias the study's findings that more children given Thimerosal-free vaccines developed autism than those who received Thimerosal-containing vaccines.

A direct comparison of children in the same age band, rather than in aggregate as the study did, yields a conflicting result.

SafeMinds compared the five- to nine-year-old groups exposed and not exposed to Thimerosal via vaccines. The exposed group had 2.3 times the number of cases as the unexposed group, with an incidence of about 1 in 500 compared to 1 in 1,500, respectively.[822]

A second flawed Danish study is Kreesten Madsen's, from 2003. For its results, researchers evaluated psychiatric records for all children born in Denmark from 1971 to 2000. The study reported that autism prevalence rose after Thimerosal's removal from vaccines in 1992. However, this conclusion is questionable, because of the study's shifting inclusion criteria. Up through 1995, the study used hospital inpatient records to register an autism diagnosis. After 1995, outpatient records were included as well. The study noted that "the proportion of outpatient to inpatient activities was about 4 to 6 times as many outpatients as inpatients with variations across time and age bands"; however, in a 2002 study also by Madsen using the same database, autism diagnoses from outpatient visits outnumbered inpatient visits by 13.5 times.[823] Therefore, it seems quite obvious that the jump in autism diagnoses seen after the Thimerosal phaseout could easily be accounted for by the inclusion of voluminous outpatient records. Oddly, the Madsen study noted that an additional analysis was run using only inpatient data, and that the same upward trend persisted, yet this critical information was not included in the study ("data not shown," in the study's words).[824]

Other autism case-counting discrepancies further put Madsen's 2003 conclusions in doubt. As noted in a separate study from 2003 using Danish patient information, prior to 1992, data in the national register used to record autism diagnoses did not include the records of a large Copenhagen clinic. This additional data accounted for about 20 percent of national cases, again artificially boosting the post-Thimerosal figures.[825] [826] Also, in 1994, a change occurred in the diagnostic criteria for inclusion in the registry as autism. Prior to 1994, inclusion was based on the *International Classification of Diseases, Eighth Revision* (*ICD-8*) diagnosis of psychosis proto-infantalis, and from 1994 onward, inclusion was based on the *ICD-10* diagnoses of infantile autism and atypical autism. The Madsen authors admitted in the paper's text, "The increase in the incidence of autism from 1990 on may be attributable to more attention being drawn to the syndrome of autism and to a change in the diagnostic criteria from the *ICD-8* to the *ICD-10* in 1994."

Of further noteworthiness, authors of the Madsen study debated about including autism incidence data for an additional available year, 2001, that showed strong decreases in the two- to four-year-old and seven- to nine-year-old cohorts. The manuscript submitted to *Pediatrics*—after rejection by the top-tier journals *The Lancet* and *JAMA*—initially contained this data.[827] [828] [829] Reviewers questioned the significance and potential reasons behind the drop in autism incidence; ultimately, the study that *Pediatrics* published did not include the 2001 data.[830]

A letter to the editor of the *Journal of American Physicians and Surgeons* in 2004 corrected for the Madsen study's inaccuracies. The result, the letter's authors found, was "significant decreases in autism incidence after 1993 among each group studied, including a dramatic 75% reduction within the 2 to 4-year-old cohort."[831]

The overall murkiness of Danish statistics keeping was well summarized in a 2004 study by coauthors of Madsen's. That study, which took the long view by looking at autism spectrum disorder prevalence during the period between 1971 and 2000, concluded that "the increasing prevalence and incidence rates during the 1990s may well be explained by changes in the registration procedures and more awareness of the disorders, although a true increase in the incidence cannot be ruled out."[832]

The story regarding autism rates in Denmark, however, does not end there. A recent 2013 study by Therese Grønborg, which had nothing to do with vaccines, gauged the recurrence rate of autism in siblings and half-siblings born from 1980 through 2004. This study drew upon the same database as the Hviid and Madsen studies, the Psychiatric Central Research Register, for the number of autism diagnoses in the country. Yet the Grønborg paper shows strikingly different statistics than the Madsen paper, and in fact contradicts the latter's claim that autism incidence rose after the Thimerosal phaseout in 1992.

According to the Madsen study, 956 children were diagnosed with autism from the years 1970 through 2000; incidence rose from well under 1 per 10,000 in the 1970s to close to 5 per 10,000 for the age range of 2 to 4 years by 2000. Puzzlingly, the Grønborg study reports 2,231 cases of autism just from 1980 through 1999, and for all ASDs, the number is 10,377; how exactly researchers, again, supposedly using the same database, found such a startlingly higher number of cases of autism (and ASDs in general) remains unclear.

Most importantly, over the period from 1995 through 2000— evaluated by both studies—the Grønborg study reports that the total number of ASD cases decreased each year, while the number of births went down at a far smaller rate. In terms of prevalence, the ASD figures declined from a high of 1.5 percent in 1994-1995, down to 1.2 by 2000-2001, and still lower in 2002-2004 to 1.0, where although the number of cases was somewhat higher than in the previous period, the number of births was comparatively much higher, bucking the fairly flat trend line of the late 1990s. The number of strictly autism cases rose over the Grønborg study's assessed period, but the prevalence leveled off at 0.4 from 1996-1997 through 2002-2004.[833] Overall, with regard to the true rates of autism in Denmark, the major discrepancies between these two studies, Madsen 2003 and Grønborg 2013 put the former's contention that autism increased post-Thimerosal in doubt.

The last country we will consider is the United Kingdom. Recently, researchers at University College London and Boston University undertook a study to update figures on the annual prevalence and incidence rates of autism in United Kingdom children. The study was actually prompted by the CDC's reporting in 2012 that the autism prevalence rate in 2008 in eight-year-old US children had rocketed to 1 in 88. This rise represented a 78 percent increase from CDC's 2004 estimate, speaking to a continued spike in prevalence witnessed through the 1990s. The researchers, however, found a different trend in the United Kingdom. Based on information in a British medical database, a fivefold increase in annual autism incidence rates in eight-year-olds occurred during the 1990s. This surge was followed by a plateauing in the early 2000s, with rates holding steady from 2004 through 2010, the last year reviewed. The authors attribute broadening diagnostic criteria and social factors, already covered in this book, to explain some of the 1990s' jump. But, they write, the "actual cause remains in large part a mystery."[834] It is notable in this context, however, that the

United Kingdom did phase out Thimerosal in 2004.[835] Admittedly, though, the full effects (if any) from this phaseout on children as old as eight, as assessed in the study, have yet to be borne out.

To recap, available epidemiological literature points to a definite rise in autism prevalence since the early 1990s, consistent through the 1990s in the United States with an increase in Thimerosal exposure through the childhood immunization schedule, and into today through maternal and childhood flu shots. As for decreased Thimerosal exposure and a reduction in prevalence, studies have not been able to convincingly settle the issue. (This book examines additional information about the dubious reliability of the Danish studies and the inherent bias of their authors in Part Four.) Case reporting inconsistencies and the increased administration of Thimerosal-containing flu vaccines to young children and pregnant women in the United States are just two of the confounding factors.

To investigate further, we now turn to a potential biological basis for Thimerosal's causing autism.

Notes

[804] http://www.cdc.gov/ncbddd/autism/data.html.

[805] http://understandingautism.columbia.edu/about.html.

[806] Parner ET, Thorsen P, Dixon G, de Klerk N, Leonard H, Nassar N, Bourke J, Bower C, Glasson EJ. A comparison of autism prevalence trends in Denmark and Western Australia. *J Autism Dev Disord*. 2011 Dec;41(12):1601-8.

[807] http://www.cdc.gov/vaccinesafety/concerns/thimerosal/thimerosal_timeline.html.

[808] http://www.cdc.gov/mmwr/preview/mmwrhtml/rr5103a1.htm.

[809] http://www.fda.gov/BiologicsBloodVaccines/SafetyAvailability/VaccineSafety/UCM096228.

[810] http://www.cdc.gov/mmwr/preview/mmwrhtml/00047346.htm.

[811] http://www.cdc.gov/mmwr/preview/mmwrhtml/rr5908a1.htm.

[812] Geier DA, Geier MR. Comparative evaluation of the effects of MMR immunization and mercury doses from thimerosal-containing childhood vaccines on the population prevalence of autism. *Med Sci Monit*. 2004; 10(3): PI33-PI39.

[813] Geier DA, Geier MR. Early downward trends in neurodevelopmental disorders following removal of thimerosal-containing vaccines. *J Am Phys Surg*. 2006; 11(1): 8-13.

[814] Geier DA, Geier MR. An assessment of downward trends in neurodevelopmental disorders in the United States following removal of thimerosal from childhood vaccines. *Med Sci Monit*. 2006;12(6):CR231-CR239.

[815] Geier DA, Kern JK, King PG, Sykes LK, Geier MR. The risk of neurodevelopmental disorders following a Thimerosal-preserved DTaP formulation in comparison to its Thimerosal-reduced formulation in the vaccine adverse event reporting system (VAERS). *J Biochem Pharmacol Res*. 2014 Jun 1;2(2):64-73.

[816] Schechter R, Grether JK. Continuing increases in autism reported to California's developmental services system: mercury in retrograde. *Arch Gen Psychiatry*. 2008 Jan;65(1):19-24.

[817] SafeMinds. *SafeMinds Critique of Schechter & Grether Paper on California's Autism DDS Data and Thimerosal Exposure*. 2008 Jan available at http://www.SafeMinds.org/government-affairs/SafeMinds-analysis-schechter-grether-01-08v2.pdf.

[818] Madsen KM, Hviid A, Vestergaard M, Schendel D, Wohlfahrt J, Thorsen P, Olsen J, Melbye M. A population-based study of measles, mumps, and rubella vaccination and autism. *N Engl J Med*. 2002 Nov 7;347(19):1477-82.

[819] Immunization Safety Review Committee Board on Health Promotion and Disease Prevention, IOM. *Final Report, Immunization Safety Review: Vaccines And Autism*. May 2004.

[820] Hviid A, Stellfeld M, Wohlfahrt J, Melbye M. Association between thimerosal-containing vaccine and autism. *JAMA*. 2003 Oct 1;290(13):1763-6.

[821] http://www.cfpr.dk/central-research-register/.

[822] Bernard, Sallie. SafeMinds. *Analysis of the Danish Autism Registry Data Base in Response to the Hviid et al Paper on Thimerosal in JAMA (October, 2003)*. 2003 Oct *available at* http://www.SafeMinds.org/research/Hviid_et_alJAMA-SafeMindsAnalysis.pdf.

[823] Madsen KM, Hviid A, Vestergaard M, Schendel D, Wohlfahrt J, Thorsen P, Olsen J, Melbye M. A population-based study of measles, mumps, and rubella vaccination and autism. *N Engl J Med*. 2002 Nov 7;347(19):1477-82.

[824] Madsen KM, Lauritsen MB, Pedersen CB, Thorsen P, Plesner AM, Andersen PH, Mortensen PB. Thimerosal and the occurrence of autism: negative ecological evidence from Danish population-based data. *Pediatrics*. 2003 Sep;112(3 Pt 1):604-6.

[825] Stehr-Green P, Tull P, Stellfeld M, Mortenson PB, Simpson D. Autism and thimerosal-containing vaccines: lack of consistent evidence for an association. *Am J Prev Med*. 2003 Aug;25(2):101-6.

[826] Blaxill, Mark; SafeMinds. *Danish Thimerosal-Autism Study in Pediatrics: Misleading and Uninformative on Autism-Mercury Link*. 2003 Sep *available at* http://www.SafeMinds.org/research/Blaxill-DenmarkAutismThimerosalPediatrics.pdf.

[827] http://www.journal-ranking.com/ranking/listCommonRanking.html?citingStart-Year=1901&externalCitationWeight=1&journalListId=370&selfCitationWeight=1.

[828] Marlene Briciet Lauritsen, "Manuscript about Thimerosal and autism," email to Poul Thorsen, Kreesten Madsen, Diana Schendel, November 13, 2002.

[829] Kreesten Meldgaard Madsen, "RE: Manuscript about Thimerosal and autism," email to Marlene Briciet Lauritsen, Poul Thorsen, Diana Schendel, November 13, 2002.

[830] Letter to Jerold F. Lucey responding to *Pediatrics* reviewer comments [No further detail available].

[831] Trelka JA, Hooker BS. More on Madsen's analysis. *J Am Phys Surg*. 2004; 9(4):101.

[832] Lauritsen MB, Pedersen CB, Mortensen PB. The incidence and prevalence of pervasive developmental disorders: a Danish population-based study. *Psychol Med*. 2004 Oct;34(7):1339-46.

[833] Grønborg TK, Schendel DE, Parner ET. Recurrence of autism spectrum disorders in full- and half-siblings and trends over time: a population-based cohort study. *JAMA Pediatr*. 2013 Oct 1;167(10):947-53. doi: 10.1001/jamapediatrics.2013.2259.

[834] Taylor B, Jick H, Maclaughlin D. Prevalence and incidence rates of autism in the UK: time trend from 2004-2010 in children aged 8 years. BMJ Open. 2013 Oct 16;3(10):e003219. doi: 10.1136/bmjopen-2013-003219.

[835] http://web.archive.org/web/20070609114311/http://www.advisorybodies.doh.gov.uk/jcvi/mins011004.htm.

Chapter 17: Animal Studies Show a Biological Basis for Thimerosal Causing Autism

With epidemiological evidence suggestive of a link between Thimerosal exposure and the risk of autism, the question turns to whether scientists can reproduce such a link in animals. Tests with human cells (though not subjects, of course) are also necessary in explicating any link. To these ends, as this chapter will review, several dozen studies have established what could indeed be a biological basis for Thimerosal causing autism.

Some particularly insightful studies have demonstrated the inducement of autism-like symptoms and pathological phenomena by exposing animals to Thimerosal.[836] The first, a 2004 study by Mady Hornig of Columbia University, assessed two different populations of mice.[837] One of these groups possessed a genetic propensity for autoimmune disease, wherein the immune system inappropriately targets the body's own tissues.[838] With adjustments for corresponding weight and age, the young mice received Thimerosal dosages at times in their maturation analogous to the exposure that human children had during their first year of life when following the 2001 US immunization schedule. The mice with autoimmune sensitivity displayed characteristics that appear with autism, including inappropriate responses in the presence of new stimulations and disruption to cells and architecture in a brain region known as the hippocampus.[839]

Three years later, a study in Peru administered to young hamsters the vaccine equivalent dosage of Thimerosal in US children through their first six months when following the 2001 immunization schedule. Compared to the controls, the Thimerosal-injected hamsters had lower body and brain weight, along with smaller stature; these traits, however, are not consistent with the accelerated head circumference and bodily growth commonly seen in boys with autism.[840] But brain damage was also evidenced in the hamsters' cerebral cortex, including again the hippocampus as well as the cerebellum, the brain's coordination center for muscle movement.[841] [842]

A 2010 pilot study (funded in part by autism organizations) involving rhesus macaque infants examined the growth of a brain region called the amygdala that is also implicated in autism etiology. The amygdala is an almond-shaped bundle of neurons known to play a pivotal role in the expression of emotions, among other functions. In macaques the amygdala is associated with the development of social and emotional behavior. Previous studies had shown the amygdala to be enlarged in children with autism. The macaque study compared monkeys either exposed or not exposed to the complete mid- to late-1990s US childhood vaccine schedule with its attendant Thimerosal load. Brain scans revealed increased amygdala volume in the vaccine-exposed animals compared to the nonexposed animals; the study also found significantly greater total brain volume at two time points for the infant macaques, consistent with the overall brain enlargement seen in many human patients with autism.[843] Also of note, another 2010 study by many of the same investigators discovered a significant delay in acquisition of neonatal reflexes in macaques given a single dose of Thimerosal-containing HepB vaccine.[844]

Other recent animal studies point to Thimerosal affecting the cerebellum. A 2010 mouse study looked at the production of certain proteins believed to play a part in detoxifying the brain from heavy metals including mercury. The expression of two such proteins spiked in the cerebellum after Thimerosal injections, and in a dose-dependent manner. The findings support the biological plausibility of how low-dose mercury may be associated with autism, according to the study authors.[845]

Studies done at Harvard Medical School funded in part by SafeMinds have provided additional information on how Thimerosal damages the development of the cerebellum. In a study by Z. L. Sulkowski in 2011, researchers administered Thimerosal to pregnant rats to simulate flu and other Thimerosal-containing vaccines that can be given to women during pregnancy and early breastfeeding. Rat pups were tested for neurodevelopmental milestones and, after being euthanized, had their cerebellar tissue examined. The results revealed aberrant oxidative stress and thyroid hormone metabolism in the cerebellum; the pups also had motor learning and auditory development issues.[846] A follow-up study the next year by A. Khan, Sulkowski, and colleagues supported the initial findings.[847]

Further studies offer other interesting angles. Michael Lawton and colleagues, for example, in 2007 reported that methylmercury and Thimerosal inhibited the growth in mouse and rat cells of neurites, the long extensions from nerve cells that connect them to each other and to organs.[848] [849] A visually compelling example of mercury causing neurodegeneration by halting and reversing neurite growth was provided in a 2001 study by University of Calgary researchers. Leong obtained time-lapse images under a microscope of snail neurons' outgrowths shriveling when exposed to mercury.[850] (See Figure 14.)

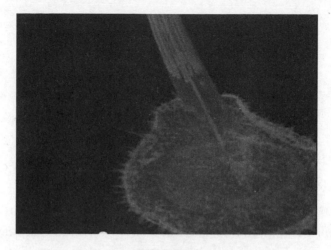

FIGURE 14
Visualization of Mercury Causing Neuronal Degradation
Credit: Christopher C. W. Leong, Naweed I. Syed, and Fritz L. Lorscheider,
University of Calgary

1. In this illustration, a neurite process (the tube at the top of the image) extends from the main cell body of a growing, healthy neuron. The amorphous, drop-like area at the end of the tube is called a growth cone, which is where structural proteins assemble to form a cell membrane.

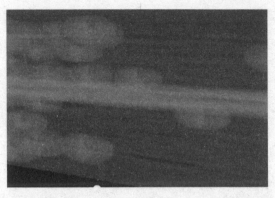

2. Two principal proteins involved in growth cone function are actin and tubulin. In this magnified view of the illustration, tubulin proteins are shown as pill-shaped units. During normal cell growth, the tubulin proteins link together end-to-end to form microtubules that surround neurofibrils.

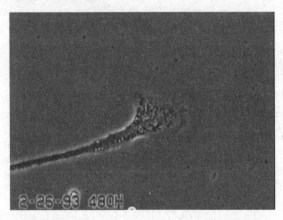

3. In this time-lapse shot from under a microscope, a neurite from a live neuron isolated from snail brain tissue is shown growing. Notably, growth cones in all animal species rely on proteins with virtually identical compositions and that have the same structural and behavioral characteristics.

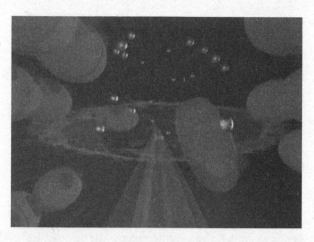

4. Returning to the illustration, when mercury is added to the cell culture, the mercury ions (shown as tiny balls) bind to sites on the tubulin, preventing the proteins from joining together. The microtubules start to break down.

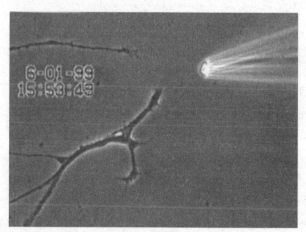

5. Now, back under the microscope, the live snail neurites are shown with mercury being added to the culture via a microinjection pipette, seen as the bright object in the upper right.

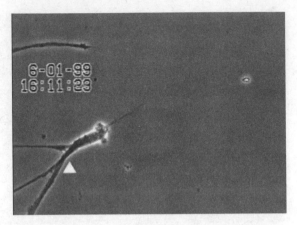

6. The mercury causes the developing neurite and its growth cone to collapse, denuding the neurofibrils, seen as the tiny filaments protruding from the detracting neurite process. The study provided the first direct evidence that low-level mercury exposure can cause this neurodegeneration in the brain.

In 2012, the Calgary researchers extended their findings from snail to rat brain cells, thus showing similar effects in mammalian cells.[851] The work confirmed previous laboratory research by Haley and Pendergrass in the mid-1990s on human brain samples.[852]

Neurodevelopmental disorders, including autism, are often accompanied by self-injurious behavior, and a factor behind this puzzling behavior could be a lessened sensitivity to pain. A 2009 study by Polish authors reported that young and adult rats that were administered Thimerosal in equivalent or greater amounts than many countries' pediatric vaccine schedules exhibited lessened pain sensitivity. Also of note, the study indicated that mercury remained in the rats' brains in significant amounts thirty days after injection.[853]

A follow-up 2010 study revealed that Thimerosal induced changes to pain-mediating opioid receptors in several brain regions in young rats. "If analogous changes occur in the brains of some children, they are likely to have profound neurological, physiological and behavioral consequences, which may be relevant for certain neurodevelopmental disorders," the researchers wrote.[854] Another 2010 study by the same Polish group went on to report widespread neuropathological changes in rats again exposed to Thimerosal at analogous levels to human pediatric vaccines. The study, the authors wrote,

> Provides clear evidence of neurotoxicity of pharmacologically relevant doses of [Thimerosal] in developing organisms, lending further support to the hypothesis implicating mercurials in paediatric neurodevelopmental disorders. On the whole, the results of this study argue for urgent removal of [Thimerosal] from all vaccines for children and pregnant women, as well as from other medicinal products and cosmetics.[855]

A 2011 study by the researchers took a broader approach. Shortly after birth, male and female rats were given a range of doses of Thimerosal and evaluated as adults for behaviors characteristically altered in autism. Rats exposed to all the ranges of Thimerosal developed locomotor impairments and exhibited anxiety and fear of novel situations. Those rats given the highest Thimerosal doses were less social as well.[856]

Notably, the male rats in this study who received the highest doses exhibited more frequent instances of antisocial activity.

In general, male rats were found to be more sensitive to certain neurochemical alterations than females. Males were also more affected than their female counterparts in the Sulkowski 2011 and Khan 2012 studies mentioned several paragraphs ago. Both of these sex-specific findings seem to agree with the pronounced skew in autism diagnoses in humans of males to females of more than four to one.[857] (See Chapter 20 for more discussion of this topic.)

Two other studies from 2012 expounded on Thimerosal's effects in the mammalian brain. Polish authors saw changes in the levels of amino acids in the prefrontal cortexes of infant rats exposed to Thimerosal that may lead to brain injury and contribute to neurodevelopmental disorders.[858] The prefrontal cortex has been dubbed the "CEO of the brain" because the region brings together information from all of the senses. In humans, the prefrontal cortex is critical for abstract thought, executive functioning, and the moderation of "proper" social behavior.[859] A Japanese study from last year also described persistent neurochemical impairments in rat brains exposed before birth to Thimerosal. The authors felt it appropriate to comment on Thimerosal use, writing, "These results indicate that embryonic exposure to thimerosal produces lasting impairment of brain monoaminergic system, and thus every effort should be made to avoid the use of thimerosal."[860]

Another characteristic of human autism with insights into its origin provided by animal research are the widespread changes in an affected individual's immune system.[861] In 2006, a study using cultured mouse cells offered a potential molecular basis behind some of the changes. Dendritic cells, which play a key role in immunological response, were shown to be exquisitely sensitive to Thimerosal, even at low concentrations.[862] The study's authors noted that resulting dysregulation of immune pathways could explain some of the genetic susceptibility of the immune system to mercury.[863]

Recent work also involving immunology has explored the "cell danger" theory of autism causation. According to this theory, environmental exposures (possibly including mercury) trigger cells to go into a defensive metabolic mode and stop communicating with each other properly. This disrupted communication manifests as autistic symptomology, and could be particularly damaging during early brain development. The concept has been tested in mice by exposing adult females to a simulated viral infection during vulnerable times in their pregnancies. These females give birth to pups with neurodevelopmental abnormalities that have features of human autism spectrum disorder.[864][865] The release of inflammatory molecules by the mother's immune system, it seems, can cause abnormal development in the eventual offspring.[866] Mercury, as has been demonstrated in prior cited studies, as well as by Renee Gardner and colleagues in 2009, affects immune function in humans.[867] Maternal infections are already a recognized risk factor for autism, so this immunological angle being studied in mice could offer important insights into autism causation.

Notes

[836] Geier DA, Kern JK, Geier MR. The biological basis of autism spectrum disorders: Understanding causation and treatment by clinical geneticists. *Acta Neurobiol Exp (Wars)*. 2010;70(2):209-26.

[837] http://www.mailman.columbia.edu/our-faculty/profile?uni=mh2092.

[838] http://www.medterms.com/script/main/art.asp?articlekey=2402.

[839] Hornig M, Chian D, Lipkin WI. Neurotoxic effects of postnatal thimerosal are mouse strain dependent. *Mol Psychiatry*. 2004 Sep;9(9):833-45.

[840] Chawarska K, Campbell D, Chen L, Shic F, Klin A, Chang J. Early generalized overgrowth in boys with autism. *Arch Gen Psychiatry*. 2011 Oct;68(10):1021-31.

[841] Laurente J, Remuzgo F, Ávalos B, Chiquinta J, Ponce B, Avendaño R, Maya L Neurotoxic effects of thimerosal at vaccines doses on the encephalon and development in 7 days-old hamsters. *An Fac Med Lima*. 2007; 68(3): 223-237 [Spanish].

[842] http://medical-dictionary.thefreedictionary.com/cerebellum.

[843] Hewitson L, Lopresti BJ, Stott C, Mason NS, Tomko J. Influence of pediatric vaccines on amygdala growth and opioid ligand binding in rhesus macaque infants: A pilot study. *Acta Neurobiol Exp (Wars)*. 2010;70(2):147-64.

[844] Hewitson L, Houser LA, Stott C, Sackett G, Tomko JL, Atwood D, Blue L, White ER. Delayed acquisition of neonatal reflexes in newborn primates receiving a thimerosal-containing hepatitis B vaccine: influence of gestational age and birth weight. *J Toxicol Environ Health A*. 2010;73(19):1298-313. doi: 10.1080/15287394.2010.484709.

[845] Minami T, Miyata E, Sakamoto Y, Yamazaki H, Ichida S. Induction of metallothionein in mouse cerebellum and cerebrum with low-dose thimerosal injection. *Cell Biology and Toxicology*. 2010; 26(2): 143-152.

[846] Sulkowski ZL, Chen T, Midha S, Zavacki AM, Sajdel-Sulkowska EM. Maternal thimerosal exposure results in aberrant cerebellar oxidative stress, thyroid hormone metabolism, and motor behavior in rat pups; sex- and strain-dependent effects. *Cerebellum*. 2012 Jun;11(2):575-86.

[847] Khan A, Sulkowski ZL, Chen T, Zavacki AM, Sajdel-Sulkowska EM. Sex-dependent changes in cerebellar thyroid hormone-dependent gene expression following perinatal exposure to thimerosal in rats. *J Physiol Pharmacol*. 2012 Jun;63(3):277-83.

[848] Lawton M, Iqbal M, Kontovraki M, Lloyd Mills C, Hargreaves AJ. Reduced tubulin tyrosination as an early marker of mercury toxicity in differentiating N2a cells. *Toxicol In Vitro.* 2007 Oct; 21(7): 1258-1261.

[849] http://medical-dictionary.thefreedictionary.com/Neurites; http://medical-dictionary. thefreedictionary.com/axon.

[850] Leong CC, Syed NI, Lorscheider FL. Retrograde degeneration of neurite membrane structural integrity of nerve growth cones following in vitro exposure to mercury. *Neuroreport.* 2001 Mar 26;12(4):733-7.

[851] Xu F, Farkas S, Kortbeek S, Zhang FX, Chen L, Zamponi GW, Syed NI. Mercury-induced toxicity of rat cortical neurons is mediated through N-methyl-D-Aspartate receptors. *Mol Brain.* 2012 Sep 14;5:30. doi: 10.1186/1756-6606-5-30.

[852] Pendergrass JC, Haley BE. *Mercury-EDTA Complex Specifically Blocks Brain-Tubulin-GTP Interactions: Similarity to Observations in Alzheimer's Disease. Status Quo and Perspective of Amalgam and Other Dental Materials. International Symposium Proceedings.* LT Friberg and GN Schrauzer, eds. Georg Thieme Verlag, Stuttgart-New York. 1995; 98-105.

[853] Olczak M, Duszczyk M, Mierzejewski P, Majewska MD. Neonatal administration of a vaccine preservative, thimerosal, produces lasting impairment of nociception and apparent activation of opioid system in rats. *Brain Research.* 2009 Nov; 1301: 143-151.

[854] Olczak M, Duszczyk M, Mierzejewski P, Bobrowicz T, Majewska MD. Neonatal administration of Thimerosal causes persistent changes in mu opioid receptors in the rat brain. *Neurochem Res.* 2010; 35(11): 1840-1847.

[855] Olczak M, Duszczyk M, Mierzejewski P, Wierzba-Bobrowicz T, Majewska MD. Lasting neuropathological changes in rat brain after intermittent neonatal administration of thimerosal. *Folia Neuropathol.* 2010;48(4):258-69.

[856] Olczak M, Duszczyk M, Mierzejewski P, Bobrowicz T, Meyzac K, Majewska MD. Persistent behavioral impairments and alterations of brain dopamine system after early postnatal administration of thimerosal in rats. *Behavioural Brain Res.* 2011 Sep 30; 223(1): 107-118.

[857] http://www.cdc.gov/NCBDDD/autism/facts.html.

[858] Duszczyk-Budhathoki M, Olczak M, Lehner M, Majewska MD. Administration of thimerosal to infant rats increases overflow of glutamate and aspartate in the prefrontal cortex: protective role of dehydroepiandrosterone sulfate. *Neurochem Res.* 2012 Feb;37(2):436-47.

[859] http://www.hhs.gov/opa/familylife/tech_assistance/etraining/adolescent_brain/ Development/prefrontal_cortex/.

[860] Ida-Eto M, Oyabu A, Ohkawara T, Tashiro Y, Narita N, Narita M. Prenatal exposure to organomercury, thimerosal, persistently impairs the serotonergic and dopaminergic systems in the rat brain: implications for association with developmental disorders. *Brain Dev.* 2012 May 31. [Epub ahead of print].

[861] Careaga M, Van de Water J, Ashwood P. Immune dysfunction in autism: a pathway to treatment. *Neurotherapeutics.* 2010 Jul;7(3):283-92.

862 http://lab.rockefeller.edu/steinman/dendritic_intro/.

863 Goth SR, Chu RA, Gregg JP, Cherednichenko G, Pessah IN. Uncoupling of ATP-mediated calcium signaling and dysregulated interleukin-6 secretion in dendritic cells by nanomolar thimerosal. *Environ Health Perspect.* 2006 Jul; 114(7): 1083-1091.

864 Naviaux RK, Zolkipli Z, Wang L, Nakayama T, Naviaux JC, Le TP, Schuchbauer MA, Rogac M, Tang Q, Dugan LL, Powell SB. Antipurinergic therapy corrects the autism-like features in the poly(IC) mouse model. *PLoS One.* 2013;8(3):e57380. doi: 10.1371/journal.pone.0057380. Epub 2013 Mar 13.

865 http://www.sciencedaily.com/releases/2013/03/130313182019.htm.

866 Meyer U, Nyffeler M, Engler A, Urwyler A, Schedlowski M, Knuesel I, Yee BK, Feldon J. The time of prenatal immune challenge determines the specificity of inflammation-mediated brain and behavioral pathology. *J Neurosci.* 2006 May 3;26(18):4752-62.

867 Gardner RM, Nyland JF, Evans SL, Wang SB, Doyle KM, Crainiceanu CM, Silbergeld EK. Mercury induces an unopposed inflammatory response in human peripheral blood mononuclear cells in vitro. *Environ Health Perspect.* 2009 Dec;117(12):1932-8. doi: 10.1289/ehp.0900855. Epub 2009 Aug 19.

Chapter 18:
A Biological Basis for Thimerosal Causing Autism in Humans

The results suggesting a link between Thimerosal and brain damage in animals support similar observation in research with human biology. We'll now review some of the compelling research suggesting a link between the mercury in Thimerosal and autism causation.

Numerous studies have shown that human neurons and nervous system support cells, called glial cells, are sensitive to Thimerosal.[868] Moreover, the different cell types are susceptible to damage in a manner that is consistent with functional changes documented in autism-affected brains on a cellular level.

A key aspect of cellular sensitivity to Thimerosal stems from a breaking down of cells' mercury-clearing pathways, exacerbating the toxicity of the heavy metal. The oxidative stress promoted by Thimerosal harms cellular structures and alters epigenetics, the expression of genes, both of which are especially critical during prenatal and early postnatal periods of development. Besides the toxicity to cells, oxidative stress and epigenetical alternations just mentioned, more studies have hinted at still other ways in which Thimerosal might instigate autism.

To begin with damage to cell types, many researchers have compared mercury's effects on human tissue in the lab using the standard cellular surrogates of neuroblastoma (neuron) and astrocytoma/glioma (glial cell). Studies have shown that not all human nervous system cells appear equally sensitive to Thimerosal, a finding that speaks to a potential pathophysiology for autism. Papers in 2005 and 2009 reported that neuroblastoma cells are significantly more sensitive to damage from mercury and Thimerosal than astrocytoma cells.[869][870] Those results followed a 2004 study by Tarja Toimela and Hanna Tahti, which showed that concentrations of organic and inorganic mercury that do not cause significant damage to astrocytoma cells have a much larger impact on neuroblastoma cells.[871] Meanwhile, Diana Vargas and colleagues in 2005 discovered in autopsies of brains of patients with autism "an active neuroinflammatory process" marked by activation of microglia and astroglia.[872]

An additional study in 2008 advances the potential importance of the preceding results. Edith López-Hurtado and Jorge Prieto examined speech production and processing areas in preserved brain specimens from eight individuals with autism and seven controls. In the brains of individuals with autism, the researchers observed significantly greater average densities of glial cells. In contrast, the overall density of neurons in these individuals with autism was found to be lower than normal, as would be expected given Thimerosal's higher capacity to damage neurons compared to glial cells. Furthermore, the researchers noted significantly increased numbers of lipofuscin-containing neurons in the brain specimens from individuals with autism.[873] Lipofuscin is a depot, or storage site, in cells for heavy metals such as mercury, as was revealed in a 1996 human brain autopsy study of a person occupationally exposed to mercury vapors.[874] The identification of elevated lipofuscin-containing neurons in brains affected by autism is therefore an important pathology finding.[875]

These results, when taken together, begin to paint a compelling portrait of how functional changes caused by mercury exposure in the brain might cause autism in some cases. As a 2010 review of these several studies noted, in discussing López-Hurtado and Prieto's 2008 work:

It is important to note that visual images obtained from the brain samples of patients diagnosed with an ASD were virtually identical in morphology [shape and structure] with those observed in co-cultures of neuroblastoma and astrocytoma cells exposure to [mercury] by Toimela and Tahti.[876]

Studies cited thus far in this chapter along with others that illuminate the brain pathology of Thimerosal exposure have also discovered significant dysfunction in cell structures called mitochondria. Mitochondria are the "power plants" of cells, generating much of the chemical energy a cell needs in order to function and carry out its myriad biological operations. These cellular structures also, for instance, play a role in mediating a cell's growth as well as its programmed death.[877] Thimerosal promotes cell death by triggering the release of certain biomolecules from mitochondria, according to various studies, including those by Samina Makani in 2002, Michelle Humphrey in 2005, Leman Yel in 2005, and Wen-Xue Li in 2012.[878] [879] [880] [881] In 2011, Abha and Ved Chauhan observed mitochondrial deficits in specific brain areas, including the cerebellum and frontal and temporal regions in autistic children.[882] In 2012, Martyn Sharpe documented Thimerosal's toxic effect on mitochondria specifically in normal, healthy human astrocyte cells.[883]

Numerous other studies, in particular by Richard Frye, have explored the consistent association of mitochondrial dysfunction with autism spectrum disorders.[884] [885] Intriguingly, the high-energy organ systems of the central nervous, muscular, and gastrointestinal systems that are affected by mitochondrial disease are also often dysfunctional in patients with autism.[886] A 2010 study has suggested that mitochondrial irregularities occur in up to 80 percent of people with autism.[887]

The Geiers in 2009 also noted mitochondrial dysfunction, cellular degeneration, and death when cultured nervous system and fetal cells were exposed to levels of Thimerosal similar to that known to be induced by fetal and early infant exposure to mercury from vaccines.[888] David Baskin, in 2003, and Michelle Herdman, in 2006, meanwhile, further described how Thimerosal induces neuronal cell death on a biomolecular level.[889] [890] A major factor is oxidative stress, in which free oxygen-containing compounds, or radicals, cause cellular injury, a mechanism investigated by a range of studies, including Chauhan and Chauhan's 2006 work.[891]

A 2011 review study on the plausibility of a mercury-autism connection from a cellular perspective noted these lines of thought, concluding:

> [Mercury] has well-known effects relating to the disruption of sulfur chemistry leading to elevated oxidative stress which, in turn, results into broader physiological/organ affects [sic], particularly to the CNS [central nervous system]. Oxidative stress was consistently elevated in autism. Although this is not unique to autism (as many disease states are associated with this biochemical characteristic), it does suggest that autism is more than just a neurological disease but also a disease which reflects dysfunction at various metabolic levels. Nevertheless, research studies identifying [mercury's] effects on glial cells and mitochondria that are consistent with findings in autistic patients, lend further support to the [mercury]-autism hypothesis.[892]

Corroborating evidence of oxidative stress's role in autism potentially stemming from Thimerosal exposure came in a 2013 study. Researchers led by Phillip Gorrindo looked at levels of F2t-Isoprostanes, a compound considered a "gold standard biomarker of oxidative stress," as the study phrased it, across four groups. These groups included children with autism and gastrointestinal problems, children with autism alone, children with gastrointestinal problems alone, and an unaffected group. The study hypothesized that children with autism and the common comorbidity of gastrointestinal dysfunction would have signs of greater overall metabolic abnormality, given that the brain and gut are both highly metabolically active regions. Indeed, the study found elevated F2t-Isoprostanes in all three affected groups, with the highest levels in the children with autism and gastrointestinal illness.[893]

Another 2013 study further ties together how Thimerosal might negatively impact mitochondrial function through oxidative stress. Sharpe, Baskin and their colleague Taylor Gist obtained samples of cells called B-lymphocytes from eleven families that included people with autism, their twins who do not have autism and also non-twin siblings. The cells were cultured in increasing levels of Thimerosal and studied for their reproduction and mitochondrial function, compared to controls. A subpopulation from four families demonstrated Thimerosal hypersensitivity. In these individuals (two twins and two siblings), the Thimerosal concentration needed to hinder their cellular reproduction was just 40 percent of the concentration that hindered the normal cells of the control group. The hypersensitive cells likewise had greater levels of markers of oxidative stress. The study concluded "certain individuals with a mild mitochondrial defect may be highly susceptible to mitochondrial specific toxins like the vaccine preservative thimerosal," a finding which as we'll see could be very important in explaining autism cases like that of Hannah Poling, covered in Chapter 21.[894]

The oxidative stress damage to various cell types wrought by Thimerosal appears largely caused by the chemical's effects on a powerful antioxidant called glutathione. Besides reining in free radicals, glutathione is also the key defense against mercury in cells because it helps remove the toxic element from the body.[895] A 2005 study by former FDA scientist Jill James evaluated two lines of cells with different levels of glutathione that were then exposed to Thimerosal. James and her coauthors found that those cells that expressed higher levels of glutathione were at a lower risk of Thimerosal toxicity.[896] The study also showed that pretreating cells with glutathione helped them survive in the presence of Thimerosal.[897]

A study published just this year coauthored by Frye and James demonstrated similar results, comparing immune system cell lines from white males with autism to normal white male cell lines. The mitochondria in the cells from the individuals with autism were known to function improperly, especially when challenged by free oxygen radicals. When the researchers subsequently exposed both cell lines to ethylmercury, the cells from the individuals with autism suffered dysfunction compared to the healthy control cells. Increasing the amount of available glutathione reduced the baseline dysfunction of the cells from individuals with autism and blunted their poor response to ethylmercury exposure. The study concluded:

> These findings suggest that the epidemiological link between environmental mercury exposure and an increased risk of developing autism may be mediated through mitochondrial dysfunction and support the notion that a subset of individuals with autism may be vulnerable to environmental influences with detrimental effects on development through mitochondrial dysfunction.[898]

That conclusion is additionally drawn from the fact that not everyone's ability to naturally produce glutathione is the same. A landmark 2004 study by James first found that many children with autism are deficient in their capacity to produce glutathione, as well as the amino acid cysteine, a building block of glutathione. The study showed that children affected by an ASD have mean blood plasma levels that are significantly lower for cysteine (a 19 percent reduction) and for glutathione (a 46 percent reduction) in comparison to normally developed children. These deficits might be innocuous unless a child is exposed to large quantities of mercury.[899][900] Since James's original study, at least eleven other studies have reported significant decreases in glutathione in the plasma of children with autism, averaging about a third lower than the level in normally developing children.[901][902][903][904][905][906][907][908][909][910][911][912]

Other findings also jibe with the idea of the buildup of mercury in the body as a biological basis for autism. Parents have often reported the worsening of symptoms after their child eats certain foods, including dairy products, chocolate, wheat, corn, sugar, apples, and bananas, according to a 1999 study by Antonino Alberti. An inability to effectively metabolize certain compounds in these foods could amplify autistic symptoms, the study proposed. Alberti documented that when compared to controls, children with autism exhibited deficits in their ability to metabolically perform sulfation, which is the addition of sulfate groups to other biological molecules.[913][914] A 2006 review study argued that this sulfation gap could contribute to the accumulation of mercury in a subset of the population, because mercury clearance depends on the binding of the metal to sulfur-containing compounds, called thiols, such as glutathione.[915][916]

With further regard to glutathione, an important process in the biochemical pathway that produces the molecule is methylation. As mentioned earlier in this book, methylation is the addition of a methyl group composed of carbon and hydrogen to a biological molecule.[917] A 2004 study by Mostafa Waly, Richard Deth and colleagues showed that Thimerosal, along with other neurodevelopmental toxins, inhibits the enzyme methionine synthase.[918] This enzyme is needed to form methionine, which in turn is essential for the methylation of fundamental biological structures such as DNA, RNA, proteins, phospholipids, and neurotransmitters. Methylation is the most important process in the epigenetic regulation, which is the selective turning "on" and "off" of genes during development and throughout an organism's lifetime. In addition to disrupting methylation, Thimerosal also limits the production of the antioxidant glutathione, whose levels are significantly lower in children with autism.[919]

A 2013 study by Christina Muratore, Deth and colleagues demonstrated that the levels of mRNA (the messenger molecule that allows genes to make proteins) for methionine synthase are significantly lower in the brain of people with autism, especially at younger ages. The authors wrote:

These novel findings suggest that rather than serving as a housekeeping enzyme, [methionine synthase] has a broad and dynamic role in coordinating metabolism in the brain during development and aging. Factors adversely affecting [methionine synthase] activity, such as oxidative stress, can be a source of risk for neurological disorders across the lifespan via their impact on methylation reactions, including epigenetic regulation of gene expression.[920]

Notably, methionine synthase is dependent on folic acid and vitamin B12. Another recent study in Norway showed that women

219

THIMEROSAL: LET THE SCIENCE SPEAK

who took folic acid supplements before and during the early part of their pregnancies were about 40 percent less likely to have a child with autism.[921] Looking back to 2004, a study published by Marvin Boris and coauthored by Jill James discovered an increased risk of ASD in people with common mutations affecting the folate/methylation cycle.[922] Deth, along with Waly, began discussing in a 2008 study how impaired methylation and increased oxidative stress could serve as a causation model for autism, triggered perhaps by an environmental exposure such as Thimerosal.[923]

Those authors and their colleagues have continued studying autism as a disorder, with many of its cases owing to disrupted epigenetic regulation during development of the central nervous system and other systems experiencing excessive oxidative stress, such as the gastrointestinal and immune systems. With regard to the brain, neurons are at far greater risk of damage from free radicals of oxygen because they have the lowest reported levels of the antioxidant glutathione in any cell type. This is despite the fact that as an organ, the brain consumes oxygen at a rate ten times higher than other tissues. The brain compensates for this lack of glutathione with antioxidant proteins that contain selenium. However, as mentioned in Part One, these selenoproteins have an extreme affinity for binding to mercury. The heavy metal binds to them and is thus retained in the brain, allowing the toxic element to accumulate and interfere with epigenetic regulation.

The gastrointestinal inflammation commonly seen in people with autism associated with oxidative stress, discussed earlier this chapter, ties into this "redox/methylation" causation theory of autism. Inflammation diminishes the body's ability to absorb selenium and cysteine, the precursor to glutathione. In a vicious cycle, more free radicals of oxygen are thus created, reducing methylation activity and altering the epigenetic patterns in intestinal epithelial cells. The epigenetic response to this inflammation is most prominent in a section of the intestines called the terminal ileum, an important area for the absorption of folic acid and vitamin B12 needed for methionine and, ultimately, methylation in the first place.

Based on the drawing of such biochemical connections, in a 2012 study, Waly, Deth, and colleagues including Mady Hornig wrote:

As a developmental disorder in which the availability of [glutathione] is reported to be reduced by almost 40%, autism can be viewed as a syndrome resulting from an imbalance between antioxidant supply and demand—essentially, a state of oxidative stress that interrupts the normal epigenetically based program of development.[924]

The disruption to normal epigenetic patterns of methylation during development caused by the increased oxidative stress in the brain through mercury exposure in the form of Thimerosal remains an intriguing and important area of research.[925]

An unrelated genetic study of interest is the finding that people with gene deletions for two types of glutathione genes are more likely to have allergic reactions to Thimerosal.[926] In addition, a 2003 study suggested that people with a certain version of a gene called apolipoprotein-E are more vulnerable to neurodegenerative disorders because they have trouble clearing mercury from their bodies.[927]

Still other studies have explored how Thimerosal is destructive to nerves. Damani Parran in 2005 described how signaling in cells induced by nerve growth factors, which are integral to neuronal survival and during development, is disrupted by Thimerosal. The effect was seen at Thimerosal concentrations lower than those that kill cells outright.[928]

Another way that the mercury in Thimerosal might be biologically responsible for setting the developing brain on a path towards autism was recently implied. In a *Nature* paper in 2013, researchers from the University of North Carolina School of Medicine demonstrated that the impairment of enzymes called topoisomerases hampers neurodevelopment.[929] It has been known that people with mutations to their topoisomerases can develop autism, as well as other neurodevelopmental disorders. Topoisomerases help unwind DNA which, due to its double helical structure, can become "overwound" during routine cellular processes. The North Carolina scientists noticed that improperly working topoisomerases particularly affected the functioning of "long" genes that occupy a lot of space on a DNA molecule. Interestingly, many autism-linked genes are extremely long. Exposing mouse- and human-derived nerve cells to a topoisomerase-inhibiting chemical resulted in the suppression of almost 50 of the more than 300 genes linked to autism. The findings therefore suggest that environmental exposures to topoisomerase-inhibitors can broadly impact neurodevelopment. Chemotherapy drugs are one kind of chemical identified as interfering with the functioning of topoisomerases.[930] However, as a separate, earlier 2008 study showed, Thimerosal is also a potent inhibitor of a mechanism of action on DNA performed by one of the two main types of topoisomerases. Taken together, the studies convey that through topoisomerase interference,

Thimerosal exposure might impact a wide set of genes that have known roles in triggering autism.[931]

A newly proposed hypothesis could offer further insight into a link between mercury exposure and autism onset. In patients with autism, clinicians have widely documented aberrant connectivity within the brain, as neural regions "talk" to each other. Hyperconnectivity—too much talking—in particular is demonstrated physically by thicker cerebral cortex layers and larger brains, outwardly manifested as the larger heads often seen in people with autism. Some autism patients as well as animals used to model the disorder, as we've discussed previously, have increased levels of a protein called brain-derived neurotrophic factor (BDNF), thought partly responsible for the phenomenon of bigger, hyperconnected brains. Organic mercury, like that in Thimerosal, also notably increases BDNF production. Authors of a 2015 study suggest testing Thimerosal out in animal brains to learn more about this possible relationship.[932]

Overall, the number of parallels between mercury's deleterious effects on neural tissue and the brain pathology in autism are striking. The biomolecular evidence presented in this chapter, along with other intriguing lines of evidence, was catalogued in a sweeping review published in 2012. The study noted some twenty distinct parallels between mercury intoxication and autism brain pathology, which, to quote the technical literature, are as follows:

(1) microtubule degeneration, specifically large, long-range axon degeneration with subsequent abortive axonal sprouting (short, thin axons); (2) dentritic overgrowth; (3) neuroinflammation; (4) microglial/astrocytic activation; (5)

brain immune response activation; (6) elevated glial fibrillary acidic protein; (7) oxidative stress and lipid peroxidation; (8) decreased reduced glutathione levels and elevated oxidized glutathione; (9) mitochondrial dysfunction; (10) disruption in calcium homeostasis and signaling; (11) inhibition of glutamic acid decarboxylase (GAD) activity; (12) disruption of GABAergic and glutamatergic homeostasis; (13) inhibition of IGF-1 and methionine synthase activity; (14) impairment in methylation; (15) vascular endothelial cell dysfunction and pathological changes of the blood vessels; (16) decreased cerebral/cerebellar blood flow; (17) increased amyloid precursor protein; (18) loss of granule and Purkinje neurons in the cerebellum; (19) increased pro-inflammatory cytokine levels in the brain (TNF-α, IFN-γ, IL-1β, IL-8); and (20) aberrant nuclear factor kappa-light-chain-enhancer of activated B cells (NF-κB).[933]

We now will explore further the practical consideration that people with autism might have diminished natural abilities to remove mercury from their bodies. If so, these people should possess significantly altered levels of mercury compared to healthy individuals. The next chapter reviews studies that pertain to this expectation.

Notes

[868] http://www.medterms.com/script/main/art.asp?articlekey=11382.

[869] James SJ, Slikker W 3rd, Melnyk S, New E, Pogribna M, Jernigan S. Thimerosal neurotoxicity is associated with glutathione depletion: protection with glutathione precursors. *Neurotoxicology.* 2005 Jan;26(1):1-8.

[870] Geier DA, King PG, Geier MR. Mitochondrial dysfunction, impaired oxidative-reduction activity, degeneration, and death in human neuronal and fetal cells induced by low-level exposure to Thimerosal and other metal compounds. *Toxicol Environ Chem.* 2009;91: 735–749.

[871] Toimela T, Tähti H. Mitochondrial viability and apoptosis induced by aluminum, mercuric mercury and methylmercury in cell lines of neural origin. *Arch Toxicol.* 2004 Oct;78(10): 565-74.

[872] Vargas DL, Nascimbene C, Krishnan C, Zimmerman AW, Pardo CA. Neuroglial activation and neuroinflammation in the brain of patients with autism. *Ann Neurol.* 2005 Jan;57(1):67-81.

[873] López-Hurtado E, Prieto JJ. A microscopic study of language-related cortex in autism. Am J Biochem. *Biotech.* 2008; 4(2): 130-145.

[874] Opitz H, Schweinsberg F, Grossmann T, Wendt-Gallitelli MF, Meyermann R. Demonstration of mercury in the human brain and other organs 17 years after metallic mercury exposure. *Clin Neuropathol.* 1996 May-Jun; 15(3): 139-144.

[875] Kern JK, Geier DA, Audhya T, King PG, Sykes LK, Geier MR. Evidence of parallels between mercury intoxication and the brain pathology in autism. *Acta Neurobiol Exp (Wars).* 2012;72(2):113-53.

[876] Geier DA, Kern JK, Geier MR. The biological basis of autism spectrum disorders: Understanding causation and treatment by clinical geneticists. *Acta Neurobiol Exp (Wars).* 2010;70(2):209-26.

[877] http://www.britannica.com/EBchecked/topic/386130/mitochondrion.

[878] Makani S, Gollapudi S, Yel L, Chiplunkar S, Gupta S. Biochemical and molecular basis of thimerosal-induced apoptosis in T cells: a major role of mitochondrial pathway. *Genes Immun.* 2002 Aug;3(5):270-8.

[879] Humphrey ML, Cole M, Pendergrass JC, Kiningham KK. Mitochondrial mediated Thimerosal-induced apoptosis in a human neuroblastoma cell line (SK-N-SH). *Neuro Toxicol.* 2005 Jun; 26(3): 407-416.

880 Yel L, Brown LE, Su K, Gollapudi S, Gupta S. Thimerosal induces neuronal cell apoptosis by causing cytochrome c and apoptosis-inducing factor release from mitochondria. *Int J Mol Med.* 2005 Dec;16(6):971-7.

881 Li WX, Chen SF, Chen LP, Yang GY, Li JT, Liu HZ, Zhu W. Thimerosal-induced apoptosis in mouse C2C12 myoblast cells occurs through suppression of the PI3K/Akt/survivin pathway. *PLoS One.* 2012;7(11):e49064. doi: 10.1371/journal.pone.0049064. Epub 2012 Nov 7.

882 Sharpe MA, Livingston AD, Baskin DS. Thimerosal-derived ethylmercury is a mitochondrial toxin in human astrocytes: possible role of Fenton chemistry in the oxidation and breakage of mtDNA. *J Toxicol.* 2012;2012:373678. doi: 10.1155/2012/373678. Epub 2012 Jun 28.

883 Chauhan A, Gu F, Essa MM, Wegiel J, Kaur K, Brown WT, Chauhan V. Brain region-specific deficit in mitochondrial electron transport chain complexes in children with autism. *J Neurochem.* 2011 Apr;117(2):209-20. doi: 10.1111/j.1471-4159.2011.07189.x. Epub 2011 Feb 24.

884 Rossignol DA, Frye RE. Mitochondrial dysfunction in autism spectrum disorders: a systematic review and meta-analysis. *Mol Psychiatry.* 2012 Mar;17(3):290-314. doi: 10.1038/mp.2010.136. Epub 2011 Jan 25.

885 Haas RH. Autism and mitochondrial disease. *Dev Disabil Res Rev.* 2010 Jun;16(2):144-53. doi: 10.1002/ddrr.112.

886 Frye RE, Rossignol DA. Mitochondrial dysfunction can connect the diverse medical symptoms associated with autism spectrum disorders. *Pediatr Res.* 2011 May;69(5 Pt 2):41R-7R.

887 Giulivi C, Zhang YF, Omanska-Klusek A, Ross-Inta C, Wong S, Hertz-Picciotto I, Tassone F, Pessah IN. Mitochondrial dysfunction in autism. *JAMA.* 2010 Dec 1;304(21):2389-96.

888 Geier DA, King PG, Geier MR. Mitochondrial dysfunction, impaired oxidative-reduction activity, degeneration, and death in human neuronal and fetal cells induced by low-level exposure to Thimerosal and other metal compounds. *Toxicol Environ Chem.* 2009 Jun;91(4):735–749.

889 Baskin DS, Ngo H, Didenko VV. Thimerosal induces DNA breaks, caspase-3 activation, membrane damage, and cell death in cultured human neurons and fibroblasts. *Toxicol Sci.* 2003 Aug;74(2):361-8. Epub 2003 May 28.

890 Herdman ML, Marcelo A, Huang Y, Niles RM, Dhar S, Kiningham KK. Thimerosal induces apoptosis in a neuroblastoma model via the cJun N-terminal kinase pathway. *Toxicol Sci.* 2006 Jul; 92(1): 246-253.

891 Chauhan A, Chauhan V. Oxidative stress in autism. *Pathophysiology.* 2006 Aug; 13(3): 171-181.

892 Garrecht M, Austin DW. The plausibility of a role for mercury in the etiology of autism: a cellular perspective. *Toxicol Environ Chem.* 2011 May;93(5-6):1251-1273. Epub 2011 May 20.

893 Gorrindo P1, Lane CJ, Lee EB, McLaughlin B, Levitt P. Enrichment of elevated plasma F2t-isoprostane levels in individuals with autism who are stratified by presence of gastrointestinal dysfunction. *PLoS One.* 2013 Jul 3;8(7):e68444. doi: 10.1371/journal.pone.0068444. Print 2013.

894 Sharpe MA1, Gist TL, Baskin DS. B-lymphocytes from a population of children with autism spectrum disorder and their unaffected siblings exhibit hypersensitivity to thimerosal. *J Toxicol.* 2013;2013:801517. doi: 10.1155/2013/801517. Epub 2013 Jun 9.

895 http://medical-dictionary.thefreedictionary.com/glutathione.

896 http://achri.archildrens.org/researchers/JamesJ.htm.

897 James SJ, Slikker W 3rd, Melnyk S, New E, Pogribna M, Jernigan S. Thimerosal neurotoxicity is associated with glutathione depletion: protection with glutathione precursors. Neurotoxicology. 2005 Jan;26(1):1-8.

898 Rose S, Wynne R, Frye RE, Melnyk S, James SJ. Increased susceptibility to ethylmercury-induced mitochondrial dysfunction in a subset of autism lymphoblastoid cell lines. J Toxicol. 2015;2015:573701. doi: 10.1155/2015/573701. Epub 2015 Jan 21.

899 James SJ, Cutler P, Melnyk S, Jernigan S, Janak L, Gaylor DW, Neubrander JA. Metabolic biomarkers of increased oxidative stress and impaired methylation capacity in children with autism. Am J Clin Nutr. 2004 Dec;80(6):1611-7.

900 Environmental Working Group. Overloaded? New Science, New Insights about Mercury and Autism in Susceptible Children. 2004 available at http://www.ewg.org/reports/autism/.

901 James SJ, Melnyk S, Jernigan S, Cleves MA, Halsted CH, Wong DH, Cutler P, Bock K, Boris M, Bradstreet JJ, Baker SM, Gaylor DW. Metabolic endophenotype and related genotypes are associated with oxidative stress in children with autism. Am J Med Genet B Neuropsychiatr Genet. 2006 Dec 5;141B(8):947-56.

902 Geier DA, Geier MR. A case series of children with apparent mercury toxic encephalopathies manifesting with clinical symptoms of regressive autistic disorders. J Toxicol Environ Health A. 2007 May 15;70(10):837-51.

903 James SJ, Melnyk S, Jernigan S, Hubanks A, Rose S, Gaylor DW. Abnormal transmethylation/transsulfuration metabolism and DNA hypomethylation among parents of children with autism. J Autism Dev Disord. 2008 Nov;38(10):1976. doi: 10.1007/s10803-008-0614-2.

904 James SJ, Melnyk S, Fuchs G, Reid T, Jernigan S, Pavliv O, Hubanks A, Gaylor DW. Efficacy of methylcobalamin and folinic acid treatment on glutathione redox status in children with autism. Am J Clin Nutr. 2009 Jan;89(1):425-30. doi: 10.3945/ajcn.2008.26615. Epub 2008 Dec 3.

905 Adams JB, Baral M, Geis E, Mitchell J, Ingram J, Hensley A, Zappia I, Newmark S, Gehn F, Rubin RA, Mitchell K, Bradstreet J, El-Dahr JM. The severity of autism is associated with toxic metal body burden and red blood cell glutathione levels. J Toxicol. 2009;2009:532640. doi: 10.1155/2009/532640. Epub 2009 Aug 26.

906 Pastural E, Ritchie S, Lu Y, Jin W, Kavianpour A, Khine Su-Myat K, Heath D, Wood PL, Fisk M, Goodenowe DB. Novel plasma phospholipid biomarkers of autism: mitochondrial dysfunction as a putative causative mechanism. Prostaglandins Leukot Essent Fatty Acids. 2009 Oct;81(4):253-64. doi: 10.1016/j.plefa.2009.06.003. Epub 2009 Jul 15.

907 Al-Gadani Y, El-Ansary A, Attas O, Al-Ayadhi L. Metabolic biomarkers related to oxidative stress and antioxidant status in Saudi autistic children. Clin Biochem. 2009 Jul;42(10-11):1032-40. doi: 10.1016/j.clinbiochem.2009.03.011. Epub 2009 Mar 21.

908 Geier DA, Kern JK, Garver CR, Adams JB, Audhya T, Nataf R, Geier MR. Biomarkers of environmental toxicity and susceptibility in autism. J Neurol Sci. 2009 May 15;280(1-2):101-8. doi: 10.1016/j.jns.2008.08.021. Epub 2008 Sep 25.

[909] Geier DA, Kern JK, Garver CR, Adams JB, Audhya T, Geier MR. A prospective study of transsulfuration biomarkers in autistic disorders. *Neurochem Res.* 2009 Feb;34(2):386-93. doi: 10.1007/s11064-008-9782-x. Epub 2008 Jul 9.

[910] Paşca SP, Dronca E, Kaucsár T, Craciun EC, Endreffy E, Ferencz BK, Iftene F, Benga I, Cornean R, Banerjee R, Dronca M. One carbon metabolism disturbances and the C677T MTHFR gene polymorphism in children with autism spectrum disorders. *J Cell Mol Med.* 2009 Oct;13(10):4229-38. doi: 10.1111/j.1582-4934.2008.00463.x.

[911] Adams JB, Audhya T, McDonough-Means S, Rubin RA, Quig D, Geis E, Gehn E, Loresto M, Mitchell J, Atwood S, Barnhouse S, Lee W. Nutritional and metabolic status of children with autism vs. neurotypical children, and the association with autism severity. *Nutr Metab (Lond).* 2011 Jun 8;8(1):34. doi: 10.1186/1743-7075-8-34.

[912] Melnyk S, Fuchs GJ, Schulz E, Lopez M, Kahler SG, Fussell JJ, Bellando J, Pavliv O, Rose S, Seidel L, Gaylor DW, James SJ. Metabolic imbalance associated with methylation dysregulation and oxidative damage in children with autism. *J Autism Dev Disord.* 2012 Mar;42(3):367-77. doi: 10.1007/s10803-011-1260-7.

[913] Alberti A, Pirronea P, Eliab M, Waring RH, Corrado Romano. Sulphation deficit in 'low-functioning' autistic children: a pilot study. *Bio Psychiatry.* 1999; 46: 420-424.

[914] http://medical-dictionary.thefreedictionary.com/sulfation.

[915] Maya L, Luna F. Thimerosal and children's neurodevelopmental disorders. *Ann Fac Med (Lima).* 2006; 67(3); 243-262 [Spanish].

[916] http://medical-dictionary.thefreedictionary.com/thiol.

[917] http://medical-dictionary.thefreedictionary.com/methylation.

[918] Waly M, Olteanu H, Banerjee R, Choi SW, Mason JB, Parker BS, Sukumar S, Shim S, Sharma A, Benzecry JM, Power-Charnitsky VA, Deth RC. Activation of methionine synthase by insulin-like growth factor-1 and dopamine: a target for neurodevelopmental toxins and thimerosal. *Mol Psychiatry.* 2004 Apr;9(4):358-70.

[919] James SJ, Cutler P, Melnyk S, Jernigan S, Janak L, Gaylor DW, Neubrander JA. Metabolic biomarkers of increased oxidative stress and impaired methylation capacity in children with autism. *Am J Clin Nutr.* 2004 Dec;80(6):1611-7.

[920] Muratore CR, Hodgson NW, Trivedi MS, Abdolmaleky HM, Persico AM, Lintas C, De La Monte S, Deth RC. Age-dependent decrease and alternative splicing of methionine synthase mRNA in human cerebral cortex and an accelerated decrease in autism. *PLoS One.* 2013;8(2):e56927. doi: 10.1371/journal.pone.0056927. Epub 2013 Feb 20.

[921] Surén P, Roth C, Bresnahan M, Haugen M, Hornig M, Hirtz D, Lie KK, Lipkin WI, Magnus P, Reichborn-Kjennerud T, Schjølberg S, Davey Smith G, Øyen AS, Susser E, Stoltenberg C. Association between maternal use of folic acid supplements and risk of autism spectrum disorders in children. *JAMA.* 2013 Feb 13;309(6):570-7. doi: 10.1001/jama.2012.155925.

[922] Boris M, Goldblatt A, Galanko J, James S. Association of 5,10-methylenetetrahydrofolate reductase (MTHFR) gene polymorphisms with autistic spectrum disorders. *J Am Phys Surg.* 2004;9:106-8.

[923] Deth R, Muratore C, Benzecry J, Power-Charnitsky VA, Waly M. How environmental and genetic factors combine to cause autism: A redox/methylation hypothesis. *Neurotoxicology*. 2008 Jan;29(1):190-201. Epub 2007 Oct 13.

[924] Waly MI, Hornig M, Trivedi M, Hodgson N, Kini R, Ohta A, Deth R. Prenatal and postnatal epigenetic programming: implications for GI, immune, and neuronal function in autism. *Autism Res Treat*. 2012;2012:190930. doi: 10.1155/2012/190930. Epub 2012 Jun 19.

[925] Deth R, Hodgson N, Trivedi M, Muratore C, Waly M. Autism: a neuroepigenetic disorder. *Autism Science Digest*. Issue 03 *available at* http://www.scribd.com/doc/78560867/Autism-A-Neuroepigenetic-Disorder-Deth-R-et-al#download.

[926] Westphal GA, Schnuch A, Schulz TG, Reich K, Aberer W, Brasch J, Koch P, Wessbecher R, Szliska C, Bauer A, Hallier E. Homozygous gene deletions of the glutathione S-transferases M1 and T1 are associated with thimerosal sensitization. *Int Arch Occup Environ Health*. 2000; 73(6): 384-388.

[927] Godfrey ME, Wojcik DP, Krone CA. Apolipoptrotein E genotyping as a potential biomarker for mercury neurotoxicity. *J Alzheimers Dis*. 2003 Jun; 5: 189-196.

[928] Parran DK, Barker A, Ehrich M. Effects of Thimerosal on NGF signal transduction and cell death in neuroblastoma cells. *Toxicol Sci*. 2005; 86(1): 132-140.

[929] King IF, Yandava CN, Mabb AM, Hsiao JS, Huang HS, Pearson BL, Calabrese JM, Starmer J, Parker JS, Magnuson T, Chamberlain SJ, Philpot BD, Zylka MJ. Topoisomerases facilitate transcription of long genes linked to autism. *Nature*. 2013 Sep 5;501(7465):58-62. doi: 10.1038/nature12504. Epub 2013 Aug 28.

[930] http://news.unchealthcare.org/news/2013/august/researchers-discover-a-potential-cause-of-autism.

[931] Wu X, Liang H, O'Hara KA, Yalowich JC, Hasinoff BB. Thiol-modulated mechanisms of the cytotoxicity of thimerosal and inhibition of DNA topoisomerase II alpha. *Chem Res Toxicol*. 2008 Feb;21(2):483-93. doi: 10.1021/tx700341n. Epub 2008 Jan 16.

[932] Koh JY, Lim JS, Byun HR, Yoo MH. Abnormalities in the zinc-metalloprotease-BDNF axis may contribute to megalencephaly and cortical hyperconnectivity in young autism spectrum disorder patients. *Mol Brain*. 2014 Sep 3;7:64. doi: 10.1186/s13041-014-0064-z.

[933] Kern JK, Geier DA, Audhya T, King PG, Sykes LK, Geier MR. Evidence of parallels between mercury intoxication and the brain pathology in autism. *Acta Neurobiol Exp (Wars)*. 2012;72(2):113-53.

Chapter 19: Correlations between Mercury Levels and Autism Levels

Before launching into this section, we will provide a brief recap of the three previous chapters to create a foundation that supports correlations between mercury levels and autism. First, epidemiological studies have suggested a correlation between mercury exposure and the rate of autism spectrum disorders. Second, animal and human cell models have demonstrated the toxic effects of low-dose mercury exposure on neural tissue. Third, Thimerosal seems to damage the ability of the body to remove mercury, and people with autism might have poor innate clearance mechanisms to begin with. A key extension of these findings in relating Thimerosal exposure to autism is to assess whether children diagnosed with autism are carrying higher mercury body burdens than their peers.

Numerous studies have shown that children with autism tend to have more mercury in their bodies than individuals who do not have autism. Research has also revealed that higher levels of bodily mercury—as well as poorer abilities to excrete mercury—are associated with more severe symptoms of autism.

Some of these studies have gauged mercury levels and clearance ability in the body through an analysis of the trace elements in hair. A study in 2003 by Amy Holmes, Mark Blaxill, and Boyd Haley reported that hair mercury levels in a group of children with autism were about eight times less than in healthy control group children. Interestingly, the study noted that the more severe a case of autism, the lower the amount of mercury present in the affected child's hair: "Within the autistic group, hair mercury levels varied significantly across mildly, moderately, and severely autistic children, with mean group levels of 0.79, 0.46, and 0.21 [parts per million], respectively." The results suggested that hair excretion patterns among infants with autism were significantly reduced relative to normal children.[934] Haley, a coauthor of the paper, adds that it is important to consider that in utero fetuses cannot excrete mercury through the production of feces or urine, so mercury levels can build up in their bodies. This study is controversial, however, because the mean hair concentration in the control group was unusually high when compared to that reported in the National Health and Nutrition Examination Survey. "These issues," wrote Hertz-Picciotto in a book chapter, "combined with absent information regarding whether cases and controls were analyzed simultaneously on the same instruments, whether the laboratory personnel were blinded, and how contamination was addressed, raise concerns about validity of the findings."[935]

Another small 2003 study by Lin-Wen Hu also found lower mercury content in the hair from individuals with autism than in the hair of healthy control individuals.[936] A 2005 study by Fido and Al-Saad in Kuwait found the opposite effect, with children affected by autism possessing higher levels of mercury and other heavy metals in their hair than did healthy subjects. However, the contradictory results could simply be a straightforward indication of higher bodily mercury burden in the autistic group.[937]

A 2010 study found further evidence. It paired age-matched groups of children with and without autism ages three to four and seven to nine years old. In the younger cohort, the children with autism had lower mercury hair concentrations than did their normally developed peers, but the opposite result was found in the older group. As the age of patients with autism increased, therefore, so did the levels of the heavy metal in their hair. The authors wrote:

> Our data seem consistent with the notion that young autistic children might be poor eliminators of heavy metals—hence showing lower mercury levels in the hair—but may retain greater amounts of mercury in their body tissues, including the brain. At adrenarche [an increase in various hormones around eight years of age] their toxin elimination capacity may improve, as reflected by higher levels of mercury in hair of older autistic children.[938 939]

A 2011 Egyptian study found that mercury and copper levels in children's hair correlated with autism severity, although zinc did not.[940] A 2012 study reported similar findings, with autism severity significantly correlating with mercury hair concentrations but not for the other metals tested, which included arsenic, cadmium, lead, chromium, cobalt, nickel, aluminum, tin, uranium, and manganese.[941] Another 2012 study on Saudi Arabian children, like the Kuwaiti study mentioned previously, found elevated hair concentrations for aluminum, arsenic, cadmium, mercury, antimony, nickel, lead, and vanadium in children with autism versus controls. Selenium levels in the autistic sample, notably, were deficient.[942] Even more recent results from studies of Middle Eastern populations include a 2014 study by Heba Yassa that analyzed hair and blood samples from 90 Egyptian children, half of whom have autism. The study reported higher levels of mercury and lead in children with autism than their unaffected peers.[943]

A 2014 study involved children in Oman who have nutritional deficiencies that promote oxidative stress. Omani children with autism had lower levels of the antioxidant glutathione and thus decreased methylation capacity, as discussed in the previous chapter, associated with elevated hair mercury levels. "Since autism in other countries is associated with similar redox and methylation deficits of non-nutritional origin," the study's draft text states, "our results strongly suggest that these metabolic factors are a fundamental feature of autism."[944]

Along with hair, many parts of the body have shown elevated mercury levels in individuals with autism, according to various studies. These include fingernails (Lakshmi Priya and Geetha 2011), blood (DeSoto and Hitlan 2007; Geier 2010; and Yassa 2014, just mentioned above), baby teeth (Adams 2007), and—though not reaching statistical significance—in the brains of children with autism, specifically the cerebellum (Sajdel-Sulkowska, 2008).[945 946 947 948 949]

The DeSoto and Hitlan study just cited bears further discussion. It was a reanalysis of a study by Patrick Ip and colleagues in 2004 that reported essentially no difference in hair and blood mercury levels between ASD-affected and healthy children. The paper categorically stated that "the results from our cohort study with similar environmental mercury exposure indicate that there is no causal relationship between mercury as an environmental neurotoxin and autism."[950] DeSoto and Hitlan pointed out statistical errors in Ip's study, which led to an erratum being published in 2007 in the journal that had published Ip's original paper. Although Ip offered corrections to their data, their erratum maintained that there was no statistically significant difference between the two groups of patients.[951]

When DeSoto and Hitlan reran the numbers, though, they instead found a statistically significant relationship between mercury levels in the blood and diagnosis of an ASD; in other words, blood mercury level could be used to predict an autism diagnosis. Also, according to the reanalysis, participants with autism were significantly more likely to have lower hair mercury levels than would be predicted as a function of their blood levels. This finding is suggestive of patients with autism being more variable and less efficient at excreting mercury. Furthermore, the revised Ip findings for blood mercury had a probability (P) value of 0.056, which is just outside the conventionally accepted threshold for statistical significance of 0.05. DeSoto and Hitlan thought Ip's firm rejection of there being any relationship between blood mercury levels and autism was therefore overstated.[952] As a final note, a separate study that Ip and colleagues also published in 2004 based on the same data set was later retracted in 2008.[953][954]

Less controversially, the screening of urine for compounds called porphyrins has also indicated high body burdens of mercury in those afflicted with autism. A 2006 study by Robert Nataf found that a majority of individuals in a large group of French children with autism excreted excess porphyrin levels compared to controls. The children's porphyrin profile was consistent with environmental heavy metal exposure, in particular mercury. Notably, children with the "mild" form of autism, Asperger's syndrome, did not have changed porphyrin profiles. Furthermore, a subgroup of children with autism in the study treated with a chelating agent that helps remove heavy metals, including mercury, from the body subsequently had their porphyrin excretion levels drop.[955]

A study conducted by the Geiers the same year on US children produced similar findings, again showing that porphyrin levels rose with autism spectrum disorder severity.[956] David Austin and Kerrie Shandley in 2008 extended the results to a third continent, Australia.[957] Seung-Il Youn in 2010 found correlations between liver detoxification and oxidative stress markers with urinary porphyrins, further supporting previous studies.[958] James Woods, who has done extensive work on porphyrins and links to mercury exposure, has also shown that some patients with autism have abnormal porphyrin profiles.[959]

More studies on the matter, such as those by David Geier in 2009 and Janet Kern in 2010, have continued to find that elevated porphyrin levels associated with mercury intoxication correlate with autism severity.[960] [961] In agreement with these findings, the 2011 study by Lakshmi Priya and Geetha, cited just prior, reported higher mercury levels in the hair and nails of children in low-functioning (more severely autistic) patients than in medium- and high-functioning patients.[962] A 2013 study found a strong association of blood levels of toxic metals, in particular cadmium and mercury, with variation in autism severity degree.[963] Another Geier study in 2009 on urinary porphyrins also noted decreased blood plasma levels of glutathione, cysteine, and sulfate in its autism-affected patient group, consistent with the diminished abilities to excrete mercury discussed in the previous chapter.[964]

As a result of findings such as these indicating a high mercury body burden for individuals with autism, some doctors and parents have tried chelation therapy to remove heavy metals from affected children. Chelation has proven successful in lowering blood and urine mercury concentrations and in some cases ameliorating the neurological effects of mercury poisoning. For example, a 1984 report from China described how a couple dozen people poisoned by ethylmercury-contaminated grain responded well to chelation.[965] A 1996 report described a forty-four-year-old man who had received Thimerosal-preserved HepB immunoglobulin following a liver transplant. After developing symptoms such as slurred speech, slow movements and tremors, doctors discovered that the patient had very high blood mercury levels. Administration of a chelating agent known as dimercaptosuccinic acid (DMSA) for five weeks restored the patient's speech and locomotor abilities.[966]

With regard to autism, studies have reported significant improvements in children by removing mercury from their bodies. A 2002 study treated ten patients with autism with thiamine tetrahydrofurfuryl disulfide (TTFD), and all but two of the patients saw a rise in their autism evaluation scores.[967] A study the next year by Jeff Bradstreet compared mercury excretion after a three-day DMSA treatment in children with ASD and a control group. The individuals with an ASD excreted roughly three times as much mercury in their urine as the control group. Furthermore, in an age- and sex-matched comparison of ASD individuals and healthy children—all of whom had been vaccinated—the ASD group excreted about five times more mercury than did the control group. With reference back to the Holmes hair study, discussed previously in this chapter, the study authors wrote:

> Our analysis shows that children who developed autistic spectrum disorders had significantly greater accumulated mercury than controls. Our results are similar to those of the retrospective study by Holmes et al. They observed that there was a significant relationship between increasingly severe autism and decreasing mercury levels in first baby haircuts in comparison to normal controls. Our results and those of Holmes et al. probably result from a decreased ability of children with autistic spectrum disorders to excrete mercury, resulting in the retention of potentially toxic mercury levels.[968]

Further evidence of chelation's benefits came in the previously cited 2014 Yassa study in Egypt. It found a "significant decline in the blood level of lead and mercury with the use of DMSA as a chelating agent," corresponding with "a decline in the autistic symptoms with the decrease in the lead and mercury level in [the] blood."[969] Although chelation has produced positive results for some people with autism, the treatment is still controversial.[970][971] As the nonprofit Autism Research Institute states:

Chelation is not a "cure" for autism. If, in the opinion of a medical doctor, the patient has an unusual heavy-metal burden, chelation might be warranted, just as it would be for a patient who does not have ASD. Additional research is needed to investigate the prevalence and underlying reasons for impaired excretion of environmental toxins, and to determine treatment efficacy.[972]

Moving on from the epidemiological and biological evidence, a final, strong piece of support for a mercury-autism connection is the gender bias in autism diagnoses, with far more males than females presenting. The next chapter will explore a possible basis for this observation.

Notes

[934] Holmes AS, Blaxill MF, Haley BE. Reduced levels of mercury in first baby haircuts of autistic children. *Int J Toxicol*. 2003 Jul-Aug; 22(4): 277-285.

[935] Hertz-Picciotto I. Large Scale Epidemiologic Studies of Environmental Factors in Autism. *Autism Spectrum Disorders*. Amaral DG, Dawson G, Geschwind DH, eds. Oxford University Press, 2011.

[936] Hu L, Bernard J, Che J. Neutron activation analysis of hair samples for the identification of autism. *Trans Am Nuclear Soc*. 2003;89:16-20.

[937] Fido A, Al-Saad S. Toxic trace elements in the hair of children with autism. *Autism*. 2005 Jul;9(3):290-8.

[938] Majewska MD, Urbanowicz E, Rok-Bujko P, Namysłowska I, Mierzejewski P. Age-dependent lower or higher levels of hair mercury in autistic children than in healthy controls. *Acta Neurobiol Exp*. 2010, 70: 196–208.

[939] http://medical-dictionary.thefreedictionary.com/adrenarche.

[940] Elsheshtawy E, Tobar S, Sherra K, Atallah S, Elkasaby R. Study of some biomarkers in the hair of children with autism. *Middle East Current Psychiatry*. 2011, 18:6-10.

[941] Geier DA, Kern JK, King PG, Sykes LK, Geier MR. Hair toxic metal concentrations and autism spectrum disorder severity in young children. *Int J Environ Res Public Health*. 2012 Dec 6;9(12):4486-97. doi: 10.3390/ijerph9124486.

[942] Blaurock-Busch E, Amin OR, Dessoki HH, Rabah T. Toxic metals and essential elements in hair and severity of symptoms among children with autism. *Maedica (Buchar)*. 2012 Jan;7(1):38-48.

[943] Yassa HA. Autism: a form of lead and mercury toxicity. *Environ Toxicol Pharmacol*. 2014 Nov;38(3):1016-24. doi: 10.1016/j.etap.2014.10.005. Epub 2014 Nov 6.

[944] Hodgson NW1, Waly MI, Al-Farsi YM, Al-Sharbati MM, Al-Farsi O, Ali A, Ouhtit A, Zang T, Zhou ZS, Deth RC. Decreased glutathione and elevated hair mercury levels are associated with nutritional deficiency-based autism in Oman. Exp Biol Med (Maywood). 2014 Mar 27.

[945] Lakshmi Priya MD, Geetha A. Level of trace elements (copper, zinc, magnesium and selenium) and toxic elements (lead and mercury) in the hair and nail of children with autism. *Biol Trace Elem Res*. 2011 Aug;142(2):148-58. Epub 2010 Jul 13.

[946] DeSoto MC, Hitlan RT. Blood levels of mercury are related to diagnosis of autism: a reanalysis of an important data set. *J Child Neurol*. 2007 Nov;22(11):1308-11.

947 Geier DA, Audhya T, Kern JK, Geier MR. Blood mercury levels in autism spectrum disorder: is there a threshold level? *Acta Neurobiol Exp (Wars)*. 2010;70(2):177-86.

948 Adams JB, Romdalvik J, Ramanujam VM, Legator MS. Mercury, lead, and zinc in baby teeth of children with autism versus controls. *J Toxicol Environ Health A*. 2007 Jun;70(12):1046-51.

949 Sajdel-Sulkowska EM, Lipinski B, Windom H, Audhya T, McGinnis W. Oxidative stress in autism: elevated cerebellar 3-nitrotyrosine levels. *Am J Biochem Biotechnol*. 2008; 4(2): 73-84.

950 Ip P, Wong V, Ho M, Lee J, Wong W. Mercury exposure in children with autistic spectrum disorder: case-control study. *J Child Neurol*. 2004 Jun; 19(6): 431-4.

951 Erratum. *J Child Neurol*. 2007 22: 1324.

952 DeSoto MC, Hitlan RT. Blood levels of mercury are related to diagnosis of autism: a reanalysis of an important data set. *J Child Neurol*. 2007 Nov; 22(11): 1308-1311.

953 Brumback, RA. The further mercurial adventures of Ip et al. *J Child Neurol*. 2008 Dec;23(12): 1497.

954 Retraction. Environmental mercury exposure in children: South China's experience. *Pediatr Int*. 2008 Aug;50(4):606.

955 Nataf R, Skorupka C, Amet L, Lam A, Springbett A, Lathe R. Porphyrinuria in childhood autistic disorder: implications for environmental toxicity. *Toxicol Appl Pharmacol*. 2006 Jul 15; 214(2): 99-108.

956 Geier DA, Geier MR. A prospective assessment of porphyrins in autistic disorders: a potential marker for heavy metal exposure. *Neurotox Res*. 2006;10:57-63.

957 Austin DW, Shandley K. An investigation of porphyrinuria in Australian children with autism. *J Toxicol Environ Health A*. 2008; 71(20): 1349-1351.

958 Youn SI, Jin SH, Kim SH, Lima S. Porphyrinuria in Korean Children with autism: correlation with oxidative stress. *J Toxicol Environ Health, Part A*. 2010; 73(10): 701-710.

959 Woods JS, Armel SE, Fulton DI, Allen J, Wessels K, Simmonds PL, Granpeesheh D, Mumper E, Bradstreet JJ, Echeverria D, Heyer NJ, Rooney JP. Urinary porphyrin excretion in neurotypical and autistic children. *Environ Health Perspect*. 2010 Oct;118(10):1450-7. Epub 2010 Jun 24.

960 Geier DA, Kern JK, Geier MR. A prospective blinded evaluation of urinary porphyrins verses the clinical severity of autism spectrum disorders. *J Toxicol Environ Health A*. 2009;72(24):1585-91.

961 Kern JK, Geier DA, Adams JB, Geier MR. A biomarker of mercury body-burden correlated with diagnostic domain specific clinical symptoms of autism spectrum disorder. *Biometals*. 2010 Dec; 23(6): 1043-1051.

962 Lakshmi Priya MD, Geetha A. Level of trace elements (copper, zinc, magnesium and selenium) and toxic elements (lead and mercury) in the hair and nail of children with autism. *Biol Trace Elem Res*. 2011 Aug;142(2):148-58. Epub 2010 Jul 13.

963 Adams JB, Audhya T, McDonough-Means S, Rubin RA, Quig D, Geis E, Gehn E, Loresto M, Mitchell J, Atwood S, Barnhouse S, Lee W. Toxicological status of children with autism

vs. neurotypical children and the association with autism severity. *Biol Trace Elem Res.* 2013 Feb;151(2):171-80. doi: 10.1007/s12011-012-9551-1. Epub 2012 Nov 29.

[964] Geier DA, Kern JK, Garver CR, Adams JB, Audhya T, Nataf R, Geier MR. Biomarkers of environmental toxicity and susceptibility in autism. *J Neurol Sci.* 2009 May 15;280(1-2):101-8.

[965] Zhang J. Clinical observations in ethyl mercury chloride poisoning. *Am J Ind Med.* 1984;5(3):251-8.

[966] Lowell JA, Burgess S, Shenoy S, Peters M, Howard TK. Mercury poisoning associated with hepatitis-B immunoglobulin. *Lancet.* 1996 Feb 17; 347(8999): 480.

[967] Lonsdale D, Shamberger RJ, Audhya T. Treatment of autism spectrum children with thiamine tetrahydrofurfuryl disulfide: a pilot study. *Neuro Endocrinol Lett.* 2002; 23: 303-308.

[968] Bradstreet J, Geier DA, Kartzinel JJ, Adams JB, Geier MR. A case-control study of mercury burden in children with autistic spectrum disorders. *J Am Phys Surg.* 2003; 8: 76-79.

[969] Yassa HA. Autism: a form of lead and mercury toxicity. Environ Toxicol Pharmacol. 2014 Nov;38(3):1016-24. doi: 10.1016/j.etap.2014.10.005. Epub 2014 Nov 6.

[970] http://legacy.autism.com/ari/editorials/ed_chelationoverview.htm.

[971] http://www.mayoclinic.com/health/autism-treatment/AN01488.

[972] http://www.autism.com/index.php/about_ari_faq.

Chapter 20:
Mercury's Elevated
Risks for Males

Any hypothesis about the environmental and genetic causes of the autism epidemic must explain the disorder's elevated risk for male children. For those afflicted with "classic" autism—that is, low and moderately functioning individuals—the male-to-female ratio is estimated at four to one. For high-functioning Asperger's syndrome cases, the sex ratio is further skewed, with around eleven males affected for one female. Other neurodevelopmental disorders have a male bias in prevalence as well, including attention deficit and hyperactivity disorder (ADHD), conduct disorder, Tourette Syndrome, dyslexia, and specific language impairment. Yet the preponderance of male versus female cases is far more pronounced in autism and Asperger's.[973]

Mercury poisoning offers a possible yet credible explanation for this observed gender divergence. Various studies have shown that both animal and human males are more susceptible to mercury toxicity than females.

Polly Sager, for instance, in 1984 discovered that cell division in the brains of young, mercury-exposed mice was inhibited more in males than females.[974] A. D. Rossi in 1997 showed that giving a low dose of mercury to pregnant rats decreased the locomotor activity of their adult male offspring but not the female pups.[975] A study by some of the same authors in 2011 indicated that male susceptibility is already evident in youth and that brain maturation is affected.[976] Meanwhile, Donald Branch in 2009 documented that high-dose Thimerosal given to seven male and seven female mice resulted in the deaths of all of the males but none of the females.[977]

Now on to human results. In a mercury-exposed population of Cree Indian children in Quebec, Gail McKeown-Eyssen observed abnormalities in muscle tone or reflexes just in boys, though the study questioned the importance of its own findings.[978] Philippe Grandjean in 1998 reported that among a group of humans exposed to mercury while in the womb via their mother's diets, boys did worse than girls did on several neuropsychological tests.[979] Vahter reviewed some of these animal and human studies in 2007, among others, and commented that "gender differences in exposure to toxic metals have been well documented" in the literature.[980]

A key reason for the heightened sensitivity to mercurials in males appears to be greater levels of the quintessential male hormone, testosterone.[981] In tissue culture experiments by Haley in 2005, testosterone amplified the neuronal toxicity of Thimerosal, whereas the classical female hormone estrogen diminished toxicity.[982]

Biochemically, it seems that testosterone acts synergistically with mercury, increasing its toxicity by preventing removal from the body. In turn, the presence of mercury disrupts hormonal pathways that then lead to the production of more testosterone and other male hormones called androgens.[983] Such a relationship is supported by findings of testosterone and other androgen levels being abnormally high in animals and humans exposed to low-dose mercury. In 1997, H. C. Freeman and G. B. Sangalang documented the phenomenon in gray seals that eat mercury-contaminated fish and shellfish.[984] A 1994 study of human workers exposed to mercury reported a correlation between serum testosterone levels and cumulative mercury exposure.[985] Other studies have reported on mercury impacting enzyme activity in a way that would be expected to raise androgen levels, such as those by James Veltman and Mahin Maines in 1986, Shawn Gerstenberger in 2000, and Faye Xu in 2002.[986 987 988]

Those results dovetail with a report of abnormally high androgen levels in patients with autism published back in 1997. Tordjman found that 1 in 3 prepubescent children diagnosed with an ASD had significantly increased plasma testosterone levels relative to control subjects. The study was prompted by the noted male bias in ASD diagnoses and observations of precocious development of secondary sexual characteristics, such as pubic hair, in prepubescent patients afflicted with autism.[989]

A 2010 study using the CDC's VSD database found evidence for this observed phenomenon of early onset of puberty. Researchers reported on significantly increased rate ratios of premature puberty in a population of children born between 1990 and 1996 who received an additional 100 microgram exposure of mercury from Thimerosal-containing vaccines.[990]

Further work on androgen levels in autistic patients includes a small study in 2010 showing elevated levels of dehydroepiandrosterone (DHEA) and serum testosterone relative to age- and sex-specific reference ranges.[991] A larger subsequent ASD patient group showed higher levels of various androgens, including serum testosterone (158 percent), serum free testosterone (214 percent), percent free testosterone (121 percent), DHEA (192 percent), and androstenedione (173 percent) in comparison with controls.[992]

DHEA is important for its role in testosterone production. Testosterone is regulated in part by the conversion of DHEA to a metabolite called dehydroepiandrosterone-sulfate (DHEA-S) by the enzyme known as HST. If less HST is available, DHEA increases and leads to more testosterone. The maintenance of HST depends on sulfation and glutathione, which, as Chapter 18 explained, are disrupted by mercury.[993] Accordingly, DHEA-S levels should be reduced in individuals with autism, assuming greater mercury body burdens than controls, and this result was indeed confirmed in a 2005 study by Strous.[994]

A finding from over sixty years ago also shows that mercury intoxication derails a developing hormonal system and leads to excessive androgen production. Young sufferers of acrodynia, or "pink disease," which is now known to have been primarily caused by the use of mercurous chloride teething powders in infants, often exhibited high levels of androgen hormones, altered adrenocortical secretion, and even pseudohermaphroditism (improper sexual organ development), according to D. B. Cheek in 1951.[995]

More recent findings not directly associated with mercury offer further insights into how hormonal balances are upset in autism. In 2006, Rebecca Knickmeyer reported that females with ASD experience menarche—their first menstrual period—an average of eight months later than healthy females. This report also noted that some women with ASD can have extremely delayed onsets. Exposure to excessive androgens in the womb was cited as one possibility for inducing the delayed menarche.[996] Although the study's findings appear to be in contradiction to the average early onset of puberty seen in Geier 2010, both studies point to increased androgen activity as a potential cause of the mistimed onsets.[997] [998] A study in 2007 by Erin Ingudomnukul, coauthored by Knickmeyer, found that women with ASDs do indeed have elevated rates of nine testosterone-related disorders, including hirsutism, irregular menstrual cycles, and severe acne.[999]

The picture is still not complete regarding why so many more males receive an autism diagnosis than females. Nor, of course, is the overall etiology of all autism cases clear. Yet, as this Part Three has aimed to show, epidemiological evidence, animal studies, human studies, and even the gender bias in autism as a sort of "nail in the coffin" all generally fit with the theory of mercury exposure from Thimerosal contributing to triggering the disorder.

Notes

973 Baron-Cohen S, Lombardo MV, Auyeung B, Ashwin E, Chakrabarti B, Knickmeyer R. Why are autism spectrum conditions more prevalent in males? *PLoS Biol.* 2011 Jun;9(6):e1001081. Epub 2011 Jun 14.

974 Sager PR, Aschner M, Rodier PM. Persistent, differential alterations in developing cerebellar cortex of male and female mice after methylmercury exposure. *Brain Res.* 1984 Jan;314(1):1-11.

975 Rossi AD, Ahlbom E, Ogren SO, Nicotera P, Ceccatelli S. Prenatal exposure to methylmercury alters locomotor activity of male but not female rats. *Exp Brain Res.* 1997 Dec;117(3):428-36.

976 Giménez-Llort L, Ahlbom E, Daré E, Vahter M, Ögren S, Ceccatelli S. Prenatal exposure to methylmercury changes dopamine-modulated motor activity during early ontogeny: age and gender-dependent effects. *Environ Toxicol Pharmacol.* 2001 Jan 1;9(3):61-70.

977 Branch DR. Gender-selective toxicity of thimerosal. *Experimental Toxicol Pathol.* 2009 Mar; 61(2): 133-136.

978 McKeown-Eyssen GE, Ruedy J, Neims A. Methyl mercury exposure in northern Quebec. II. Neurologic findings in children. *Am J Epidemiol.* 1983 Oct;118(4):470-9.

979 Grandjean P, Weihe P, White RF, Debes F. Cognitive performance of children prenatally exposed to "safe" levels of methylmercury. *Environ Res.* 1998 May;77(2):165-72.

980 Vahter M, Åkesson A, Lidén C, Ceccatellia S, Berglund M. Gender differences in the disposition and toxicity of metals. *Environ Res.* 2007 May; 104(1): 85-95.

981 http://medical-dictionary.thefreedictionary.com/testosterone.

982 Haley BE. Mercury toxicity: Genetic susceptibility and synergistic effects. *Med Veritas.* 2005; 2: 535-542.

983 Geier DA, Kern JK, Geier MR. The biological basis of autism spectrum disorders: Understanding causation and treatment by clinical geneticists. *Acta Neurobiol Exp (Wars).* 2010;70(2):209-26.

984 Freeman HC, Sangalang GB. A study of the effects of methyl mercury, cadmium, arsenic, selenium, and a PCB, (aroclor 1254) on adrenal and testicular steroidogenesesin vitro, by the gray seal Halichoerus grypus. *Arch Environ Contam Toxicol.* 1977; 5(1): 369-383.

985 Barregård L, Lindstedt G, Schütz A, Sällsten G. Endocrine function in mercury exposed chloralkali workers. *Occup Environ Med.* 1994; 51: 536-540.

⁹⁸⁶ Veltman JC, Maines MD. Alterations of heme, cytochrome P-450, and steroid metabolism by mercury in rat adrenal. *Arch Biochem Biophys.* 1986 Aug 1; 248(2): 467-478.

⁹⁸⁷ Gerstenberger SL, Heimler I, Smies R, Hutz RJ, Dasmahapatra AK, Tripoli V, Dellinger JA. Minimal endocrine alterations in rodents after consumption of lake trout (Salvelinus namaycush). *Arch Environ Contamin Toxicol.* 2000; 38(3): 371-376.

⁹⁸⁸ Xu F, Suiko M, Sakakibara Y, Pai TG, Liu MC. Regulatory effects of divalent metal cations on human cytosolic sulfotransferases. *J Biochem.* 2002 Sep;132(3):457-62.

⁹⁸⁹ Tordjman S, Ferrari P, Sulmont V, Duyme M, Roubertoux P. Androgenic activity in autism. *Am J Psychiatry.* 1997 Nov; 154(11): 1626-17.

⁹⁹⁰ Geier DA, Young HA, Geier MR. Thimerosal exposure and increasing trends of premature puberty in the Vaccine Safety Datalink. *Indian J Med Res.* 2010;131:500-7.

⁹⁹¹ Geier DA, Geier MR. A clinical and laboratory evaluation of methionine cycle-transsulfuration and androgen pathway markers in children with autistic disorders. *Horm Res.* 2006;66(4):182-8. Epub 2006 Jul 5.

⁹⁹² Geier DA, Geier MR. A prospective assessment of androgen levels in patients with autistic spectrum disorders: biochemical underpinnings and suggested therapies. *Neuro Endocrinol Lett.* 2007 Oct;28(5):565-73.

⁹⁹³ Geier DA, Kern JK, Geier MR. The biological basis of autism spectrum disorders: Understanding causation and treatment by clinical geneticists. *Acta Neurobiol Exp (Wars).* 2010;70(2):209-26.

⁹⁹⁴ Strous RD, Golubchik P, Maayan R, Mozes T, Tuati-Werner D, Weizman A, Spivak B. Lowered DHEA-S plasma levels in adult individuals with autistic disorder. *Eur Neuropsychopharmacol.* 2005 May;15(3):305-9.

⁹⁹⁵ Cheek DB, Hetzel BS, Hine DC. Evidence of adrenal cortical function in pink disease. *Med J Aust.* 1951 Jul 7; 2(1): 6-8 *as described in* Geier DA, Kern JK, Geier MR. The biological basis of autism spectrum disorders: Understanding causation and treatment by clinical geneticists. *Acta Neurobiol Exp (Wars).* 2010;70(2):209-26.

⁹⁹⁶ Knickmeyer RC, Wheelwright S, Hoekstra R, Baron-Cohen S. Age of menarche in females with autism spectrum conditions. *Dev Med Child Neurol.* 2006 Dec;48(12):1007-8.

⁹⁹⁷ Geier DA, Geier MR. A prospective assessment of androgen levels in patients with autistic spectrum disorders: biochemical underpinnings and suggested therapies. *Neuro Endocrinol Lett.* 2007 Oct;28(5):565-73.

⁹⁹⁸ Geier DA, Young HA, Geier MR. Thimerosal exposure and increasing trends of premature puberty in the Vaccine Safety Datalink. *Indian J Med Res.* 2010;131:500-7.

⁹⁹⁹ Ingudomnukul E, Baron-Cohen S, Wheelwright S, Knickmeyer R. Elevated rates of testosterone-related disorders in women with autism spectrum conditions. *Horm Behav.* 2007 May;51(5):597-604. Epub 2007 Feb 8.

Chapter 21:
The Hannah Poling Case, the Vaccine Court, and Genetic Predisposition for Autism

We conclude Part Three by reviewing the National Vaccine Injury Compensation Program (VICP) and cases of interest before it, such as that of Hannah Poling. In this controversial case, vaccines were first implicated in a VICP decision for involvement in the onset of autism, specifically for a child with a mitochondrial disorder. The particular pathology might explain a significant number of autism cases, given that recent studies have suggested that mitochondrial disorders occur in a majority of autism patients. Overall, the

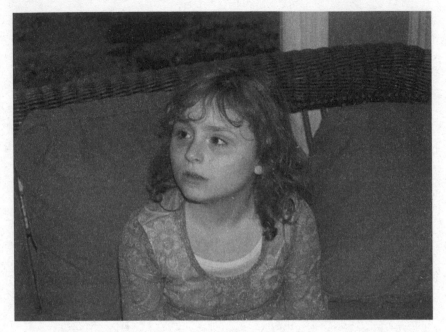

Hannah Poling around the time of the VICP decision. Credit: Terry Poling

Poling case serves as a powerful example of a relatively clear-cut link between Thimerosal-containing vaccines and significant brain damage.

Born in December 1998, Hannah met developmental milestones through the first year-and-a-half of her life. In July 2000, she received five vaccination shots covering nine diseases: diphtheria, pertussis, tetanus, Haemophilus influenzae, measles, mumps, rubella, polio, and varicella. Two days later, Hannah became feverish, lethargic, and irritable. Over the next several months, Hannah continued to suffer from fevers and diarrhea, among other ailments, and lost social and language skills. By early 2001, she had been diagnosed with "regressive encephalopathy with features consistent with an autistic spectrum disorder, following normal development." ("Encephalopathy" broadly means a disorder of the brain, but when considered by the VICP it has specific clinical presentations, as we will discuss further below.)[1000] Later in 2001, tests revealed that Hannah had a mitochondrial disorder. Although Hannah's condition did improve with treatment, her doctor noted in 2004 that Hannah would continue to need services in speech, occupational, physical, and behavioral therapy.[1001]

Hannah's parents, believing her injury to be a result of vaccinations, submitted a claim in 2002 to the "Vaccine Court," the popular name given to the Office of Special Masters of the US Court of Federal Claims, which administers the VICP.[1002 1003] The VICP had been congressionally created in 1986 to serve as a venue "whereby persons allegedly suffering injury or death as a result of the administration of certain compulsory childhood vaccines may petition the federal government for monetary damages," according to the VICP's website.[1004 1005] In March 2008, Hannah's parents went public with the decision—rendered by the Department of Health and Human Services (HHS) in November 2007—to concede that Hannah's injuries were vaccine-induced.[1006 1007] The court issued a compensatory award in 2010.[1008]

The Poling case garnered significant media attention, in part because Hannah's parents are Jon Poling, a neurologist trained at Johns Hopkins, and Terry Poling, a registered nurse and attorney.[1009 1010] Although Jon Poling did not disclose it at the time, he had authored a 2006 case study describing his daughter's fully diagnosed autism and mitochondrial dysfunction as well.[1011] The published study, however, was not factored into the Vaccine Court's proceedings.[1012 1013]

More significantly, the case stood out for being the first autism adjudication deemed by the VICP as "compensable." Since the VICP's creation, petitioners have filed nearly 16,000 petitions as of March 4, 2015, over 5,600 of which involve autism. To date, the VICP has awarded close to $2.9 billion in over 4,000 instances where the child died or suffered permanent injury and brain damage caused by vaccines.[1014]

In 2002, a surge of hundreds of autism claims—which expanded to thousands over the next two years—prompted the VICP to establish the Omnibus Autism Proceeding (OAP). The OAP evaluated three theories for vaccines causing autism by selecting three "test cases" in the program to help in the assessment of each theory. These three theories of "general causation," the phrase used in the VICP documents, were as follows: "(1) that MMR [measles, mumps, and rubella] vaccines and thimerosal-containing vaccines can combine to cause autism; (2) that thimerosal-containing vaccines can alone cause autism; and, (3) that MMR vaccines alone can cause autism." (A conclusion on the third theory was never presented because the evidence relevant to that theory was reviewed under the first theory.)[1015]

After years of hearings and review, in February 2009, the program's special masters ruled against the petitioners in the three test cases of the joint MMR-Thimerosal causation theory, thus closing that avenue for compensation through the VICP. In March 2010, the test cases for the second causation theory of Thimerosal-containing vaccines alone were also ruled against. As a result, the 4,700 or so claims at the time before the VICP of autism causation were dismissed en masse.[1016]

The Poling case, interestingly, was to be one of the three Thimerosal test cases reviewed under the second theory prior to HHS and the Department of Justice conceding it.[1017] Andrew Zimmerman—then at the Kennedy Krieger Institute, now at Massachusetts General Hospital—provided expert testimony regarding Hannah's condition as well as that of a child named Michelle Cedillo, whose petition ended up serving as one of the eventually dismissed test cases.[1018] Zimmerman stated that the cause for Hannah's "regressive encephalopathy" was an "underlying mitochondrial dysfunction, exacerbated by vaccine-induced fever and immune stimulation that exceeded metabolic energy reserves."[1019] Given that Hannah demonstrably had autism—Zimmerman was a coauthor of Jon Poling's 2006 study stating as much—Zimmerman's testimony in effect said that vaccines caused Hannah's condition. In the Cedillo case, however, Zimmerman's testimony differed considerably. He rejected any link between mercury exposure and autism and blamed genetics for Cedillo's neurodevelopmental deficits.[1020] The Cedillo case's testimony fit, conveniently and thoroughly, with the government's position that Thimerosal does not cause autism.

Other children might very well have developed autism for the same reasons Hannah did. The mitochondrial disorder that, according to the government, predisposed Poling to her condition is apparently asymptomatic; prior to vaccination, Hannah was an "alert and active" child, her pediatrician observed. Although she did experience chronic ear infections, she was healthy, and she did not suffer from lethargy or other obvious deficits of energy.[1021]

In a press briefing on March 6, 2008, about the leaked Poling decision—though case-specific details could not be discussed—CDC director Julie Gerberding characterized Hannah's case as a "really very special situation in a child who was genetically predisposed" and that "we need to have an open mind about causes of autism even if they're rare or unusual causes of autism."[1022] According to an article by Kirby, however, a conference call held a few days later suggested that Hannah's case might not be so unusual. During the March 11, 2008, call between CDC vaccine safety officials, vaccine safety research experts, and a health insurance trade organization, a doctor discussed an unpublished study of thirty children with autism, including Hannah, who had regressed. All of them had mild mitochondrial dysfunction as well as elevations or imbalances in the same liver enzymes and amino acids as Hannah experienced. Participants on the call also speculated that as many as 2 percent, or 1 in 50 people, may possess a genetic mutation for mild mitochondrial dysfunction.[1023]

Participants also discussed Portuguese research by Guiomar Oliveira showing notable correlations between autism and mitochondrial disease. Studies in 2005 and 2007 detected mitochondrial disorders in 7.2 percent of a population, "suggesting that this might be one of the most common disorders associated with autism."[1024][1025] A small study referenced previously in Part Three and published since the Poling decision pegs the percent at a far higher figure. The 2010 study reported that eight out of the ten children with autism it examined had biological markers for mitochondrial dysfunction.[1026] Also important to note is that low levels of mercury toxicity could actually induce mitochondrial dysfunction accompanied by oxidative stress, as suggested by studies cited in this book.[1027]

In the 2007 Poling decision and subsequent decision documents, HHS medical personnel would not fully concede to an autism diagnosis. The 2007 Poling case text stated that the vaccinations Hannah received on July 19, 2000, "significantly aggravated an underlying mitochondrial disorder, which predisposed her to deficits in cellular energy metabolism, and manifested as a regressive encephalopathy with features of autism spectrum disorder."[1028 1029 1030]

Besides such indirect language, the VICP's online public statistics records went to additional lengths to disavow any link between autism and vaccine exposure, as might be implied by the Poling concession. A VICP "Data & Statistics" web page has historically presented information regarding adjudications, awards paid, a list of vaccines reported as sources of claimed injuries, and so on (see Figure 15).

In the "Adjudications" section, a chart had listed the total case numbers by year since 1989 under two overarching columns of "Non-Omnibus Autism Proceeding" (essentially, non-autism claims) and "Omnibus Autism Preceding" (autism claims). The single compensable OAP case through fiscal year 2010—Hannah Poling's—received a double asterisk next to it in the chart, directing readers to a nearby statement that said: "HHS has never concluded in any case that autism was caused by vaccination."[1031] Another case deemed compensable in fiscal year 2012 also received this double asterisk, likewise shown in Figure 15. Over the last few years, several more cases that were once part of the OAP have similarly been conceded. Rather than continuing to list compensable autism cases online with this double asterisk, sometime in the spring of 2013, the online Data & Statistics page for the VICP

II. Adjudications [1]

Fiscal Year	Non-Omnibus Autism Proceeding			Omnibus Autism Proceeding			Total
	Compensable	Dismissed	Sub-Total	Compensable*	Dismissed	Sub-Total	
FY 1989	9	12	21	0	0	0	21
FY 1990	100	33	133	0	0	0	133
FY 1991	141	447	588	0	0	0	588
FY 1992	166	487	653	0	0	0	653
FY 1993	125	588	713	0	0	0	713
FY 1994	162	446	608	0	0	0	608
FY 1995	160	575	735	0	0	0	735
FY 1996	162	408	570	0	0	0	570
FY 1997	189	198	387	0	0	0	387
FY 1998	144	181	325	0	0	0	325
FY 1999	98	139	237	0	0	0	237
FY 2000	125	104	229	0	0	0	229
FY 2001	86	87	173	0	0	0	173
FY 2002	104	99	203	0	4	4	207
FY 2003	56	78	134	0	21	21	155
FY 2004	62	122	184	0	111	111	295
FY 2005	60	70	130	0	51	51	181
FY 2006	69	82	151	0	109	109	260
FY 2007	83	86	169	0	34	34	203
FY 2008	147	80	227	0	55	55	282
FY 2009	134	44	178	0	187	187	365
FY 2010	179	79	258	1**	214	215	473
FY 2011	259	106	365	0	1,265	1,265	1,630
FY 2012	254	144	398	1**	2,292	2,293	2,691
FY 2013	92	31	123	0	221	221	344
Totals	3,166	4,726	7,892	2	4,564	4,566	12,458

*May include case(s) that were originally filed and processed as an OAP cases but in which the final adjudication does not include a finding of vaccine-related autism.

**HHS has never concluded in any case that autism was caused by vaccination.

FIGURE 15

changed formats, no longer dividing the Adjudications section into the two non-autism and autism columns, and thus doing away with double asterisks for OAP cases. (The VICP's newly formatted statistics are now compiled in a PDF document available via a new web page.)[1032]

A further review of the VICP offers some insight into the sort of splitting of hairs when it has come to acknowledging autism versus other forms of vaccine-induced brain damage. The Health Resources and Services Administration (HRSA), which manages the VICP under HHS, maintains a Vaccine Injury Table. This table lists and explains injuries and conditions that are presumed to be caused by vaccines. Petitioners who do not meet these eligibility criteria must prove that the administered vaccine caused the injury or condition. Although HRSA has refused to include autism among the compensable brain injuries for any vaccine, the agency does accept the term "encephalopathy," used in the Poling case, for instance. "Encephalopathy" on the Vaccine Injury Table refers generally to a decreased or absent response to the environment—for example, through a lack of eye contact—and is often associated with seizure activity.[1033]

Interviews by the book's author with a lawyer who has practiced before the Vaccine Court, along with a close observer of the court, have revealed that the surrogate terms "encephalopathy" or "seizure disorder" appear more acceptable to the court than "autism." Accordingly, lawyers file cases using these popular euphemisms for "autism" based on the far higher probability of their clients, the petitioners, ultimately being compensated.[1034][1035] In a *CBS News* piece in September 2010, Sharyl Attkisson reported on this trend, writing:

Children who end up with autistic symptoms or autism have won vaccine injury claims over the years—as long as they highlighted general, widely-accepted brain damage; not autism specifically. But when autism or autistic symptoms are alleged as the primary brain damage, the cases are lost . . . some families who believe vaccines caused autism in a loved one are circulating these words of advice: use "encephalopathy" in vaccine court and you're more likely to win. Argue "autism" and you're sure to lose.[1036]

A 2011 study published in *Pace Environmental Law Review* has supported this claim of positive adjudications with regard to encephalopathy as a sort of stand-in for autism. The preliminary study showed that children in 83 out of some 200 sample cases awarded damages for vaccine-induced encephalopathy have also been diagnosed with autism. In other words, the study revealed a 41.5 percent rate of autism among VICP awardees claiming that their children were neurologically damaged by vaccines.[1037]

Also cited in this study is a February 2009 email response to journalist and author David Kirby by an HRSA communications officer named David Bowman. The response indirectly admitted to encephalopathy acting as a compensable finding in place of autism:

The government has never compensated, nor has it ever been ordered to compensate, any case based on a determination that autism was actually caused by vaccines. We have compensated cases in which children exhibited an encephalopathy, or general brain disease. Encephalopathy may be accompanied by a medical progression of an array of symptoms including autistic behavior, autism, or seizures.

Some children who have been compensated for vaccine injuries may have shown signs of autism before the decision to compensate, or may ultimately end up with autism or autistic symptoms, but we do not track cases on this basis.

The Bowman response was apparently meant to dispel any connection between vaccine exposure and autism development, yet the "encephalopathy" that supposedly separates the two seems more, in fact, like a bridge linking them.

To close this book chapter and part, we will briefly review the language used in cases recently and subsequently settled after Hannah Poling and the *Pace Environmental Law Review* study. These cases' files serve to further document this ongoing phenomenon of "autism" being unspeakable in compensations, despite its presence in the very subjects compensated by the VICP.

In December 2012, several such decisions were issued. One case was that of Elias Tembenis, originally part of the OAP, but later decided outside of this proceeding. According to the petitioners, Tembenis came down with Pervasive Developmental Disorder (otherwise called PDD-NOS), an autism spectrum disorder, among other developmental disorders and epilepsy, following a DTaP vaccination. Tembenis received the shot in December 2000, so the vaccine could plausibly have contained Thimerosal. The child eventually died at age seven. The VICP ruled that the vaccine exposure was indeed the cause of Tembenis's epilepsy and death, resulting in a substantial compensation. The autism spectrum disorder component of the case, however, was not cited by the VICP in rendering compensation.[1038][1039][1040]

Another example is that of Emily Paige Lowrie. A July 2000 DTaP vaccine triggered, in her expert witness doctor's words as recorded in the VICP files, "encephalopathy characterized by speech delay and probable global development delay that occurred in the setting of temporal association with immunizations as an acute encephalopathy" and "paroxysmal episodes," or seizure-like event.[1041] In a *Huffington Post* story in 2013, Emily's mother said that her daughter also had PDD-NOS.[1042] The case was compensated for over a million dollars.[1043] Based on the preceding evidence offered in this book chapter, it might have worked to the petitioner's advantage in Emily's case that autism spectrum disorder terminology was not used by her doctor in official court filings.

Yet another case decided recently shows that it is not just claims surrounding potentially Thimerosal-containing vaccines that cannot invoke "autism," despite it being a clinical feature in vaccine-injured children. Ryan Mojabi's parents claimed he had developed autism and asthma following an encephalopathy due to vaccines and in particular measles, mumps, and rubella (MMR), administered between March 2003 and February 2005. The case was awarded nearly $970,000. The decision did not address the asthma or autism claims directly, instead allowing that Mojabi suffered a Table-defined injury of "encephalitis"—a term used interchangeably on the Table with "encephalopathy"—"within five to fifteen days" of receipt of an MMR vaccine in December 2013.[1044]

The preceding discussion of the VICP speaks to some of the controversy that surrounds government health agencies' handling of the autism epidemic. Next, in Part Four, we will turn to the evidence of negligence, and even malfeasance, at the CDC in its scientific accounting and public handling of the Thimerosal-preserved vaccine issue and neurodevelopmental disorders.

Notes

1000 http://www.ninds.nih.gov/disorders/encephalopathy/encephalopathy.htm.

1001 Transcript, United States Court of Federal Claims Office of Special Masters. Nov 9, 2007 *available at* http://www.huffingtonpost.com/david-kirby/the-vaccineautism-court-d_b_88558. html.

1002 United States Court of Federal Claims Office of Special Masters. Attorneys' Fees and Costs; Reasonable Amount Requested to which Respondent Does Not Object. No. 02-1466V. Jan 28, 2011. http://www.uscfc.uscourts.gov/sites/default/files/CAMPBELL-SMITH.POLING012811.pdf.

1003 http://en.wikipedia.org/wiki/Vaccine_court.

1004 http://www.uscfc.uscourts.gov/vaccine-programoffice-special-masters.

1005 http://www.hrsa.gov/vaccinecompensation/index.html.

1006 Offit PA. Vaccines and autism revisited—the Hannah Poling case. *N Engl J Med.* 2008 May 15;358(20):2089-91.

1007 http://www.nytimes.com/2008/03/08/us/08vaccine.html.

1008 United States Court of Federal Claims Office of Special Masters. MMR Vaccine; Thimerosal-Containing Vaccines; Autism Spectrum Disorder; Finding of Entitlement; Damages Decision Based on Proffer. July 21, 2010. http://www.uscfc.uscourts.gov/sites/default/files/CAMPBELLSMITH.%20DOE77082710.pdf.

1009 http://www.athensneuro.com/medicalstaff.html#poling.

1010 http://www.cnn.com/2008/HEALTH/conditions/03/06/vaccines.autism/.

1011 Poling JS, Frye RE, Shoffner J, Zimmerman AW. Developmental Regression and Mitochondrial Dysfunction in a Child with Autism. *J Child Neurol.* 2006 Feb; 21(2): 170–172.

1012 Poling JS. Correspondence on "Developmental Regression and Mitochondrial Dysfunction in a Child with Autism." *J Child Neurol.* 2008 Sep 23(9): 1089.

1013 Brumback RA. The appalling Poling saga. *J Child Neurol.* 2008 Sep;23(9):1090-1; author reply 1089-90.

1014 http://www.hrsa.gov/vaccinecompensation/data.html.

1015 http://www.uscfc.uscourts.gov/sites/default/files/vaccine_files/autism.background.2010. pdf.

[1016] United States Court of Federal Claims Office of Special Masters. Autism Update—September 29, 2010 *available at* http://www.uscfc.uscourts.gov/sites/default/files/autism/autism%20 update%209%2029%2010.pdf

[1017] Holland M, Conte L, Krakow R, Colin L. Unanswered questions from the Vaccine Injury Compensation Program: a review of compensated cases of vaccine-induced brain injury. *Pace Envtl. L. Rev.* 2011; 28:480.

[1018] http://health.usnews.com/doctors/andrew-zimmerman-336535.

[1019] Andrew Zimmerman, letter to Cliff Shoemaker, November 30, 2007.

[1020] Andrew Zimmerman, letter to USDOJ/Civil Torts Branch/OCVL, April 24, 2007.

[1021] Transcript, United States Court of Federal Claims Office of Special Masters. Nov 9, 2007 *available at* http://www.huffingtonpost.com/david-kirby/the-vaccineautism-court-d_b_88558.html.

[1022] http://www.cdc.gov/media/transcripts/2008/t080307.htm

[1023] http://www.huffingtonpost.com/david-kirby/the-next-big-autism-bomb-_b_93627.html.

[1024] Oliveira G, Diogo L, Grazina M, Garcia P, Ataíde A, Marques C, Miguel T, Borges L, Vincente AM, Oliveira CR. Mitochondrial dysfunction in autism spectrum disorders: a population-based study. *Dev Med Child Neurol.* 2005; 47(3): 185-189.

[1025] Oliveira G, Ataíde A, Marques C, Miguel TS, Coutinho AM, Mota-Vieira L, Gonçalves E, Lopes NM, Rodrigues V, Carmona da Mota H, Vicente AM. Epidemiology of autism spectrum disorder in Portugal: prevalence, clinical characterization, and medical conditions. *Dev Med Child Neurol.* 2007 Oct;49(10):726-33.

[1026] Guilivi C, Zhang Y-F, Omanska-Klusek A, Ross-Inta C, Wong S, Hertz-Picciotto I, Tassone F, Pessah IN. Mitochondrial dysfunction in autism. *JAMA.* 2010;304(21):2389-2396.

[1027] Boyd Haley, correspondence with book researchers.

[1028] Transcript, United States Court of Federal Claims Office of Special Masters. Nov 9, 2007 *available at* http://www.huffingtonpost.com/david-kirby/the-vaccineautism-court-d_b_88558.html.

[1029] United States Court of Federal Claims Office of Special Masters. MMR Vaccine; Thimerosal-Containing Vaccines; Autism Spectrum Disorder; Finding of Entitlement; Damages Decision THIMEROSAL: LET THE SCIENCE SPEAK 218 Based on Proffer. July 21, 2010 *available at* http://www.uscfc.uscourts.gov/sites/default/files/ CAMPBELLSMITH.%20 DOE77082710.pdf.

[1030] United States Court of Federal Claims Office of Special Masters. Attorneys' Fees and Costs; Reasonable Amount Requested to which Respondent Does Not Object. No. 02-1466V. Jan 28, 2011 *available at* http://www.uscfc.uscourts.gov/sites/default/files/CAMPBELL-SMITH. POLING012811.pdf.

[1031] http://web.archive.org/web/20130228053911/http://www.hrsa.gov/vaccinecompensation/statisticsreports.html.

[1032] http://www.hrsa.gov/vaccinecompensation/data.html.

[1033] http://www.hrsa.gov/vaccinecompensation/vaccinetable.html.

1034 Robert F. Kennedy, Jr., telephone interview with Bob Krakow [date unavailable]

1035 Robert F. Kennedy, Jr., telephone interview with Louis Conte [date unavailable]

1036 http://www.cbsnews.com/8301-31727_162-20016356-10391695.html.

1037 Holland M, Conte L, Krakow R, Colin L. Unanswered questions from the Vaccine Injury Compensation Program: a review of compensated cases of vaccine-induced brain injury. *Pace Envtl. L. Rev.* 2011; 28:480.

1038 http://www.uscfc.uscourts.gov/sites/default/files/opinions/LORD.TEMBENIS073112.pdf.

1039 http://www.uscfc.uscourts.gov/sites/default/files/opinions/MEROW.TEMBENIS101912.pdf.

1040 http://www.uscfc.uscourts.gov/sites/default/files/opinions/LORD.TEMBENIS112910.pdf.

1041 http://www.uscfc.uscourts.gov/sites/default/files/opinions/CAMPBELL-SMITH.LOWRIE%2010-26-2012.pdf.

1042 http://www.huffingtonpost.com/david-kirby/post2468343_b_2468343.html.

1043 http://www.uscfc.uscourts.gov/sites/default/files/opinions/CAMPBELL-SMITH.LOWRIE.12.3.2012.pdf.

1044 http://www.uscfc.uscourts.gov/sites/default/files/opinions/CAMPBELL-SMITH.MOJABI-PROFFER.12.13.2012.pdf.

PART FOUR:

CONFLICTS OF INTEREST IN POLICYMAKING AND REGULATION

Chapter 22:
The CDC's and Other Agencies' Conflicts of Interest

In 1997, concern over the toxicity of mercury led Congress to pass a law called the Food and Drug Administration (FDA) Modernization Act. The Act required the FDA to review the use of mercury in pediatric vaccines, foods, and other products. The FDA found that the mercury level in the childhood vaccine schedule surpassed safety guidelines set by the Environmental Protection Agency (EPA).[1045][1046][1047] On a precautionary basis, the US Public Health Service (USPHS) and the American Academy of Pediatrics (AAP) issued a joint statement in July 1999 calling for the removal of Thimerosal-containing vaccines "as soon as possible."[1048]

Behind the scenes, the FDA's work raised alarms in that agency and others. In a July 1999 email memo to Lawrence Bachorik, the Food and Drug Administration's (FDA) senior advisor for communications, Peter Patriarca, then the director of the FDA Division of Viral Products and FDA liaison to the AAP Committee on Infectious Diseases, wrote that "the greatest point of vulnerability on this issue is that the systematic review of thimerosal in vaccines by the FDA could have been done years ago. . . . The calculations done by FDA are not complex."[1049] [1050] [1051] He added, "I'm not sure if there will be an easy way out of the potential perception that the FDA, CDC and immunization policy bodies may have been 'asleep at the switch' re: thimerosal until now."[1052]

In separate emails in June 1999, Patriarca shared a list of "pros and cons" he wrote up regarding the USPHS/AAP joint statement, then in preparation, with CDC and National Immunization Program colleagues. As a con, Patriarca described how the public would ask why the FDA had not required manufacturers to remove Thimerosal from their products: "We must keep in mind that the dose of ethyl mercury was not generated by 'rocket science': conversion of the % thimerosal to actual [micrograms] of mercury involves 9th grade algebra. What took the FDA so long to do the calculations? Why didn't CDC and the advisory bodies do these calculations while rapidly expanding the childhood immunization schedule?" Patriarca went on to write about the potential for perceived lack of due diligence regarding the expanded vaccine regimen: "It will also raise questions about various advisory bodies about aggressive recommendations for use [of Thimerosal in childhood vaccines]."[1053] [1054] [1055]

Many members on the advisory bodies who review vaccine science have financial ties to the vaccine industry. The agencies compromised by these conflicts include the following: (a) the CDC, the agency charged with investigating medical disease issues, preventing disease, promoting vaccines and vaccination programs, ensuring that certain vaccines are safe once in use, making recommendations for FDA-approved vaccines, and, together with the Secretary of the Department of Health and Human Services (HHS), making guidelines for vaccination of certain populations and surveying vaccine safety; (b) the FDA, the agency charged with overseeing the regulation-compliant vaccine development process, licensing the manufacturers of vaccines, approving vaccines and their labeling, monitoring the vaccine makers' compliance with the applicable "current good manufacturing practice" regulations for vaccines, and monitoring the safety of FDA-approved vaccines; and (c) the Institute of Medicine (IOM), which examines policy issues for the National Academy of Sciences (NAS), as well as at the request of federal and private organizations, including the CDC and HHS National Vaccine Program Office.[1056 1057 1058 1059 1060 1061 1062]

Of these agencies, the CDC is particularly compromised. By recommending a vaccine for mass use and setting the vaccination timing for initial doses as well as booster doses, the CDC has the extraordinary power to guarantee a market and profits to the vaccine makers. Oftentimes, the people who make these decisions within the CDC have a financial stake in the decisions' outcomes.

According to a July 2003 report by investigative journalist Mark Benjamin that appeared in United Press International (UPI), members of the CDC's Advisory Committee on Immunization Practices (ACIP) often share vaccine patents, own stock in vaccine companies, receive payment for research or to monitor vaccine trials, and receive vaccine-maker funding for their academic departments. Furthermore, each year, the CDC itself receives money from the vaccine makers from licensing agreements and for work on collaborative projects, and the CDC's scientists regularly leave the agency to work for vaccine manufacturers.[1063] One prominent example is Julie Gerberding, who after serving as director of the CDC for seven years became the president of Merck Vaccines in January 2010.[1064]

A *New York Times* story from December 2009 painted a similar picture. An HHS inspector general's report found that 64 percent of the experts serving on advisory panels in 2007 to evaluate vaccines for flu and cervical cancer had potential conflicts of interest that the CDC never disclosed, identified, or resolved.[1065]

To look at an example in detail, consider the officials on a committee that recommended the Thimerosal-preserved HepB vaccination for infants in 1991.[1066] At that time, the chairperson of the CDC's Advisory Committee on Immunization Practice (ACIP) was Samuel Katz. He had helped develop a measles vaccine manufactured by Merck, which was also the manufacturer of the HepB vaccine that was seeking ACIP's recommendation for widespread use in newborn children.[1067] When Katz chaired the ACIP committee, he was also a paid consultant for Merck, Wyeth, and other vaccine makers, according to the UPI report.

Another ACIP member of note at that time was Neal Halsey, director of the Institute of Vaccine Safety at Johns Hopkins University and a former CDC employee.[1068] Halsey has received salary support and grants for the Institute of Vaccine Safety from several vaccine companies.[1069] According to UPI's 2003 report, Halsey's Institute for Vaccine Safety at Johns Hopkins University was funded by vaccine manufacturers, including Merck and what was then Wyeth, now part of Pfizer.[1070] An *ABC News* article from 1999 reported that a Johns Hopkins' spokesperson said that the Institute receives funds from Merck, SmithKline Beecham, North American Vaccines, Connaught/Pasteur Merrieux, and Wyeth-Lederle.[1071]

A further, starker example involves the approval of a rotavirus vaccine. In late 1998, ACIP recommended the vaccine, then known as Wyeth Lederle's RotaShield, for use in young babies despite concerns about the potential risk of intussusception, a serious condition in which one part of the bowel slides inside another part, causing a blockage that can require surgery and can even lead to death.[1072][1073][1074] Unfortunately, those concerns turned out to be well founded. As a 2000 study noted, "By the beginning of October 1999, 101 confirmed and presumed cases of intussusception had been reported to VAERS [the Vaccine Adverse Event Reporting System]. The rate of reporting increased greatly after the July 1999 announcement of the temporary postponement of rotavirus vaccination. Fifty-two patients required surgery, nine required bowel resection and one patient died."[1075] On October 22, 1999, ACIP voted to no longer recommend RotaShield, and after less than a year on the market, the vaccine was withdrawn.[1076][1077] An August 2001 report by the House Government Reform Committee found that "four out of eight CDC advisory committee members who voted to approve guidelines for the rotavirus vaccine in June 1998 had financial ties to the pharmaceutical companies that were developing different versions of the vaccine."[1078]

One of the members of the CDC's ACIP was Paul Offit, currently chief of the Division of Infectious Diseases and director of the Vaccine Education Center at Children's Hospital of Philadelphia (CHOP).[1079][1080] Offit shared a patent for another rotavirus vaccine called RotaTeq, then in development by Merck. While on ACIP, Offit voted to approve the competitor Wyeth's

RotaShield vaccine and recused himself from the vote to take back its recommended use.[1081] Even so, the creation of a market for rotavirus vaccine did serve to potentially financially benefit Offit. He acknowledged in the UPI report that he would make money if the Merck RotaTeq vaccine obtained approval, which it did in February 2006.[1082] In a 2008 *Newsweek* article, Offit acknowledged receiving a portion of the $182 million CHOP earned by selling its interest in future royalties for the vaccine; an

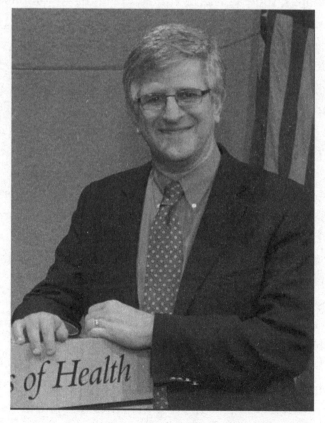

Paul Offit. Credit: public domain

investigation by *Age of Autism* estimated the minimum amount received by Offit as $29 million.[1083][1084]

Offit has been a principal defender of Thimerosal-containing vaccines.[1085][1086][1087] He told this book's author in 2005 that he believed it had been a mistake to precipitously remove Thimerosal from vaccines. Offit also said that he was offended by Kennedy's suggestion that a scientist's direct financial stake in CDC approval might bias his judgment. "It's offensive to say that physicians and clinicians and public health people are in the pocket of industry and thus are making decisions that they know are unsafe for children, Bobby. It's just not the way it works. It isn't. It couldn't, because when people are given the kind of responsibility that happens at the ACIP or CDC, they can't do that. That's why they don't do that."[1088]

Nevertheless, the mere existence of extensive government and industry ties makes a conflict of interest that much more likely. Those in suitably empowered positions to probe the ties, such as congressional members, have criticized what they have seen. In May 2003, the Congressional Subcommittee on Human Rights and Wellness issued a report titled "Mercury in Medicine—Are We Taking Unnecessary Risks?"[1089] The report takes its name from a hearing that took place before the subcommittee-containing Committee on Government Reform back in July 2000 about Thimerosal's continued presence at that time in childhood vaccinations during the long phaseout period.[1090]

The 2003 report was the culmination of multiple hearings during a congressional investigation spanning three years. Among its findings, the report stated, "The CDC in general and the National Immunization Program in particular are conflicted in their duties to monitor the safety of vaccines, while also charged with the responsibility of purchasing vaccines for resale as well as promoting increased immunization rates." The Congressional report faulted the CDC for "bias against theories regarding vaccine-induced autism," and funding researchers "who also worked for vaccine manufacturers to conduct population-based epidemiological studies." The report concluded that:

> Thimerosal used as a preservative in vaccines is likely related to the autism epidemic. This epidemic in all probability may have been prevented or curtailed had the FDA not been asleep at the switch regarding the lack of safety data regarding injected Thimerosal and the sharp rise of infant exposure to this known neurotoxin. Our public health agencies' failure to act is indicative of institutional malfeasance for self protection and misplaced protectionism of the pharmaceutical industry.[1091]

Congressman Dan Burton (R-Indiana), who chaired the subcommittee that wrote the report and who has an autistic grandson, commented further on the matter.[1092] In 2003, he told UPI, "CDC routinely allows scientists with blatant conflicts of interest to serve on influential advisory committees that make recommendations on new vaccines . . . while these same scientists have financial ties, academic affiliations and other vested interests in the products and companies for which they are supposed to be providing unbiased oversight."[1093]

Congressman Dave Weldon (R-Florida), also a member of the subcommittee, offered the following comments on the CDC in 2004:[1094]

The CDC has a built-in conflict of interest that is likely to bias any reviews. CDC is tasked with promoting vaccination, ensuring high vaccination rates, and monitoring the safety of vaccines. They serve as their own watchdog—neither common nor desirable when seeking unbiased research. . . . Unfavorable safety reports lead to lower vaccination rates. An association between vaccines and autism would also force CDC officials to admit that their policies irreparably damaged thousands of children. Who among us would easily accept such a conclusion about ourselves? Yet this is what the CDC is asked to do. Also, the relationship between the CDC and vaccine manufacturers has become extremely close. If a conflict of interest does not exist here, then we certainly have the appearance of one.[1095]

This intrinsic conflict of interest has continued to draw criticism, even from within the Department of Health and Human Services' own oversight entity, the Office of the Inspector General (OIG). A 2009 report by the HHS OIG investigated the CDC's compliance with ethics requirements in 2007 for its so-called special government employees. These are people temporarily employed by the CDC to serve on committees advising the federal government on issues such as immunization recommendations. The rules call for the CDC to obtain confidential financial disclosure reports from these employees, covering their assets, sources of income, and non-income-earning activities. The forms must be reviewed for completeness and all conflicts of interest must be identified and resolved before employees can serve on committees. The OIG found, however, that "for almost all special Government employees,

CDC did not ensure that financial disclosure forms were complete in 2007." Fully 97 percent of employees' confidential financial disclosure reports contained at least one omission, and "most of the forms had more than one type of omission." More problematically, "CDC did not identify or resolve potential conflicts of interest for 64 percent of special Government employees in 2007," the report also found. "Permitting such participation [on committees] could compromise the integrity of the committees' work if committees make recommendations to the Government that do not best serve the public's interest," the OIG report cautioned.[1096]

Amidst this persistent culture of ignored and overlooked conflicts of interest, in 1999, CDC employee Thomas Verstraeten began work on a study whose initial findings suggested a severe lapse by certain federal agencies in performing their basic duties.

Notes

[1045] Baker JP. Mercury, vaccines, and autism: one controversy, three histories. *Am J. Public Health*. 2008; 98:244-253.

[1046] Offit PA, Jew RK. Addressing parents' concerns: do vaccines contain harmful preservatives, adjuvants, additives, or residuals? *Pediatrics*. 2003 Dec;112(6 Pt 1):1394-7.

[1047] http://www.fda.gov/RegulatoryInformation/Legislation/FederalFoodDrugand-CosmeticActFDCAct/SignificantAmendmentstotheFDCAct/FDAMA/default.htm.

[1048] Joint statement of the American Academy of Pediatrics (AAP) and the United States Public Health Service (USPHS). *Pediatrics*. 1999 Sep;104(3 Pt 1):568-9.

[1049] http://www.biologicsconsulting.com/assets/1/15/Patriarca_Peter.pdf.

[1050] http://www.fda.gov/AboutFDA/WhatWeDo/History/Overviews/ucm095305.htm.

[1051] http://pediatrics.aappublications.org/cgi/collection/committee_on_infectious_diseases.

[1052] Peter Patriarca, "Re: Q and As," email to Lawrence Bachorik, Norman Baylor, Elaine Esber, Karen Goldenthal, Leslie Ball, Carolyn D. Deal, July 2, 1999.

[1053] Peter Patriarca, "Re: 'vaccine preservative WG,'" email to Martin Myers, ajs2@cdc.gov, ezg0@cdc.gov, June 29, 1999.

[1054] Peter Patriarca, "FW: 'vaccine preservative WG,'" email to Roger Bernier and Jose Cordero, June 29, 1999.

[1055] United States. Mercury in medicine report. *Congressional Record*. Washington: GPO, May 21, 2003: 1011-1030.

[1056] http://www.cdc.gov/globalhealth/GDDER/optcenter/.

[1057] http://www.cdc.gov/features/StopMosquitoes/.

[1058] http://www.cdc.gov/vaccines/who/teens/downloads/vaccine-resources.pdf.

[1059] http://www.cdc.gov/vaccinesafety/index.html.

[1060] http://www.cdc.gov/vaccines/acip/about.html.

[1061] http://www.fda.gov/biologicsbloodvaccines/developmentapprovalprocess/biologicslicen-seapplicationsblaprocess/ucm133096.htm.

[1062] Stratton K, Gable A, McCormick MC, eds.; Immunization Safety Review Committee, Board on Health Promotion and Disease Prevention, Institute of Medicine. *Immunization Safety Review: Thimerosal-Containing Vaccines and Neurodevelopmental Disorders*. The National Academies Press. Washington, DC. October 1, 2001.

1063 http://www.upi.com/Odd_News/2003/07/21/UPI-Investigates-The-vaccine-conflict/UPI-44221058841736/.

1064 http://investing.businessweek.com/research/stocks/people/person.asp?person-Id=52514649&ticker=MRK&previousCapId=288502&previousTitle=Merck%20%26%20Co.%20Inc.

1065 http://www.nytimes.com/2009/12/18/health/policy/18cdc.html?_r=1&.

1066 http://www.cdc.gov/mmwr/preview/mmwrhtml/00033405.htm.

1067 http://www.cdc.gov/vaccines/acip/meetings/downloads/min-archive/min-feb11.pdf.

1068 http://www.vaccinesafety.edu/Aboutus.htm.

1069 http://www.path.org/vaccineresources/files/Halsey_Vaccine_Safety.pdf.

1070 http://web.archive.org/web/20031227033815/http://more.abcnews.go.com/sections/living/SecondOpinion/secondopinion_53.html.

1071 http://www.pfizer.com/home/.

1072 http://www.cdc.gov/mmwr/preview/mmwrhtml/rr5802a1.htm.

1073 http://www.cdc.gov/mmwr/preview/mmwrhtml/00056669.htm.

1074 http://www.nlm.nih.gov/medlineplus/ency/article/000958.htm.

1075 Delage G. Rotavirus vaccine withdrawal in the United states; the role of postmarketing surveillance. *Can J Infect Dis*. 2000 Jan;11(1):10-2.

1076 http://www.cdc.gov/vaccines/vpd-vac/rotavirus/vac-rotashield-historical.htm.

1077 http://www.cdc.gov/mmwr/preview/mmwrhtml/rr5802a1.htm.

1078 http://www.whale.to/v/staff.html.

1079 http://www.chop.edu/doctors/offit-paul-a.html.

1080 http://www.paul-offit.com/resume.html.

1081 http://www.ageofautism.com/2009/02/voting-himself-rich-cdc-vaccine-adviser-made-29-million-or-more-after-using-role-to-create-market.html.

1082 http://www.fda.gov/BiologicsBloodVaccines/Vaccines/ApprovedProducts/ucm142303.htm.

1083 http://www.thedailybeast.com/newsweek/2008/10/24/stomping-through-a-medical-mine-field.html.

1084 http://www.ageofautism.com/2009/02/voting-himself-rich-cdc-vaccine-adviser-made-29-million-or-more-after-using-role-to-create-market.html.

1085 Offit PA. Thimerosal and vaccines—a cautionary tale. *N Engl J Med*. 2007 Sep 27;357(13):1278-9.

1086 http://www.boston.com/news/globe/ideas/articles/2007/06/03/at_risk_vaccines/.

1087 http://www.npr.org/2011/01/07/132740175/paul-offit-on-the-anti-vaccine-movement.

[1088] Robert F. Kennedy, Jr., telephone interview with Paul Offit, May 4, 2005.

[1089] United States. Mercury in medicine report. *Congressional Record*. Washington: GPO, May 21, 2003: 1011-1030.

[1090] http://www.gpo.gov/fdsys/pkg/CHRG-106hhrg72722/html/CHRG-106hhrg72722.htm.

[1091] United States. Mercury in medicine report. *Congressional Record*. Washington: GPO, May 21, 2003: 1011-1030.

[1092] http://bioguide.congress.gov/scripts/biodisplay.pl?index=b001149.

[1093] http://www.upi.com/Odd_News/2003/07/21/UPI-Investigates-The-vaccine-conflict/UPI-44221058841736/.

[1094] http://bioguide.congress.gov/scripts/biodisplay.pl?index=w000267.

[1095] http://www.iom.edu/~/media/Files/Activity%20Files/PublicHealth/ImmunizationSafety/IOMWeldonFinal2904.pdf.

[1096] https://oig.hhs.gov/oei/reports/oei-04-07-00260.pdf.

Chapter 23: The Verstraeten Study: Links between Thimerosal and Neurological Damage

The Vaccine Safety Datalink Team study on Thimerosal, with Thomas Verstraeten as its lead author (which we shall refer to as the Verstraeten study), has raised significant controversy. The study's final results, which eventually were published in *Pediatrics* in November 2003, differed markedly from earlier runs of the data. At least six different analyses of the data took place over four years, and with each run, the risk of a child developing neurodevelopmental disorders including autism tended to diminish.[1097] This chapter will review the first three rounds of data analysis and more of the reaction to the results.

280

Verstraeten's early results, as well as various emails between concerned parties, were not presented to the public. The unveiling of these items occurred through subsequent Freedom of Information Act (FOIA) requests by parents and, in particular, by an anti-Thimerosal group called SafeMinds.[1098][1099] Verstraeten provoked alarm, this book contends, within the vaccine industry community when his initial analyses showed possible causative links between Thimerosal exposure and neurological damage. The documents obtained through FOIA suggest that government health agencies made an effort to "water down" Verstraeten's findings and obscure the associations.[1100]

The rationale behind these actions appears to be twofold. Officials expressed concern over a potential loss in public confidence in—and thus adherence to—vaccination recommendations, which could lead to the return of many deadly and debilitating childhood diseases long held in check.[1101][1102][1103] Less honorably, however, health officials also seem to have expressed concern over how the vaccine industry would fare if some of its products were revealed as having been responsible for perhaps a large proportion of the steady rise in neurodevelopmental disorders, including autism, in previous decades and through today.[1104]

A sampling of emails between involved parties speaks to these motivations. In a November 29, 1999, email to Robert Davis, an epidemiologist who would be a coauthor on Verstraeten's 2003 article, and Frank DeStefano, project director of the VSD, Verstraeten shared some of his initial analysis on Thimerosal exposure and medical outcomes.[1105][1106] He wrote, "After running, rethinking, rerunning, and rethinking . . . for about two weeks now I should touch base with you I think to see whether you can agree with what I've come up with so far. I'll attach the SAS [statistical software] programs hoping you or one of your statisticians can detect major flaws before I jump to conclusions."[1107] In the email, Verstraeten did not report significantly higher, so-called risk ratios for the majority of possible outcomes, but in an email with additional early analyses to the same colleagues on December 17, some of the risk ratios were quite elevated. Verstraeten wrote in this email that "all the harm is done in the first month [of life]." Verstraeten titled this second email "It just won't go away."[1108]

Davis's involvement in the study is concerning because he had previously received funding from Merck, GlaxoSmithKline, and Wyeth (now Pfizer).[1109] [1110] All three companies produced Thimerosal-containing vaccines and have stood as defendants in Thimerosal-related lawsuits.[1111] [1112] [1113] The CDC has never explained why it allowed the deeply industry-tied Davis to be involved with the Verstraeten study.

The study itself was a "retrospective cohort study"; it attempted to assess epidemiologically whether sets of children exposed to differing cumulative amounts of Thimerosal by a certain young age were more or less likely to have detrimental outcomes. The earliest known analysis and review of data by Verstraeten and colleagues took place sometime in 1999. The first public knowledge of this earliest analysis only came to light in November 2013, as revealed in a single-page document obtained through FOIA by Congressman Posey's office.[1114] The document is a study abstract prepared for an Epidemic Intelligence Service conference by the CDC in 1999, authored by Verstraeten, Davis and DeStefano and a fourth author. It is not known whether the abstract, or a full study of some sort, was in fact presented, or who saw it. The abstract is entitled "Increased risk of developmental neurologic impairment after high exposure to thimerosal-containing vaccine in first month of life." The study authors reviewed the computerized health records in the VSD of more than 400,000 infants born between 1991 and 1997 records at four HMOs. The two groups compared in the study were children who received more than 25 micrograms in their first month of life and an unexposed group. The relative risk for a child in the exposed group developing a neurologic development disorder by the age of six was 1.8, or almost twice that of the unexposed group. The relative risk for autism stood much higher at 7.6, as well as for "nonorganic sleep disorders" at 5.0; speech disorders registered an increased relative risk of 2.1.[1115]

The study designs from there on out would grow more complicated, with differing Thimerosal exposure categories at different times of life and the introduction of various study inclusion (and exclusion) criteria, for example. The subsequent analyses also included additional neurodevelopmental disorders, such as attention deficit disorder (ADD), attention-deficit hyperactivity disorder (ADHD), and tics, and drew mainly or entirely from VSD data from two HMOs for children born from 1992 to 1997.

Verstraeten communicated the next known run of the data by email to his colleagues at the CDC in December 1999. He made a number of comparisons, including between the following exposure groups: children who in their first month received 0, 12.5, more than 12.5, 25, and more than 25 micrograms of mercury from vaccines; children who in their first three months received 50 micrograms, and those who received more or less than 50 micrograms; children who in their first three months received less than

12.5 micrograms, and those who received 12.5, 50, 75, and more than 75 micrograms. Verstraeten also looked at the effects of incremental monthly increases of mercury of between 5 and more than 10 micrograms in the first three months.

The group that was most exposed demonstrated markedly elevated chances of developing neurodevelopmental disorders, compared to the least-exposed group. The group of children who were exposed to more than 25 micrograms of mercury in their first month was 11.35 times more likely to be diagnosed with autism, nearly four times more likely to be diagnosed with ADD, and about twice as likely to have developmental speech or language disorders. Verstraeten also calculated that, compared with babies exposed to less than 12.5 micrograms of mercury in their first three months, babies exposed to 75 micrograms of mercury or more in their first three months were 2.19 times more likely to be diagnosed with autism, and 2.84 and 1.20 times more likely to be diagnosed with ADD and speech and language disorder, respectively.[1116]

A third data run followed on the heels of this second go-through. Verstraeten, along with his colleagues, wrote up a second analysis of the VSD data in a confidential document in late February 2000. In his second report, Verstraeten described a two-and-a-half-fold (2.48) increased risk of autism for children who received the most mercury (more than 62.5 micrograms) by three months of age compared with those who received 37.5 micrograms or less. Increased risks were also noted for speech disorder, stuttering, and attention deficit disorder in children compared to the lowest Thimerosal exposure category, though all these individual outcomes were not deemed statistically significant. Notably, Verstraeten excluded from the revised analysis children born to hepatitis B–positive mothers who were exposed to Thimerosal-preserved HepB immunoglobulin shots during the study period, as these subjects "were more likely to have higher exposure and outcome levels." The report authors wrote in conclusion that "this analysis does not rule out that receipt of thimerosal-containing vaccine in children under three months of age may be related to an increased risk of neurologic developmental disorders. Specific conditions that may warrant detailed study include autism, dyslalia, misery and unhappiness disorder, and attention deficit disorder."[1117]

A fourth analysis of the VSD data took place over the next few months. By June 2000, Verstraeten, Davis, DeStefano, and the VSD team had prepared the analysis for publication in a study titled "Risk of Neurologic and Renal Impairment Associated with Thimerosal-Containing Vaccines." The study examined cumulative mercury exposure at one, two, three, and six months of age for more than 109,000 children born between 1992 and 1997.[1118] In this third run, the relative risk for developing autism came out to 1.69 for the children who received the most mercury (more than 62.5 micrograms) by three months of age, compared with those received 37.5 micrograms or less. Although lower than the 2.48 for the comparable group in the second run, this finding still showed a 69 percent increased risk of autism.

Instead of publishing the article, Verstraeten shared his findings in June 2000 at a secret meeting with a select group of fifty-three individuals at the Simpsonwood United Methodist Church's Conference and Retreat Center near Atlanta, Georgia.[1119] [1120] [1121] The meeting was held without public notice, and organizers did not plan to release any information about Verstraeten's study publicly until the Advisory Committee on Immunization Practices

THIMEROSAL: LET THE SCIENCE SPEAK

(ACIP) meeting later that month. Attendees included numerous high-ranking CDC and FDA representatives, such as Vito Caserta, chief medical officer for the National Vaccine Injury Compensation Program (VICP), as well as some state public health officials and vaccine officials from other nations and the World Health Organization (WHO). Representatives of the vaccine makers SmithKline Beecham (now GlaxoSmithKline), Merck, Wyeth (now Pfizer), and Aventis Pasteur (now Sanofi Pasteur) also attended, all of whom had been named defendants in lawsuits by the parents of children with an autism diagnosis.[1122] [1123] [1124] [1125] [1126]

SafeMinds obtained a transcript of the discussions at Simpsonwood and has since presented this information in press releases, on its website, and during Congressional testimony. What emerged in those Simpsonwood discussions was a striking disparity of beliefs and purposes in reaction to the analyses provided by Verstraeten and his colleagues. Some thought that the study did not reveal anything and questioned whether it should have been done in the first place. Others, however, saw strong evidence of Thimerosal's dangers and thought there was reason for concern. Some other attendees thought that the evidence was weak but that more research should be done because of the potentially widespread consequences.[1127]

Verstraeten introduced his research as "the study that nobody thought we should do," and summarized his findings by saying, "We have found statistically significant relationships between" Thimerosal exposure and neurological disorders.[1128] Verstraeten noted that the data actually understated the connection between Thimerosal and conditions such as speech delays and ADD, because many of the children considered in the study were "just not old enough to be diagnosed."[1129] Although Verstraeten did not specifically address the effect of their cohort's ages on the Thimerosal-autism link, autism is typically not diagnosed until an affected child is several years old, with more recent improvements having lowered the typical age of diagnosis to about four years.[1130]

This issue was just one of many discussed by meeting participants. Over the course of the two-day meeting, differing viewpoints emerged amongst its attendees about whether the preliminary results did in fact suggest potential neurological harm from Thimerosal, or the opposite, of no association whatsoever.

Verstraeten recounted at the conference that the relationship between Thimerosal and autism and other neurologic disorders reflected in the VSD data had prompted him to review the large body of research studies linking mercury to brain damage. He apparently read at least some of the then-available studies previously referenced in this book. "When I saw this and I went back through the literature," Verstraeten said, "I was actually stunned by what I saw because I thought it is plausible."[1131]

CDC statistician Philip Rhodes, among others, took on the task of analyzing Verstraeten's data and making recommendations about what the information could and could not show.[1132][1133] By including children born prematurely, whom Verstraeten had excluded from the study, Rhodes noted that this "further brings things down" in terms of a correlation between Thimerosal exposure and speech disorders, for instance. But the inclusion of a subset of prematurely born children "brings it back up a little bit," Rhodes said. "So you can push. I can pull. But there has been substantial movement from this very highly significant result, down to a fairly marginal result."[1134] Rhodes later said that "the data

THIMEROSAL: LET THE SCIENCE SPEAK

doesn't lead me to conclusively say that nothing is going on, but beyond a certain level there is not a lot going on."[1135]

Verstraeten acknowledged the flexibility of the data in linking Thimerosal exposure to neurologic disorders. "You can look at this data and turn it around," he said. "I can come up with very high risks. I can come up with very low risks, depending on how you turn everything around. You can make it go away for some and then it comes back for others." In an echo of his December 17, 1999, email to Robert Davis, Verstraeten said that "the bottom line is . . . our signal will simply not just go away."[1136]

Paul Stehr-Green, associate professor of epidemiology at the University of Washington and lead author of a key study that came out after Simpsonwood that we will review shortly, thought the data were not demonstrative of a link.[1137 1138] "In terms of strength of association, even though I think there was evidence to form an association, I think at best they demonstrate weak elevated risks for some of these outcomes," Stehr-Green said. "The levels of exposure in this study were likely lower than exposure levels in other studies where no effect was observed, so that kind of mitigates against biological plausibility."[1139]

After two days of reviewing the study, though, some scientists and regulators at Simpsonwood seemed convinced by Verstraeten's epidemiological data that Thimerosal-preserved vaccines could cause harm. William Weil, representing the American Academy of Pediatrics, said to the attendees that "the number of dose-related relationships are linear and statistically significant. You can play with this all you want. They are linear. They are statistically significant." Weil went on to say:

The increased incidence of neurobehavioral problems in children in the past few decades is probably real. . . . I work in the school system where my effort is entirely in special education and I have to say the number of kids getting help in special education is growing nationally and state by state at a rate we have not seen before. So there is some kind of an increase. We can argue about what it is due to. . . . The rise in the frequency of neurobehavioral disorders . . . is much too graphic. We don't see that kind of genetic change in 30 years.[1140]

Earlier at the conference, Weil had gotten into a discussion regarding a threshold exposure to mercury, where he said the following about the theory that Thimerosal could cause neurologic harm:

I think what you are saying is in terms of chronic exposure. I think the other alternative scenario is that this is repeated acute exposures, and like many repeated acute exposures, if you consider a dose of 25 micrograms on one day, then you are above the threshold. At least we think you are, and then you do that over and over to a series of neurons where the toxic effect may be the same set of neurons or the same set of neurological processes, it is conceivable that the more mercury you get, the more effect you are going to get.[1141]

Richard Johnston, an immunologist and pediatrician from the University of Colorado, was concerned enough to worry about his own family members. "My gut feeling?" he said. "Forgive this personal comment, but I . . . do not want [my] grandson to get a Thimerosal-containing vaccine until we know better what is going on. It will probably take a long time. In the meantime . . . I think I want that grandson to only be given Thimerosal-free vaccines."[1142]

Robert Brent, a pediatrician at the Alfred I. duPont Hospital for Children in Delaware, also considered the data worrisome and vocalized a concern evidently shared with others in the room: "The medical/legal findings in this study, causal or not, are horrendous and therefore it is important that the suggested epidemiological, pharmacokinetic and animal studies be [performed] . . . we are in a bad position from the standpoint of defending any lawsuits if they were initiated and I am concerned."[1143] [1144]

John Clements, an advisor to the WHO on infant and childhood immunizations and a supporter of Thimerosal-containing vaccines in developing nations, rebuked those members of the group who had allowed Verstraeten's research to proceed.[1145] Clements said, "This study should not have been done at all, because the outcome of it could have, to some extent, been predicted." Even if the committee at Simpsonwood ultimately decided that there were no association between Thimerosal-containing vaccines and neurodevelopmental disorders, Clements warned that the information "through freedom of information [laws] will be taken by others and will be used in other ways beyond the control of this group." He said further that "now . . . the research results have to be handled."[1146]

The meeting closed with a discussion about how to keep the information from the public. "We have been privileged so far, that, given the sensitivity of information, we have been able to manage to keep it out of, let's say, less responsible hands," said

Robert (Bob) Chen, then chief of Vaccine Safety and Development at the CDC's National Immunization Program and now chief of the Immunization Safety Branch in the same CDC program.[1147][1148] "Consider this embargoed information," Roger Bernier, the associate director for Science at the CDC's National Immunization Program (NIP), announced at the meeting's close, building on his earlier statement: "We have asked you to keep this information confidential . . . [while we] . . . consider these data in a certain protected environment."[1149]

Notes

[1097] SafeMinds. *What do epidemiological studies really tell us?* *available at* http://www.safeminds.org/news/documents/Vaccines%20and%20Autism.%20Epidemiology%20Rebuttal.pdf.

[1098] http://www.putchildrenfirst.org/chapter5.html.

[1099] http://www.safeminds.org/about/mission-and-goals.html.

[1100] SafeMinds. What do epidemiological studies really tell us? available at http://www.safeminds.org/news/documents/Vaccines%20and%20Autism.%20Epidemiology%20Rebuttal.pdf.

[1101] Ruth Etzel, "Message from Ruth Etzel, M.D.," email to Lauri Hall, Ray Koteras, Hope Hurley, Roger Suchyta, July 2, 1999.

[1102] Transcript of Scientific Review of Vaccine Safety Datalink Information, held at Simpsonwood Retreat Center. Norcross, Georgia. June 7-8, 2000. Page 252, available at: http://www.autismhelpforyou.com/HG%20IN%20VACCINES%20-%20Simpsonwood%20-%20Internet%20File.pdf.

[1103] Transcript of IOM Immunization Safety Review Committee Closed Session, held at National Academy of Sciences. Washington, DC. January 12, 2001. Page 72, available at http://www.putchildrenfirst.org/media/6.4.pdf.

[1104] United States. Mercury in medicine report. Congressional Record. Washington: GPO, May 21, 2003: 1011-1030.

[1105] http://www.kpchr.org/research/public/investigators.aspx?InvID=3.

[1106] Simpsonwood meeting transcript, page 13.

[1107] Thomas Verstraeten, "Thimerosal analysis," email to Robert Davis and Frank DeStefano, November 29, 1999.

[1108] Thomas Verstraeten, "It just won't go away," email to Robert Davis and Frank DeStefano, December 17, 1999.

[1109] http://www.iom.edu/~/media/Files/Activity%20Files/PublicHealth/ImmunizationSafety/Davis.pdf.

[1110] http://www.pfizer.com/about/history/2000_present.jsp.

[1111] http://www.sec.gov/Archives/edgar/data/310158/000095012310074336/y83714e10vq.htm.

[1112] http://www.sec.gov/Archives/edgar/data/1131399/000102123104000207/b744172-20f.htm.

[1113] http://www.sec.gov/Archives/edgar/data/5187/000000518703000044/0000005187-03-000044.txt.

[1114] Brian S. Hooker, correspondence with book researchers.

[1115] Thomas M. Verstraeten, R. Davies [sic], D. Gu, F. DeStefano. *Increased risk of developmental neurologic impairment after high exposure to thimerosal-containing vaccine in first month of life.* EIS Class Year of Entry: 1999.

[1116] Thomas Verstraeten, "It just won't go away," email to Robert Davis and Frank DeStefano, December 17, 1999.

[1117] Verstraeten T, Davis R, DeStefano F. *Thimerosal VSD Study Phase I Update*, February 29, 2000.

[1118] Verstraeten T, Davis R, and DeStefano F. *Risk of Neurologic and Renal Impairment Associated with Thimerosal-Containing Vaccines.* June 1, 2000.

[1119] Simpsonwood meeting transcript, pages 1, 3-8, 14, 19, 113.

[1120] http://simpsonwoodumc.org/index.php?/about/directions/.

[1121] http://www.cdc.gov/vaccinesafety/concerns/thimerosal/thimerosal_timeline.html.

[1122] Simpsonwood meeting transcript, pages 4-7.

[1123] http://www.gsk.com/about-us/our-history.html.

[1124] http://en.sanofi.com/our_company/history/history.aspx.

[1125] http://www.pfizer.com/about/history/2000_present.jsp.

[1126] http://www.sec.gov/Archives/edgar/data/1121404/000095012304013372/y03590b5e424b5.htm.

[1127] Simpsonwood meeting transcript, pages 25-30, 83-91, 102, 211, 223-225, 236-242, 251-252, 256-257.

[1128] Simpsonwood meeting transcript, pages 31, 40-41.

[1129] Simpsonwood meeting transcript, pages 42-43.

[1130] http://www.cdc.gov/ncbddd/autism/data.html.

[1131] Simpsonwood meeting transcript, page 162.

[1132] Simpsonwood meeting transcript, pages 8, 93-112.

[1133] http://www.sph.emory.edu/cms/departments_centers/bios/faculty/index.php?Network_ID=RSPH_PRhodes.

[1134] Simpsonwood meeting transcript, page 102.

[1135] Simpsonwood meeting transcript, page 160.

[1136] Simpsonwood meeting transcript, page 153.

[1137] http://sph.washington.edu/faculty/fac_bio.asp?url_ID=Stehr-Green_Paul.

[1138] Stehr-Green P, Tull P, Stellfeld M, Mortenson PB, Simpson D. Autism and thimerosal-containing vaccines: lack of consistent evidence for an association. Am J Prev Med. 2003 Aug;25(2):101-6.

[1139] Simpsonwood meeting transcript, pages 220-221.

[1140] Simpsonwood meeting transcript, pages 208-209.

[1141] Simpsonwood meeting transcript, pages 74-75.

[1142] Simpsonwood meeting transcript, pages 5, 199-200.

[1143] Simpsonwood meeting transcript, pages 6, 229.

[1144] http://jdc.jefferson.edu/robert_brent/cv.pdf.

[1145] http://www.clem.com.au/john/pdfs/JohnClementsCV.pdf.

[1146] Simpsonwood meeting transcript, pages 247-248.

[1147] Simpsonwood meeting transcript, pages 4, 256.

[1148] http://www.sph.emory.edu/ih/TEST/rchen.html.

[1149] Simpsonwood meeting transcript, pages 5, 113, 256.

Chapter 24:
The CDC's and the IOM's Response to Verstraeten's Findings

Following the Simpsonwood meeting, the CDC took what appears to be a comprehensive approach in countering Verstraeten's findings. Agency officials took steps to countermand his results with other studies, dilute Verstraeten's findings still further, and prevent additional public access to the Verstraeten data sets.

The first part of this response began in September 2000, when the CDC and the NIH requested that the nongovernmental Institute of Medicine (IOM) assess the link between Thimerosal and neurological disorders.[1150][1151][1152] The CDC sponsored the review at a cost of about $2 million, including costs for travel, research, and staff, and attended IOM meetings.[1153][1154] The CDC's involvement in the review represents a clear conflict of interest. The organization serves as the primary advocate for Thimerosal-preserved flu vaccines for children and pregnant women, and was responsible for the expanded childhood vaccine schedule in the 1990s that added Thimerosal-preserved vaccines for HepB and Hib.[1155 1156 1157 1158 1159]

The IOM's Immunization Safety Review Committee met for an organizational meeting in January 2001 to discuss the task before it.[1160] Before any research was evaluated, the committee members and IOM staff exchanged comments regarding their shared goal. The members wanted to provide recommendations to the CDC on the kinds of studies and decisions that would be needed to evaluate and ensure the safety of vaccines, as well as how to communicate risks associated with vaccines.[1161] According to a transcript of the organizational meeting obtained by parents of children with autism, one committee member, Michael Kaback of the pediatrics department of the University of California, San Diego, stated:[1162 1163]

> We have got a dragon by the tail here. At the end of the line, what we know is—and I agree—that the more negative that presentation [the conversation between physician and parent about vaccines] is, the less likely people are to use vaccination, immunization, and we know what the results of that will be. We are kind of caught in a trap. How we work our way out of the trap, I think is the charge.[1164]

Marie McCormick, chair of the Immunization Safety Review Committee, was more frank, noting that the CDC "wants us to declare, well, these things are pretty safe on a population level."[1165] [1166] Although the review process had not formally begun, as this meeting was organizational in nature, she expressed confidence that "we are not ever going to come down that [autism] is a true side effect of [vaccine exposure]."[1167]

A potential conflict of interest for McCormick is worth noting. The IOM stated in its report that, "given the sensitive nature of the present immunization safety review study," the organization "felt it was especially critical to establish strict criteria for committee membership. These criteria prevented participation by anyone with financial ties to vaccine manufacturers or their parent companies, previous service on major vaccine-advisory committees, or prior expert testimony or publications on issues of vaccine safety."[1168] McCormick told this book's author in 2005 that she receives no money from the pharmaceutical companies.[1169] Records show, however, that the Harvard School of Public Health where McCormick works has received generous support from Pfizer, Novartis, ASISA, and other major pharmaceutical companies.[1170][1171]

Kathleen Stratton, a member of IOM staff and study director of the Immunization Safety Review Committee, reiterated some of McCormick's message by expressing *a priori* support for the US vaccine program.[1172] According to the January organizational meeting transcript, Stratton said:

We said this before you got here, and I think we said this yesterday. The point of no return, the line we will not cross in public policy, is pull the vaccine, change the schedule. We could say it is time to revisit this, but we would never recommend that level. Even recommending research is recommendations for policy. We wouldn't say compensate, we wouldn't say pull the vaccine, we wouldn't say stop the program.[1173]

As part of the ongoing IOM deliberations, Verstraeten presented a fifth analysis of his VSD data in July 2001.[1174] In this latest run, the researchers focused on the original two HMO patient groups and studied them separately.[1175 1176] The first HMO, referred to as HMO A, had a final study cohort of around 15,000 patients, far less than the second, HMO B, which had a final study cohort of about 115,000 patients.[1177] HMO A therefore had far less power statistically than HMO B in potentially revealing neurodevelopmental disorders associated with Thimerosal.

A number of other discrepancies between HMOs A and B stood out, according to Verstraeten. These included possible biases in HMO B such as health care underutilization bias by parents, which could have led to underascertainment of cases of neurodevelopmental disorders, and variations in Thimerosal exposure for the studied children.[1178] Ultimately, the results between the two HMOs were not "consistent," Verstraeten noted, which he viewed as evidence against there being an injurious effect from Thimerosal. On the other hand, Verstraeten pointed out that certain findings did support a Thimerosal effect. These findings included overall biological plausibility, a dose-response relationship, and a high statistical significance of relative risks—that is, the chance of developing a disorder—for certain outcomes.[1179]

Autism, however, was not one of the statistically significant outcomes. In HMO A, only nineteen patients had autism, far fewer than the threshold of fifty needed for analysis based on statistical power calculations.[1180] When patient groups for both HMOs were combined, for a total of 169 cases of autism, the relative risk of developing the disorder turned out to be 1.52 for the group exposed to the highest level of Thimerosal at three months of age. The result was not statistically significant, though, because the margin of error for the relative risk figure fell just below 1.0. While the autism signal was effectively buried during all this reshuffling of data, Verstraeten still found Thimerosal exposure statistically significantly linked for other disorders, including stammering and sleep disorders in HMO A, and stammering, tics, attention deficit disorder, language delay, and speech delay in HMO B.[1181][1182]

In a maneuver that critics have seen as an attempt to nullify even those results, for the fifth analysis, Verstraeten included VSD data from a third, independent HMO (HMO C). This so-called Phase II portion of the study reevaluated possible associations in HMO C between the most common neurodevelopmental disorders and Thimerosal exposure screened for in HMOs A and B. Because autism risk had been previously found not to be related to Thimerosal exposure, the researchers did not evaluate this outcome in HMO C. The Phase II results found no statistical significance for attention deficit disorder and speech and language delay, in effect canceling out prior signals for most neurodevelopmental disorders in the study. The study yielded a generally "neutral" result, meaning the findings neither supported nor undermined a link between Thimerosal exposure and neurological damage. The relationship between Thimerosal exposure and outcomes such as stammering that were found in the other HMOs could not be studied, because there were not enough children in HMO C.[1183]

The inclusion of HMO C data is intrinsically questionable based on the quality of the HMO selected, Harvard Pilgrim, with a population based mostly in Massachusetts.[1184] Although

Harvard Pilgrim had received high national rankings from media outlets in the late 1990s, the HMO was actually close to collapsing financially and had to go into an emergency receivership by the state of Massachusetts in early 2000. An article in the *Journal of Law, Medicine & Ethics* discussed one of the major causes of the HMO's insolvency as "creaky information technology architecture" that presented a "logistical and transactions cost nightmare."[1185] As described by Congressman Dave Weldon (R-Florida), Harvard Pilgrim's "computer records had been in shambles for years, it had multiple computer systems that could not communicate with one another, and it used a health care coding system totally different from the one used across the VSD."[1186] Weldon argued that the allegedly poor recordkeeping at Harvard Pilgrim, along with its alternate coding, rendered this third HMO as broadly incomparable with HMOs A and B.[1187 1188]

In addition, the final cohort size from HMO C was only 17,547 children, close in size to HMO A and similarly not as strong in its statistical power as the far larger HMO B. Paper coauthor Davis expressed concern about HMO C's lack of statistical power to fellow coauthor DeStefano in a June 26, 2000 email, stating:

With regards to the HP [Harvard Pilgrim, HMO C] study, we need to be alittle [sic] careful, since the main question will be whether or not it had adequate power to detect an association that was only found when we lumped GHC [HMO A] and NCK [HMO B] together (and even then I think it was driven primarily by NCK data).[1189]

In terms of presentation, the evolving Verstraeten study used a potentially misleading means of graphically conveying some of its provisional results at the time. On page 47 in the PowerPoint presentation to the IOM committee, Verstraeten provided a graph showing the relative risk of autism associated with various Thimerosal exposure levels at three months of age. Instead of a conventional y axis with linear unit increases—one, two, three, and so on—the researchers employed a logarithmic scale, with units increasing exponentially from 0.1 (below the x axis) to 1 to 10. By doing so, the 1.52 relative risk figure associated with the highest Thimerosal dose of 62.5 micrograms or greater did not appear to rise as sharply, and thus dramatically, off of the x axis as it would have if linear increments were used and the y axis was not extended unnecessarily all the way to 10. In other words, using a log scale "flattened" the results visually, possibly disguising their salience to a viewer not familiar with such a scale.

The following Figures 16 through 19 bear this out. The first, Figure 16, is the exact chart used by Verstraeten, which he styled as a line, or "fever," chart. These charts are designed to show changes in a single variable over time, though in this case the style of chart is used inappropriately; the lines connecting the data points are essentially meaningless. To set up a comparison, the next chart, Figure 17, similarly displays the Verstraeten information in a log scale y axis. The third, Figure 18, plots the data points using a linear y axis scale. The fourth and final, Figure 19, a bar chart, offers another way to compare how the log and linear scales showcase the same data.

Relative risk associated with exposure at 3 months of age: <u>Autism</u>

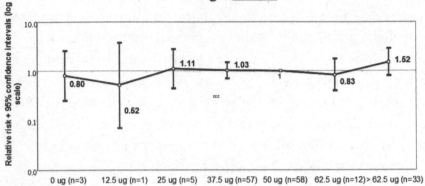

FIGURE 16

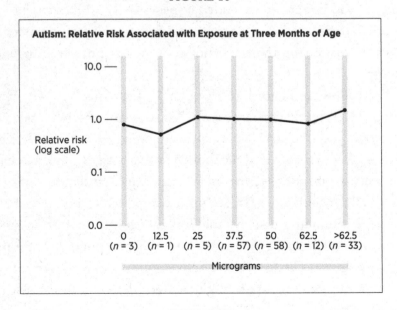

FIGURE 17

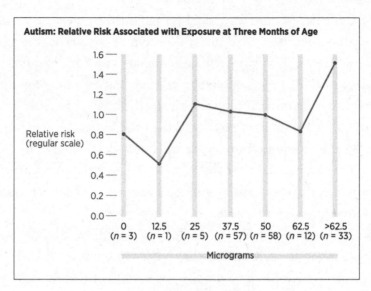

FIGURE 18

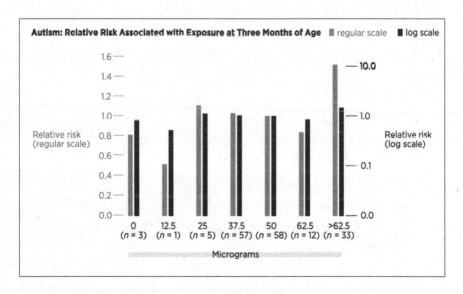

FIGURE 19

At any rate, in pure statistical terms, the 95 percent confidence intervals—error bars, essentially—shown as the vertical ranges in the Verstraeten chart for each Thimerosal exposure level cross the value of one. This means that the relative risks are not statistically significant; that is, none are statistically different from one. Yet it is notable that Verstraeten baselined the relative risk of one not at 0 micrograms of Thimerosal exposure, but at 50 micrograms, which could have served to lower the relative risk associated with autism. A more clear-cut approach would have been to compare children with no exposure to those with any exposure.

With Verstraeten's revised findings in hand, the IOM went on to issue a report in October 2001 on Thimerosal and neurodevelopmental disorders, including autism. Ultimately, the IOM committee "found inadequate evidence to accept or reject a causal relationship between thimerosal-containing vaccines and neurodevelopmental disorders." But the committee did allow that the hypothesis of a link was "biologically plausible." As the Executive Summary stated:

> The committee concludes that although the hypothesis that exposure to thimerosal-containing vaccines could be associated with neurodevelopmental disorders is not established and rests on indirect and incomplete information, primarily from analogies with methylmercury and levels of maximum mercury exposure from vaccines given in children, the hypothesis is biologically plausible.

The IOM report recommended the use of Thimerosal-free DTaP, Hib, and HepB vaccines in the United States, "despite the fact that there might be remaining supplies of thimerosal-containing vaccine available." The IOM report further recommended that with regard to other Thimerosal-containing vaccines such as DT and influenza that "full consideration be given by appropriate professional societies and government agencies to removing thimerosal from vaccines administered to infants, children, or pregnant women in the United States." The IOM also recommended additional research on the topic. Specifically, the IOM called for studies on the epidemiology of Thimerosal- and non-Thimerosal-containing vaccines and neurological disorders, as well as basic clinical science on ethylmercury exposure.[1190]

As it turned out, studies in Europe were already being conducted to look at the relationship between vaccines and neurodevelopmental outcomes. However, these four studies would rely on European populations, not the relevant US population, for reasons explored in the next chapter.

Notes

[1150] http://www7.nationalacademies.org/ocga/testimony/autsim.asp.

[1151] http://www.iom.edu/About-IOM.aspx.

[1152] Kathleen Stratton, Alicia Gable, and Marie C. McCormick, eds.; Immunization Safety Review Committee, Board on Health Promotion and Disease Prevention, Institute of Medicine. *Immunization Safety Review: Thimerosal-Containing Vaccines and Neurodevelopmental Disorders.* The National Academies Press. Washington, DC. October 1, 2001.

[1153] http://www.iom.edu/Reports/2001/Immunization-Safety-Review-Thimerosal—Containing-Vaccines-and-Neurodevelopmental-Disorders.aspx.

[1154] Department of Health and Human Services, Public Health Service, Centers for Disease Control and Prevention, Inter/Intra Agency-Agreement (IAA), Payable Agreements (CDC is Procuring Agency). CDC IAA#: 00FED17358. *Vaccine Safety Review Panel.* September 9, 2000.

[1155] http://www.cdc.gov/flu/protect/vaccine/thimerosal.htm.

[1156] http://www.cdc.gov/vaccines/acip/about.html.

[1157] http://www.cdc.gov/flu/protect/children.htm.

[1158] http://www.cdc.gov/flu/protect/vaccine/qa_vacpregnant.htm.

[1159] http://www.cdc.gov/mmwr/preview/mmwrhtml/00038256.htm.

[1160] IOM Immunization Safety Review Committee January 2001 meeting, age 8.

[1161] IOM Immunization Safety Review Committee January 2011 meeting, pages 16-17, 23, 32.

[1162] SafeMinds. What do epidemiological studies really tell us? available at http://www.safeminds.org/news/documents/Vaccines%20and%20Autism.%20Epidemiology%20Rebuttal.pdf.

[1163] http://www.pediatrics.ucsd.edu/Faculty/Pages/default.aspx.

[1164] IOM Immunization Safety Review Committee January 2001 meeting, page 33.

[1165] http://iom.edu/Global/Directory/Detail.aspx?id=0000052790.

[1166] IOM Immunization Safety Review Committee January 2001 meeting, page 34.

[1167] IOM Immunization Safety Review Committee January 2001 meeting, page 95.

[1168] Stratton K, Gable A, and McCormick MC, eds.; Immunization Safety Review Committee, Board on Health Promotion and Disease Prevention, Institute of Medicine. Immunization Safety Review: Thimerosal-Containing Vaccines and Neurodevelopmental Disorders. The National Academies Press. Washington, DC. October 1, 2001.

[1169] Robert F. Kennedy, Jr., telephone interview with Marie McCormick, April 27, 2005.

[1170] http://www.hsph.harvard.edu/faculty/marie-mccormick/.

[1171] http://www.hsph.harvard.edu/research/pharma-epi/pharmaco-funding-opportunities/.

[1172] http://www.iom.edu/Staff/Kathleen-R-Stratton.aspx.

[1173] IOM Immunization Safety Review Committee January 2001 meeting, page 69.

[1174] Verstraeten T. *Neurodevelopmental and Renal Toxicity of Thimerosal-Containing Vaccines: A Two-Phased Analysis of Computerized Databases.* PowerPoint presentation to the Institute of Medicine. July 2001.

[1175] National Academy of Sciences Institute of Medicine Immunization Safety Review Committee. *Thimerosal-Containing Vaccines and Neurodevelopmental Outcomes.* Public Meeting. Cambridge, Massachusetts. July 16, 2001. Transcript, page 85.

[1176] IOM Immunization Safety Review Committee July 2001 meeting, page 92.

[1177] IOM Immunization Safety Review Committee July 2001 meeting, pages 85-86.

[1178] IOM Immunization Safety Review Committee July 2001 meeting, pages 87, 92.

[1179] IOM Immunization Safety Review Committee July 2001 meeting, pages 94-95.

[1180] IOM Immunization Safety Review Committee July 2001 meeting, page 84.

[1181] Verstraeten T. *Neurodevelopmental and Renal Toxicity of Thimerosal-Containing Vaccines: A Two-Phased Analysis of Computerized Databases.* PowerPoint presentation to the Institute of Medicine. July 2001.

[1182] SafeMinds. *What do epidemiological studies really tell us?* available at http://www.safeminds.org/news/documents/Vaccines%20and%20Autism.%20Epidemiology%20Rebuttal.pdf.

[1183] IOM Immunization Safety Review Committee July 2001 meeting, pages 94-95.

[1184] https://www.harvardpilgrim.org/.

[1185] Dave Weldon, letter to Julie Gerberding, October 31, 2003 available at http://www.autismhelpforyou.com/EXPERT%20PAPER%20-%20Weldon%20To%20CDC%20-%20Internet%20File.pdf.

[1186] Miller FH, Miller WW. Lessons to be learned from Harvard pilgrim HMO's fiscal roller coaster ride. *J Law Med Ethics.* 2000 Sep; 28(3): 287–304.

[1187] IOM Immunization Safety Review Committee July 2001 meeting, page 90.

[1188] SafeMinds. *What do epidemiological studies really tell us?* available at http://www.safeminds.org/news/documents/Vaccines%20and%20Autism.%20Epidemiology%20Rebuttal.pdf.

[1189] Robert Davis, "RE: thimerosal: model in Davis RL et al (fwd)," email to Frank DeStefano, June 26, 2000.

[1190] Stratton K, Gable A, and McCormick MC, eds.; Immunization Safety Review Committee, Board on Health Promotion and Disease Prevention, Institute of Medicine. *Immunization Safety Review: Thimerosal-Containing Vaccines and Neurodevelopmental Disorders.* The National Academies Press. Washington, DC. October 1, 2001.

Chapter 25: The CDC's and IOM's Reliance on Flawed European Studies

At the Simpsonwood meeting mentioned a couple chapters ago, pediatrician Robert Brent urged investigators "to get other populations to study," arguing, "I do not think reanalysis of this [American] data is going to be as helpful as we would hope."[1191] Following Brent's call for studies of "other populations," a number of researchers—almost all financially allied with CDC and the vaccine industry—collected data on cases of autism in Denmark, Sweden, and the United Kingdom.[1192 1193 1194 1195] The IOM would come to rely on four studies of foreign populations in these countries (with the exception of one study that included a California cohort) for its later statements disavowing a link between Thimerosal and autism. We will refer to these studies by their lead authors, which are as follows: Hviid 2003 (Denmark); Madsen 2003 (Denmark);

Stehr-Green 2003 (California, Denmark, Sweden); and Andrews 2004 (United Kingdom). These studies all have major flaws that place their conclusions in doubt.

The CDC might already have been planning to use epidemiology from Europe to disprove Thimerosal-autism causation as early as IOM meetings held in January 2001, prior to the report issued later that year. This information came to light during a federal court case, *Easter v. Aventis Pasteur*, wherein a Texas woman sued pharmaceutical companies on the claim that Thimerosal had caused her son's autism.[1196] In barely legible handwritten notes that emerged from the 2001 IOM meeting presented by the plaintiffs, a committee member wrote, "Other countries—looked at issue because of nature of other countries? CDC-project with Denmark on autism." Another committee member made this notation: "'What we care most about' → Consistent body of epi evid that consis shows no assoc."[1197]

It appears that at least one high-ranking public health official viewed the point of the CDC studies as not to explore, study, or assess connections between Thimerosal and neurodevelopmental disorders, but to "rule out" any links and give cover to official statements on Thimerosal's safety. In May 2001, Gordon Douglas, director of strategic planning for the Vaccine Research Center at NIH, said to a Princeton University gathering, "Four current studies are taking place at the CDC in collaboration with NIH to rule out the proposed link between immunizations and autism, immunizations and possible developmental regression, inflammatory bowel disease and the MMR vaccine, and Thimerosal and the risk of autism."[1198] In addition to his federal duties as a leading public health official, Douglas formerly served as president of Merck's vaccination program.[1199] In that capacity in 1991, he had received a warning from Maurice Hilleman, described in Part One, that six-month-old children administered the US vaccination shots would have mercury exposures about 87 times the Swedish safety standard.[1200] Merck, however, continued to make a Thimerosal-preserved HepB vaccine (Recombivax) until the US Public Health Service called on vaccine manufacturers to eliminate mercury in vaccines in 1999.[1201]

We will look first at the choice of countries for epidemiological research regarding Thimerosal and neurodevelopmental disorders. In Denmark, children first received vaccinations at around five weeks of age, instead of at birth and at two months as in the United States. In addition, Denmark discontinued the use of Thimerosal-preserved early-childhood vaccines in 1992. Prior to this date, the total mercury dose a Danish child could receive was 125 micrograms—about half of the 237.5 microgram maximum exposure American children could have had in accordance with the CDC-recommended schedule of routine childhood inoculations in the 1990s.[1202]

For children represented in the additional Swedish data in Stehr-Green 2003 and in the United Kingdom in Andrews 2004, the mercury exposure level was 75 micrograms, also far lower than the US level.[1203] [1204] Researchers, including Sarah Parker and colleagues in 2004, have raised this dosing disparity and the differing vaccination schedules as a limitation affecting the general applicability of these several studies to the United States.[1205] "It's as if a researcher trying to study the involvement of mosquitoes on malaria conducted his research in Minnesota instead of Panama," Boyd Haley said to this book's author.[1206]

A second major issue with the selection of Denmark is the fact that Danish statistics collection for autism spectrum disorders (ASDs) contained an anomaly that could have made ASDs appear more common after the Thimerosal 1992 phaseout. Before that year, Danish public health authorities counted autism only for hospital inpatients, defined as people who stay in the hospital overnight or come to the hospital every day for evaluation and treatment. In 1995, the national registry began registering outpatient cases of autism as well. These outpatient cases, as reported in Madsen 2003, outnumbered inpatient cases by between four and six times. Danish researchers tried to get around this shortcoming by stating that autism rates did not decline between 1991 and 1993, when all autism cases were inpatient. But the value of this shorter period is limited because it only included a single year after Thimerosal-containing vaccines were discontinued (in 1992). The authors also stated generally that they took this administrative change into account, but they did not publish these data.[1207][1208]

Other factors also contributed to an apparent rise in autism after Thimerosal's phaseout in Denmark. In 1994, Denmark began using a broader definition of autism made available in the *International Classification of Diseases* manual published by the WHO.[1209][1210][1211] Furthermore, prior to 1992, the data in the Danish registry excluded cases diagnosed in one of Copenhagen's largest clinics, which accounted for approximately 20 percent of all Danish autism cases.[1212] All of these factors likely contributed to a deceptive rise in autism rates following the ban on Thimerosal in Denmark, which could have been exploited by biased researchers seeking to discount a Thimerosal-autism link.

As previously described in Part Three, two researchers at Autism Healing Network, Jeffrey Allen Trelka and Brian S. Hooker, criticized the 2003 Madsen study in a 2004 letter to the editor of the *Journal of American Physicians and Surgeons*. The letter stated that "Madsen's collection of inpatient treatment data since 1971 was tainted by adding outpatient activities after 1994." The letter went on to say that this evidence suggests that "the 2003 Madsen analysis is at best indeterminate regarding the effect of discontinuing the use of thimerosal-containing vaccines on autism incidence." When correcting for the inaccuracies of the Madsen study, the authors of the letter calculated that autism incidence had actually decreased significantly after 1993, "including a dramatic 75% reduction within the 2- to 4-year-old cohort." The Madsen errors "could have been easily avoided through proper accounting of the existing data in the Danish registry," the letter concluded.[1213]

Stehr-Green 2003 did acknowledge that "several external events in Denmark . . . may have spuriously increased the apparent number of autism cases," including the fact that cases from the Copenhagen clinic were not included, that only inpatient cases were included before 1995, and that the diagnostic criteria changed in 1993. The Swedish portion of Stehr-Green's study, however, also had many of the same limitations. The authors collected data only on children hospitalized for autism. Even though they were comparing apples to apples in terms of the autism prevalence before and after the use of Thimerosal in vaccines, the authors could have missed a large majority of the autism cases, and, as they point out, the rate of inpatient diagnosis could have changed over the course of the study period. Moreover, as noted previously, Swedish children were exposed to even less Thimerosal than were their Danish neighbors;

most children in Sweden received 75 micrograms of Thimerosal until 1992, when the use of Thimerosal-containing vaccines was similarly discontinued.[1214] Madsen 2003 also acknowledged this last confounding factor for the Danish data in his study, writing that "our data cannot, of course, exclude the possibility that thimerosal at doses larger than used in Denmark may lead to neurodevelopmental damage."[1215]

In the 2005 *Easter v. Aventis Pasteur* federal court case, wherein a Texas woman sued pharmaceutical companies on the claim that Thimerosal had caused her son's autism, the pharmaceutical industry's own expert witness conceded that the Danish studies were flawed. Philip S. Wang from Harvard Medical School acknowledged in a report submitted as evidence that the "dramatic" rise in autism reported in Sweden and Denmark after Thimerosal was removed from vaccines "most likely reflect[ed] changes in diagnostic practices and the availability of services for autism."[1216 1217]

It is worth commenting that, despite the possibly spurious increase in ASD cases in Denmark in the 1990s, some studies suggest that overall prevalence in the country is lower than in the United States. Denmark removed Thimerosal from its DTaP vaccine in 1992 and continues to have a recommended early childhood vaccination schedule.[1218] In a 2011 study, Parner reported an ASD prevalence in Denmark for children born between 1994 and 1999 as nearly 7 in 1,000, less than the 20 per 1,000 (or 1 in 50) prevalence estimate most recently issued by the CDC for the United States.[1219 1220] Notably, a 2010 Danish study by Maimburg reported a far lower prevalence of 1 in 1,272 for ASD (plus two rare conditions grouped under the category of "pervasive developmental disorder") for children born between 1994 and 2004.[1221] Most recently in 2013, a study by Grønborg reported that prevalence declined from a high of 1.5 percent in 1994-1995, down to 1.2 by 2000-2001, and still lower in 2002-2004 to 1.0.[1222]

Despite their countries' researchers finding that Thimerosal presented no harm to children, Denmark and Sweden have not gone back to using the preservative in vaccines. In the United Kingdom, even in light of similar findings discounting a Thimerosal-autism link in a study by Nick Andrews in 2004 and another by Jon Heron and Jean Golding in 2004, British health authorities began replacing Thimerosal-preserved vaccines with Thimerosal-free combination vaccines in September of 2004 anyway.[1223 1224 1225 1226]

The Andrews study was published in *Pediatrics* in September 2004 after being presented to the IOM earlier that year. The study's conclusion that there is "no evidence that thimerosal exposure via DTP/DT vaccines causes neurodevelopmental disorders" is predicated on a technically flawed data analysis. With regard to autism data, the study used a nontransparent, multivariate regression technique, which introduced a well-known issue called multicollinearity. The study had two independent variables—Thimerosal exposure levels and year of birth—that were "correlated" with each other because Thimerosal exposures went up with time. Problematically, these variables compete with each other to explain the outcome effect; in other words, the inclusion of the time variable reduces the significance of the exposure variable. Without a separate analysis of each independent variable, the true relationships between exposure and autism prevalence and year of birth and prevalence cannot be ascertained with statistical confidence.[1227]

A final major underlying defect of the European studies in general was that the authors did not confirm their statistical power, according to an article written by Luis Maya and Flora Luna, medical doctors in Lima, Peru. "Statistical power" refers to the probability that a test will reject a null hypothesis when the null hypothesis is false. In the case of the European studies, statistical power analysis would be used to determine the minimum sample size needed to detect a certain effect, such as Thimerosal exposure and autism diagnoses. Although the authors of Hviid 2003 do report statistically significant differences in terms of increases in autism rates over the years of the study, it is possible that these studies overall lacked the power to detect differences in the rates of autism as they related to Thimerosal exposure.[1228]

The Danish, Swedish, and United Kingdom results, along with a revised version of Verstraeten's study (which will be discussed in a later chapter), were relied on in a subsequent IOM report published in May 2004 (also discussed in a chapter thereafter). The report concluded that there is no link between autism and Thimerosal exposure. When this book's author spoke to the IOM panel chair of both the 2001 and 2004 reports, Marie McCormick, in April 2005, she seemed to be unaware or dismissive of the defects in the European studies' methodologies. "They stopped Thimerosal," she said, referring to the two Scandinavian nations, "and the incidence of autism continued to increase."

When I asked her if the European studies lacked relevancy because they examined Thimerosal doses that were significantly less than those given American children, she responded that children examined in the United Kingdom study had doses in the middle range of those received by American children, and were therefore "not completely out of the ballpark."[1229] As noted previously, children in the Andrews 2004 study received 75 micrograms of Thimerosal during their first four months of life compared to the 187.5 micrograms potentially given to US kids during the same period.[1230]

In emails exchanged between Thomas Verstraeten and Robert Chen at the CDC with Elizabeth Miller, second author of the then-unfolding Andrews study, in June 2001, Verstraeten expressed his concern that these Thimerosal exposures might be too low to be relevant. He wrote:

> The maximum exposure is indeed relatively low if that was the only T containing vaccine used. My estimate would be that you need at least >50 [micrograms] by 3 months or >100 by 6 months to see an effect if there is one, which you barely make (50 at 2 mo and 75 at 4 mo in the UK). . . . I hate to say this, but given these concerns, it may not be worth doing this after all.[1231] [1232]

Furthermore, American children could have received a large single-day dose of 62.5 micrograms of mercury around two months of age, whereas British children received no more than 25 micrograms in a single day. The Scandinavian vaccine schedules were also spread out and generally administered to older children when their brains were less vulnerable.[1233] Neal Halsey, referenced previously, told the author of this book that it was this giant, so-called "bolus dose" that most shocked and frightened him because of its obvious potential to damage a developing child's brain.[1234]

I posed similar questions to Kathleen Stratton, who was the study director of both the 2004 and the 2001 IOM reports. I asked her how the committee could have acted on flawed European studies and not taken into account the considerable clinical, biological, and epidemiological studies that contradict them. She told me, "The committee didn't think they were badly flawed."[1235]

A number of other scientists and concerned individuals, in addition to those already mentioned, have raised serious criticisms of the European studies. Joachim Mutter of University Hospital Freiburg, Germany, in 2005 criticized the Danish and United Kingdom studies, recounting in detail the numerous methodological flaws in Madsen 2003.[1236] Bernard Rimland, founder of the Autism Research Institute, wrote a letter in 2004 to the editor of *JAMA*, which published Hviid's 2003 study. Rimland pointed out the conflicts of interest facing Hviid and his coauthors, writing:

In their article on the association between thimerosal-containing vaccines and autism, Dr. Hviid and colleagues acknowledged their affiliations with the Statens Serum Institut, Copenhagen, Denmark, but did not disclose that the institute is a for-profit, state-owned enterprise with roughly $120 million in annual revenue. According to its 2002 Annual Report, vaccines present approximately one half of Staten Serum Institut's revenues and more than 80% of its profits. Furthermore, Statens Serum Institut manufactured the now discontinued monocomponent pertussis vaccine that contained thimerosal under investigation in their study. They were also the providers of diphtheria and tetanus components of a major thimerosal-containing diphtheria and tetanus toxoids and acellular pertussis vaccine (DTaP) vaccine sold in the United States.[1237][1238]

Various other such conflicts of interest cast additional doubt on the integrity of the European studies relied on by the IOM.

Stehr-Green's study, for example, was financed in part by the CDC and the Statens Serum Institut.[1239]

Kreesten Madsen's potential conflict comes on a more personal, direct basis.[1240] For example, CDC employees Coleen Boyle, Diana Schendel, and Jose Cordero all provided "comments and advice during preparation of the manuscript," and are thanked as such in the Acknowledgments section of Madsen's paper.[1241] [1242] [1243] Of greater concern—and not disclosed in the paper—in June 2001, Madsen exchanged emails with Diane Simpson, the then-acting deputy director of the National Immunization Program for the CDC. The emails are somewhat suspicious in nature and content as they reveal lines of communication between the CDC and at least one researcher who would go on to author a study arguing against a Thimerosal-autism link. As revealed in a FOIA request by parents of autistic children, Simpson contacted Madsen and asked, "Our primary question is: did the [autism] rates increase dramatically from the late 1980's [sic] into the 1990s as they did here in the United States. A quick answer to that question would mean a great deal to us here!!! (even without the specific numbers)." Madsen replied that he did not believe the autism rates rose in 1980s and not before 1993. Simpson inquired further about autism rates after 1993, and Madsen replied that changed diagnostic codes and inclusion of outpatient data included after 1995 could be behind a post-1993 rise. As put forth previously in this chapter, this potentially spurious rise in autism cases after Denmark banned Thimerosal in 1992 offered a way of "cherry picking" epidemiological data from overseas to dispel an apparent Thimerosal-autism link that surfaced in Verstraeten's data sets.[1244] [1245]

A distinctly complicated case is that of Poul Thorsen, a coauthor of the Madsen study. Thorsen, who was trained as a psychiatrist, developed a long-term relationship with the CDC after he worked there as a visiting scientist in the 1990s. He successfully pushed for CDC funds to go to governmental agencies in Denmark to study autism and vaccines, among other research efforts. Between 2000 and 2009, the CDC awarded more than $11 million toward this effort. Thorsen returned to Denmark in 2002 and became the principal investigator for the grant. Allegations of misuse of the funds emerged in 2009, and in 2011, a federal grand jury in Georgia indicted Thorsen for wire fraud and money laundering of more than $1 million from the CDC.[1246][1247][1248][1249] Despite this fraud, the CDC has refused to examine the veracity of the studies that Thorsen participated in.

The next example involves Elizabeth Miller, mentioned previously as a researcher involved in the United Kingdom studies considered by the IOM. When she presented her results to the IOM in February 2004, Miller admitted that "my department does, on occasion, do collaborative work which has commercial sponsorship."[1250] She did not specifically disclose, however, that she had received funding to study vaccines from North American Vaccine (now Baxter Healthcare), Wyeth-Lederle Vaccines, Chiron Biocine, and SmithKline Beecham.[1251][1252][1253] Miller has coauthored many studies assuring the public of vaccine safety, for example in *Pediatrics*, in violation of that journal's supposedly strict conflicts of interest disclosure requirements.[1254][1255][1256]

At this time, we will take a chapter to discuss similar concerning lapses at *Pediatrics*, a highly regarded journal and publisher of many of the major studies in the autism and vaccine debate.

Notes

[1191] Simpsonwood meeting transcript, pages 6, 249.

[1192] Hviid A, Stellfeld M, Wohlfahrt J, Melbye M. Association between thimerosal–containing vaccine and autism. *JAMA*. 2003 Oct 1;290(13):1763-6.

[1193] Madsen KM, Lauritsen MB, Pedersen CB, Thorsen P, Plesner A-M, Andersen PH, Mortenson PB. Thimerosal and the occurrence of autism: negative ecological evidence from Danish population-based data. *Pediatrics*. 2003 Sep;112(3 Pt 1):604-6.

[1194] Stehr-Green P, Tull P, Stellfeld M, Mortenson PB, Simpson D. Autism and Thimerosal-containing vaccines, lack of consistent evidence for an association. *Am J Prev Med*. 2003 Aug;25(2):101-6.

[1195] Andrews N, Miller E, Grant A, Stowe J, Osborne V, Taylor B. Thimerosal exposure in infants and developmental disorders: a retrospective cohort study in the United kingdom does not support a causal association. *Pediatrics*. 2004 Sep;114(3):584-91.

[1196] http://articles.latimes.com/2005/feb/08/business/fi-vaccine8.

[1197] Vera Easter, Individually and as Next Friend of Jordan Delaney Easter, Plaintiffs, vs. Aventis Pasteur, Inc., et al, Defendants. Plaintiff's Response in Opposition to Defendants' Daubert Motion. No. 5:03-CV-141 (TJW). United States District Court for the Eastern District of Texas Marshall Division. January 31, 2005.

[1198] Oller JW Jr, Oller SD. *Autism: The Diagnosis, Treatment, and Etiology of the Undeniable Epidemic*. Burlington, Massachusetts: Jones & Bartlett Publishers, 2009.

[1199] http://nihrecord.od.nih.gov/newsletters/08_08_2000/appoint.htm.

[1200] Maurice Hilleman, "Vaccine Task Force Assignment Thimerosal (Merthiolate) Preservative—Problems, Analysis, Suggestions for Resolution," memo to Gordon Douglas, March 27, 1991.

[1201] http://www.fda.gov/BiologicsBloodVaccines/Vaccines/ApprovedProducts/ucm110129.htm.

[1202] Hviid A, Stellfeld M, Wohlfahrt J, Melbye M. Association between thimerosal–containing vaccine and autism. *JAMA*. 2003 Oct 1;290(13):1763-6.

[1203] Stehr-Green P, Tull P, Stellfeld M, Mortenson PB, Simpson D. Autism and Thimerosal-containing vaccines, lack of consistent evidence for an association. *Am J Prev Med*. 2003 Aug;25(2):101-6.

[1204] Andrews N, Miller E, Grant A, Stowe J, Osborne V, Taylor B. Thimerosal exposure in infants and developmental disorders: a retrospective cohort study in the United Kingdom does not support a causal association. *Pediatrics*. 2004 Sep;114(3):584-91.

[1205] Parker S, Todd J, Schwartz B, Pickering L. Thimerosal-containing vaccines and autistic spectrum disorder: a critical review of published original data. *Pediatrics*. 2004;114(3):793-804.

[1206] Robert F. Kennedy, Jr., telephone interview with Boyd Haley, April 9, 2005.

[1207] Madsen KM, Lauritsen MB, Pedersen CB, Thorsen P, Plesner A-M, Andersen PH, Mortenson PB. Thimerosal and the occurrence of autism: negative ecological evidence from Danish population-based data. *Pediatrics*. 2003 Sep;112(3 Pt 1):604-6.

[1208] Hviid A, Stellfeld M, Wohlfahrt J, Melbye M. Association between thimerosal–containing vaccine and autism. *JAMA*. 2003 Oct 1;290(13):1763-6.

[1209] Madsen KM, Lauritsen MB, Pedersen CB, Thorsen P, Plesner A-M, Andersen PH, Mortenson PB. Thimerosal and the occurrence of autism: negative ecological evidence from Danish population-based data. *Pediatrics*. 2003 Sep;112(3 Pt 1):604-6.

[1210] http://www.who.int/classifications/icd/en/GRNBOOK.pdf.

[1211] Larsson HJ, Eaton WW, Madsen KM, Vestergaard M, Olesen AV, Agerbo E, Schendel D, Thorsen P, Mortenson PB. Risk factors for autism: perinatal factors, parental psychiatric history, and socioeconomic status. *Am J Epidemiol*. 2005 May 15;161(10):916-25; discussion 926-8.

[1212] Stehr-Green P, Tull P, Stellfeld M, Mortenson PB, Simpson D. Autism and Thimerosal-Containing Vaccines, Lack of Consistent Evidence for an Association. *Am J Prev Med*. 2003 Aug;25(2):101-6.

[1213] Trelka JA, Hooker BS. More on Madsen's analysis. *J Am Phys Surg*. 2004; 9(4):101.

[1214] Stehr-Green P, Tull P, Stellfeld M, Mortenson PB, Simpson D. Autism and Thimerosal-containing vaccines lack of consistent evidence for an association. *Am J Prev Med*. 2003; 25(2): 101-106.

[1215] Madsen KM, Lauritsen MB, Pedersen CB, Thorsen P, Plesner A-M, Andersen PH, Mortenson PB. Thimerosal and the occurrence of autism: negative ecological evidence from Danish population-based data. *Pediatrics*. 2003 Sep;112(3 Pt 1):604-6.

[1216] http://nihrecord.od.nih.gov/newsletters/2009/09_18_2009/milestones.htm.

[1217] Vera Easter, Individually and as Next Friend of Jordan Delaney Easter, Plaintiffs, vs. Aventis Pasteur, Inc., et al, Defendants. Plaintiff's Response in Opposition to Defendants' *Daubert* Motion. No. 5:03-CV-141 (TJW). United States District Court for the Eastern District of Texas Marshall Division. January 31, 2005.

[1218] http://www.euvac.net/graphics/euvac/vaccination/denmark.html.

[1219] Parner ET, Thorsen P, Dixon G, de Klerk N, Leonard H, Nassar N, Bourke J, Bower C, Glasson EJ. A comparison of autism prevalence trends in Denmark and Western Australia. *J Autism Dev Disord*. 2011 Dec;41(12):1601-8.

[1220] http://www.cdc.gov/media/releases/2013/a0320_autism_disorder.html.

[1221] Maimburg RD, Bech BH, Vaeth M, Møller-Madsen B, Olsen J. Neonatal jaundice, autism, and other disorders of psychological development. *Pediatrics*. 2010 Nov;126(5):872-8. Epub 2010 Oct 11.

1222 Grønborg TK, Schendel DE, Parner ET. Recurrence of autism spectrum disorders in full- and half-siblings and trends over time: a population-based cohort study. *JAMA Pediatr.* 2013 Oct 1;167(10):947-53. doi: 10.1001/jamapediatrics.2013.2259.

1223 Andrews N, Miller E, Grant A, Stowe J, Osborne V, Taylor B. Thimerosal exposure in infants and developmental disorders: a retrospective cohort study in the United Kingdom does not support a causal association. *Pediatrics.* 2004 Sep;114(3):584-91.

1224 Heron J, Golding J, ALSPAC study team. Thimerosal exposure in infants and developmental disorders: a prospective cohort study in the United Kingdom does not support a causal association. *Pediatrics.* 2004 Sep;114(3):577-83.

1225 Bedford H, Elliman D. Misconceptions about the new combination vaccine. *BMJ.* 2004 Aug 21;329(7463):411-2.

1226 http://web.archive.org/web/20070609114311/http://www.advisorybodies.doh.gov.uk/jcvi/mins011004.htm.

1227 Brian S. Hooker, correspondence with book researchers.

1228 Maya L, Luna F. Thimerosal and children's neurodevelopmental disorders. *An Fac Med Lima.* 2006; 67(3): 243-262 [Spanish].

1229 Robert F. Kennedy, Jr., telephone interview with Marie McCormick, April 27, 2005.

1230 Andrews N, Miller E, Grant A, Stowe J, Osborne V, Taylor B. Thimerosal exposure in infants and developmental disorders: a retrospective cohort study in the United Kingdom does not support a causal association. *Pediatrics.* 2004 Sep;114(3):584-91.

1231 Thomas Verstraeten, "RE: UK vaccine schedule and thimerosal exposure," email to Robert Chen, June 26, 2001.

1232 Robert Chen, "FW: UK vaccine schedule and thimerosal exposure," email to Elizabeth Miller, June 26, 2011.

1233 Geier DA, Geier MR. A two-phased population epidemiological study of the safety of thimerosal containing vaccines: a follow-up analysis. *Med Sci Monit.* 2005 Apr;11(4):CR160-170. Epub 2005 Mar 24.

1234 Robert F. Kennedy, Jr., telephone interview with Neal Halsey, May 2005.

1235 Robert F. Kennedy, Jr., telephone interview with Kathleen Stratton, April 28, 2005.

1236 Mutter J, Naumann J, Schneider R, Walach H, Haley B. Mercury and autism: accelerating evidence? *Neuro Endocrinol Lett.* 2005 Oct;26(5):439-46.

1237 Rimland B. Association between thimerosal-containing vaccine and autism. *JAMA.* 2004 Jan 14;291(2):180; author reply 180-1.

1238 http://www.ssi.dk/Service/Kontakt/Medarbejdere/Person.aspx?id=f8e82303-cdf5-42eb-879b-9d8800af6e1e.

1239 Stehr-Green P, Tull P, Stellfeld M, Mortenson PB, Simpson D. Autism and Thimerosal-containing vaccines lack of consistent evidence for an association. *Am J Prev Med.* 2003; 25(2): 101-106.

1240 http://dk.linkedin.com/pub/kreesten-meldgaard-madsen/5/143/184.

1241 http://www.cdc.gov/ncbddd/AboutUs/biographies/Boyle.html.

[1242] http://www.autism-insar.org/about/membership-directory/diana-schendel.

[1243] http://www.linkedin.com/pub/jose-f-cordero/10/ab6/155.

[1244] http://www.putchildrenfirst.org/chapter5.html.

[1245] http://www.putchildrenfirst.org/media/5.9.pdf.

[1246] http://www.reuters.com/article/2011/04/13/us-crime-research-funds-idUS-TRE73C8JJ20110413.

[1247] http://www.justice.gov/usao/gan/press/2011/04-13-11.html.

[1248] http://www.huffingtonpost.com/robert-f-kennedy-jr/time-for-cdc-to-come-clea_b_16550.html.

[1249] http://www.ageofautism.com/2010/03/poul-thorsens-mutating-resume.html.

[1250] Transcript. Immunization Safety Review Committee, Vaccines and Autism. February 9, 2004. Institute of Medicine of the National Academy of Sciences. Washington, DC. *available at* http://www.putchildrenfirst.org/media/6.16.pdf.

[1251] Committee on Safety of Medicines Declaration of Interests. *Medicines Act 1968 Advisory Bodies Annual Reports 2001. available at* http://wayback.archive.org/web/20040408205314/http://www.mca.gov.uk/aboutagency/regframework/csm/csmdoi01.pdf.

[1252] http://pediatrics.aappublications.org/content/114/3/584.abstract/reply.

[1253] http://www.bmj.com/content/335/7618/480?tab=responses.

[1254] http://www.ncbi.nlm.nih.gov/pubmed?term=Elizabeth%20Miller%20AND%20vaccine.

[1255] Andrews N, Miller E, Grant A, Stowe J, Osborne V, Taylor B. Thimerosal exposure in infants and developmental disorders: a retrospective cohort study in the United Kingdom does not support a causal association. *Pediatrics.* 2004 Sep;114(3):584-91.

[1256] http://pediatrics.aappublications.org/site/misc/policies.xhtml.

Chapter 26: The American Academy of Pediatrics' Conflicts of Interest

Pediatrics is the principal publication of the American Academy of Pediatrics (AAP), which has its own heavy conflicts.[1257] The AAP has consistently supported regular childhood immunizations even though it solicits and receives significant funding from vaccine companies, currently including Sanofi Pasteur and Merck.[1258 1259 1260]

The AAP receives substantial financial support from Thimerosal-preserved vaccine producers in the form of advertising revenues and funding for conferences, grants, and construction of its headquarters.[1261] Such financial ties could explain why the journal overlooked its own bias policies and did not require Verstraeten, Thorsen, Miller, and others to reveal their conflicts of interest when publishing articles purportedly addressing Thimerosal's safety. Relations with its financial backers could also explain why

Pediatrics consistently refuses to print letters critical of articles supporting the present orthodoxy of vaccine safety, including Thimerosal-containing products.

An example is the letter cited previously by Trelka and Hooker criticizing Madsen's 2003 study.[1262] The letter originally had been submitted to *Pediatrics*, the journal that eventually published the Madsen study after its rejection by more prestigious journals.[1263] According to Hooker, Madsen and his coauthors were given an opportunity to respond to Trelka and Hooker's comments but chose not to; nor did they contact the *Pediatrics* editor-in-chief, Jerold Lucey, or his staff regarding the raised issues. Lucey made the editorial decision not to publish the letter and stated that the 2004 IOM report—discussed later in this Part—made the letter a "moot point."[1264]

In 2008, David Ayoub, a radiologist at the Memorial Medical Center in Springfield, Illinois, and an assistant professor at Southern Illinois University School of Medicine, outlined some of the conflicts as he sees them within the AAP:[1265]

The AAP has played an important role in perpetuating the misconception that current research refutes the Thimerosal-autism link. Three key papers have been published in the AAP trade journal *Pediatrics*: Madsen (Danish epidemiological study); the Verstraeten study, of Simpsonwood fame, and Fombonne (Quebec epidemiological study). The editor-in-chief Dr. Jerald [sic] Lucey received numerous, substantiated criticisms of each of these studies, but has created an effective roadblock in disallowing any criticisms to be published in the letter to the editor section of the journal.

His response to thoughtful and reasonable criticisms has been unprofessional, illogical and insulting. My own letter to Lucey criticizing the Fombonne study was not even allowed to be published on the less publically visible online forum, even though we had obtained a copy of the Fombonne database and vaccine records from several parents proving Fombonne's work fraudulent.

Why would the organization most influential in pediatric healthcare in America turn its back to our concerns and pleas? That is not a challenging question. The AAP reports annual revenues of about $70 million, but only one fourth comes from membership dues. Their website lists extensive corporate donors, none more generous than the vaccine makers. Their journal *Pediatrics* generates about $10,000 per page for a drug ad, translating into $200,000 monthly. Even more money is generated for reprint orders, often six figures, that are distributed to pediatricians without of course the criticisms.

When I attended the AAP's National Convention in Washington D.C. in 2005, I attended as many talks I could [on] two topics that interested me—diagnosis and treatment of learning disabilities and two, vaccine safety. From the meeting brochure I made the following observations:

First, 16 speakers contributed to 18 lectures in these categories. According to the AAP's meeting brochure and my own knowledge of the presenters, 15 of 16 speakers had strong connections to the pharmaceutical industry, including the CDC. One Harvard physician claimed 42 different financial arrangements with 14 different pharmaceutical companies! My . . . when does he find the time to vaccinate anyone? It is no wonder that the message delivered by AAP and industry influenced professionals to attending pediatricians was crystal clear: there is no vaccine link![1266]

It is not surprising, then, given AAP's pharmaceutical industry ties and history that the organization has recently expressed its continued support for the use of Thimerosal in multidose vaccines. The AAP published multiple articles in *Pediatrics* online in December 2012 endorsing the World Health Organization's (WHO) recommendation exempting Thimerosal from the Minamata Convention on Mercury, an international treaty calling for the elimination of avoidable mercury exposure approved in January 2013.[1267 1268 1269 1270 1271 1272 1273]

Notes

[1257] http://pediatrics.aappublications.org/site/misc/about.xhtml.

[1258] http://pediatrics.aappublications.org/content/127/2/387.full.

[1259] http://www.chop.edu/service/vaccine-education-center/vaccine-schedule/history-of-vaccine-schedule.html.

[1260] http://www.aap.org/en-us/about-the-aap/corporate-relationships/Pages/Friends-of-Children-Fund-President%27s-Circle.aspx.

[1261] http://www.cbsnews.com/stories/2008/07/25/cbsnews_investigates/main4296175.shtml?tag=mncol;lst;2.

[1262] Trelka JA, Hooker BS. More on Madsen's analysis. *J Am Phys Surg*. 2004; 9(4):101.

[1263] http://www.journal-ranking.com/ranking/listCommonRanking.html?citingStartYear=1901&externalCitationWeight=1&journalListId=370&selfCitationWeight=1.

[1264] Brian S. Hooker, correspondence with book researchers.

[1265] http://www.zoominfo.com/#!search/profile/person?personId=19022963&targetid=profile.

[1266] http://adventuresinautism.blogspot.com/2008/02/dr-david-ayoub-calls-out-aap.html.

[1267] http://www.unep.org/newscentre/Default.aspx?DocumentID=2702&ArticleID=9373&l=en.

[1268] Orenstein WA, Paulson JA, Brady MT, Cooper LZ, Seib K. Global vaccination recommendations and thimerosal. *Pediatrics*. 2013 Jan;131(1):149-51. doi: 10.1542/peds.2012-1760. Epub 2012 Dec 17.

[1269] Cooper LZ, Katz SL. Ban on Thimerosal in draft treaty on mercury: why the AAP's position in 2012 is so important. *Pediatrics*. 2013 Jan;131(1):152-3. doi: 10.1542/peds.2012-1823. Epub 2012 Dec 17.

[1270] King K, Paterson M, Green SK. Global justice and the proposed ban on thimerosal-containing vaccines. *Pediatrics*. 2013 Jan;131(1):154-6. doi: 10.1542/peds.2012-2976. Epub 2012 Dec 17.

[1271] http://www.aap.org/en-us/about-the-aap/aap-press-room/pages/AAP-Endorses-WHO-Statement-on-Thimerosal-in-Vaccines.aspx.

[1272] http://www.unep.org/hazardoussubstances/MercuryNot/MercuryNegotiations/tabid/3320/language/en-US/Default.aspx.

[1273] http://www.unep.org/hazardoussubstances/Portals/9/Mercury/Documents/Overarching%20Framework.pdf.

Chapter 27:
Governmental Action
That Has Defended
Thimerosal

In addition to the too-close ties reviewed thus far between the CDC, the vaccine industry, certain researchers, and the AAP, proponents of Thimerosal's safety have also had backing among others in the executive, legislative, and judicial branches of the government. Early in the last decade was the critical period when Thimerosal was being phased out of childhood vaccines and government health authorities had not yet declared there to be no link between the chemical and neurodevelopmental disorders. At that time, individuals in Congress and possibly the White House influenced and contributed to the developing controversy. More recently, the Supreme Court issued a ruling in the important Bruesewitz v. Wyeth case that has further restricted the ability of parents to seek damages for children allegedly injured by vaccines.[1274]

In November 2002, congressional members made moves to apparently protect a prominent vaccine maker from Thimerosal-related lawsuits. The Republican leadership in the House of Representatives inserted the so-called "Eli Lilly" rider into the massive Homeland Security bill under consideration at that time.[1275] The rider specifically gave pharmaceutical giant Eli Lilly protection from liability for injuries caused by Thimerosal.[1276] All Thimerosal cases were to be transferred to the National Vaccine Injury Compensation Program's (VICP) special "Vaccine Court," created by statute in 1988.[1277] In this court, compensation for pain and suffering is capped—although compensation for medical care and lost earnings is not capped—and discovery, or the time to gather evidence, is limited.[1278 1279 1280 1281 1282]

The rider meant billions to the drug industry in general and Eli Lilly in particular. The action was so secretive that even a Republican congressional leader, Dan Burton, whose committee had jurisdiction over the Homeland Security bill and who had held hearings on Thimerosal's dangers, was shocked to learn of its inclusion.[1283 1284]

One of the major players in the Eli Lilly rider controversy was Senator Bill Frist (R-Tennessee), who went on to become majority leader in 2003. In March 2002, Frist had sponsored legislation with provisions identical to the rider, though the bill had stalled in committee.[1285 1286] Shortly after Frist introduced the legislation that eventually led to the Lilly rider, his political action committee received $10,000 from the Pharmaceutical Research and Manufacturers of America, a pharmaceutical industry trade organization.[1287 1288]

As the 2002 midterm elections cycle wore on, Eli Lilly wound up donating $226,250 to the National Republican Senatorial Campaign

Committee (NRSC), chaired by Frist, whereas the company gave about half that to the Democratic Senatorial Campaign Committee (DSCC).[1289] The pharmaceutical company also enriched the senator personally by purchasing 5,000 copies of his book on bioterrorism.[1290] Overall the pharmaceutical industry was the largest single contributor to the NRSC, donating about $4 million. Frist alone received $265,000 prior to his work to pass legislation to protect Eli Lilly.[1291] For the 2002 national election, along with other pharmaceutical companies, Eli Lilly gave significantly more money to Republican candidates than to Democratic candidates for federal office—about three-quarters of its $1.6 million in donations, according to the Center for Responsive Politics.[1292]

Oddly, no lawmaker (including Frist), lobbyist, or administration employee initially took credit for the rider's inclusion. The mystery of the rider swirled until Keith "Dick" Armey (R-Texas) later confirmed in 2002 he had inserted the provision.[1293] Media reports had suspected involvement by the White House, where a former Eli Lilly executive, Mitch Daniels (now president of Purdue University), then served as director of the Office of Management and Budget.[1294] The Executive Branch had further connections to Eli Lilly. President George W. Bush appointed the company's chairman and chief executive, Sidney Taurel, in June 2002 to serve on a presidential council advising on domestic security.[1295 1296]

The Bush Administration supported the vaccine industry in other ways. In November 2002, Department of Justice lawyers asked a special master of the VICP to have documents related to the approximately 1,000 cases of vaccine injuries sealed, effectively preventing the documents from being used for future civil cases outside the Vaccine Court. In a *Reuters* article, attorney Jeff Kim with Gallagher

THIMEROSAL: LET THE SCIENCE SPEAK

Boland Meiburger & Brosnan, a firm representing about 400 families of autistic children who received the MMR vaccine, "accused the government of trying to lower 'a shroud of secrecy over these documents' in order to protect vaccine manufacturers, who he said were 'the only entities' that would benefit if the documents are sealed."[1297]

After the midterm elections, the Homeland Security bill with the Lilly rider passed both houses, and President Bush signed it on November 25, 2002.[1298] Under bipartisan pressure from members of both the House and Senate, however, Congress repealed the provision in a spending bill passed in February 2003. Burton was quick to write in a letter to every member of Congress that "these provisions do not belong in the Homeland Security Act," while Congressman Henry Waxman (D-California) wrote to Daniels that the provision was "something that the White House wanted" and Senator Debbie Stabenow (D-Michigan) posed the question on the Senate floor, "Don't families and their children merit due process under the law?"[1299]

Despite the controversy, Frist returned to the issue in 2005 with a new bill that he introduced ostensibly to combat terrorism. Called the Public Readiness and Emergency Preparedness Act (PREPA), the bill protected pharmaceutical manufacturers from liability for potential side effects and injury related to vaccines and other "countermeasures" deployed during a declared public health emergency, such as a bioterror attack or influenza outbreak. The bill's supporters argued this legal protection was necessary to motivate pharmaceutical companies to create and stockpile countermeasures against public health threats; detractors saw the bill as a giveaway to the drug industry. President Bush signed the bill into law on December 30, 2005.[1300]

The law ultimately extended liability protection to manufacturers, distributors, and program planners of countermeasures as well as qualified persons who prescribe, administer, or dispense countermeasures; in essence, the entire vaccine and healthcare establishment was granted legal immunity for vaccines administered in a declared public health emergency.[1301] These vaccines include those preserved with Thimerosal. The federal law could preempt state laws against Thimerosal use, which by the mid-2000s had passed in California, Delaware, Illinois, Iowa, Missouri, and New York (in most cases applying only to young children and pregnant women); such laws had also been introduced in other states.[1302] [1303]

The Supreme Court recently handed down a decision that protects vaccine makers from civil lawsuits. In February 2011, the court issued its opinion in *Bruesewitz v. Wyeth*. The case concerned a claim by the parents of Hannah Bruesewitz (not to be confused with Hannah Poling, discussed in Chapter 21) that their child had become disabled after receiving a DTP vaccine made by Lederle Laboratories, now owned by Wyeth. The VICP—the "Vaccine Court"—had denied the Bruesewitzes' claim in 2003 per residual seizure disorder not being one of the injuries designated as compensable.[1304] Afterward, Hannah's parents sued Lederle in Pennsylvania state court on grounds that the company was subject to strict liability for negligent design of the vaccine under Pennsylvania common law. "Design defect" is one of the three major types of recognized legal product liability. Wyeth moved the suit to a district court, which ruled that the language of 42 USC § 300aa-22 in the VICP statute "preempts all design-defect claims against vaccine manufacturers brought by plaintiffs who seek compensation for injury or death caused by vaccine side effects."[1305] The Supreme Court upheld this finding, and, "in so doing, it likely closed the door on thousands of claims by parents alleging a link between vaccines and childhood autism," according to the *Supreme Court of the United States (SCOTUS) Blog*.[1306]

The ruling, this book contends, is at odds with the congressional intent to preserve the right of the vaccine-injured to pursue a civil trial after lawfully entering and exiting the Vaccine Court, as the Bruesewitz family did. In this manner, the bar to civil trials enacted in the VICP is unconstitutional for its disagreement with the plain language of the Seventh Amendment of the Constitution of the United States of America, which reads:

> In Suits at common law, where the value in controversy shall exceed twenty dollars, the right of trial by jury shall be preserved, and no fact tried by a jury, shall be otherwise re-examined in any Court of the United States, than according to the rules of the common law.[1307]

Rather than rule in favor of Wyeth, the Supreme Court justices, sworn to uphold the Constitution, should have stayed a decision and instructed the legislative and executive branches of the federal government to revise the law to restore the constitutional Seventh Amendment common law right to a trial by jury in civil courts. Or, the Supreme Court should have simply declared the VICP unconstitutional. In doing so, the court could have allowed citizens to seek justice for a vaccine injury in the same manner as any other drug injury is treated in the federal and state courts.

In closing this chapter, it's worth noting that in Italy, where citizens claiming injury from vaccines do have the right to seek redress in civil court, several recent rulings there have found in the plaintiffs' favor. As in the US, the Italian government maintains a national vaccine injury compensation program, run by the Ministry of Health. The program likewise addresses cases of alleged harm from recommended and compulsory vaccines, rather than expose the pharmaceutical industry to lawsuits.[1308]

Among the most recent rulings is one handed down by a civil court in Milan in September 2014. The Ministry had initially rejected a claim made on behalf of an infant male who developed autism following the administration of three doses of a Thimerosal-containing vaccine over a six-month span in 2006. The infant's family proceeded to sue the Ministry. Based on the testimony of medical experts, the impartial court concluded that the infant's autism was likely a result of the vaccine exposure, coupled with an underlying genetic susceptibility. A particularly strong piece of evidence in the plaintiff's favor was a 1,271 page document from the vaccine manufacturer, GlaxoSmithKline, describing a range of adverse effects and outcomes from the vaccine in question, including five cases of autism. GlaxoSmithKline's report stated nevertheless that "[t]he benefit/risk profile" of the vaccine, called Infanrix hexa, "continues to be favourable." The Ministry has appealed the Milan court's decision, and a final say will not be in for perhaps a few years.[1309]

Other cases involving both Thimerosal-containing vaccines and the measles, mumps, and rubella (MMR) vaccine, which does not contain Thimerosal, have been decided in favor of the plaintiffs. These include tribunals in the cities of Busto Arsizio in 2009, Urbino in 2011, Rimini in 2012 (reversed on appeal, however, and involving MMR), Milan again in 2012, and Pesaro in

2013. In these cases in general, the courts have stated that scientific certainty of a link between vaccine administration and injury, such as autism, is not inherently possible. Rather, based on the testimony of court appointed experts, the courts found "reliable" and "reasonable scientific probability" that a causal link exists—an appropriate and measured evaluation of the available evidence, such as timing of the appearance of symptoms shortly after vaccine administration and the biological plausibility of mercury exposure and other vaccine elements triggering neurological injury.[1310][1311]

More vaccine injury cases are pending before Italian courts.[1312] The several rulings just cited suggest that if "normal" courts in the US were allowed to hear government-rejected vaccine injury claims, jurists might also disagree with certain adjudications of the country's national vaccine compensation program.

Notes

[1274] http://www.supremecourt.gov/opinions/10pdf/09-152.pdf.

[1275] http://www.nytimes.com/2002/11/29/us/a-capitol-hill-mystery-who-aided-drug-maker.html.

[1276] Jonathan Weisman. A homeland security whodunit in massive bill, someone buried a clause to benefit drug maker Eli Lilly. *Washington Post.* November 28, 2002.

[1277] Business Wire. *Law Firms Continue Thimerosal Litigation.* November 26, 2002.

[1278] http://www.cdc.gov/vaccines/pubs/pinkbook/downloads/appendices/F/vicp-def.pdf.

[1279] http://www.hrsa.gov/vaccinecompensation/index.html.

[1280] http://nationalvaccineinjurylawyer.com/faq.asp.

[1281] http://dash.harvard.edu/bitstream/handle/1/9453695/Davenport,_Katherine_NVICP.pdf?sequence=2.

[1282] http://central-pennsylvania.legalexaminer.com/miscellaneous/vaccine-injury-compensation-program-the-need-for-more-discovery.aspx?googlcid=293804.

[1283] Kirby D. *Evidence of Harm: Mercury in Vaccines and the Autism Epidemic: A Medical Controversy.* New York: St. Martin's Press, 2005.

[1284] http://www.cbsnews.com/stories/2002/12/12/eveningnews/main532886.shtml.

[1285] http://bioguide.congress.gov/scripts/biodisplay.pl?index=f000439.

[1286] Kirby D. *Evidence of Harm: Mercury in Vaccines and the Autism Epidemic: A Medical Controversy.* New York: St. Martin's Press, 2005.

[1287] http://centerjd.org/sites/default/files/Impact%20Politics&Money.pdf.

[1288] http://www.phrma.org/about/phrma.

[1289] http://www.consumerwatchdog.org/healthcare/nw/nw002949.php3.

[1290] Kirby D. *Evidence of Harm: Mercury in Vaccines and the Autism Epidemic: A Medical Controversy.* New York: St. Martin's Press, 2005.

[1291] http://centerjd.org/sites/default/files/Impact%20Politics&Money.pdf.

[1292] http://www.opensecrets.org/bigpicture/topcontribs.asp?cycle=2002&Format=Print.

[1293] http://www.cbsnews.com/news/the-man-behind-the-vaccine-mystery/.

[1294] http://www.purdue.edu/president/p12/about/index.html.

[1295] http://www.nytimes.com/2002/11/29/us/a-capitol-hill-mystery-who-aided-drug-maker.html.

[1296] http://www.forbes.com/profile/sidney-taurel/.

[1297] Zwillich T. US government asks court to seal vaccine records. *Reuters*. November 26, 2002.

[1298] http://articles.cnn.com/2002-11-25/politics/homeland.security_1_new-department-homeland-security-head-department?_s=PM:ALLPOLITICS.

[1299] Kirby D. *Evidence of Harm: Mercury in Vaccines and the Autism Epidemic: A Medical Controversy*. New York: St. Martin's Press, 2005.

[1300] Copper BK. Notes and comments. "High and dry?" The Public Readiness and Emergency Preparedness Act and liability protection for pharmaceutical manufacturers. *J Health Law*. 2007 Winter;40(1):65-105.

[1301] http://www.phe.gov/Preparedness/legal/prepact/Pages/prepqa.aspx.

[1302] http://en.wikipedia.org/wiki/Public_Readiness_and_Emergency_Preparedness_Act.

[1303] http://www.ama-assn.org/amednews/2006/04/24/hll20424.htm.

[1304] http://healthland.time.com/2011/02/24/bruesewitz-v-wyeth-what-the-supreme-court-decision-means-for-vaccines/.

[1305] http://www.supremecourt.gov/opinions/10pdf/09-152.pdf.

[1306] http://www.scotusblog.com/?p=114239.

[1307] http://www.archives.gov/exhibits/charters/bill_of_rights_transcript.html.

[1308] http://www.ageofautism.com/2015/01/recent-italian-court-decisions-on-vaccines-and-autism.html.

[1309] http://www.ageofautism.com/2015/01/recent-italian-court-decisions-on-vaccines-and-autism.html.

[1310] Review and translation of Italian court documents by white paper researchers.

[1311] http://www.ageofautism.com/2015/01/recent-italian-court-decisions-on-vaccines-and-autism.html.

[1312] http://www.independent.co.uk/life-style/health-and-families/health-news/italian-court-reignites-mmr-vaccine-debate-after-award-over-child-with-autism-7858596.html.

Chapter 28:
The Final, Published
Verstraeten Study

As work proceeded on the four European studies in the early 2000s, the Verstraeten study was being prepared for publication. A sixth and final analysis took place before the study entered the public record, appearing in the journal *Pediatrics* in November 2003.[1313]

For the fifth analysis, described previously, a third HMO's data was analyzed as Phase II of the study. In the sixth analysis, the statistically significant neurodevelopmental disorders found in HMO A (tics, with a relative risk of 1.89) and in HMO B (language delay, at three months with a relative risk of 1.13 and at seven months with a relative risk of 1.07), were not found in HMO C. Even though these neurodevelopmental outcomes persisted in the data from HMOs A and B, because of Phase II, the Verstraeten team reasoned that they had found no consistent significant associations between Thimerosal-containing vaccines and neurodevelopmental outcomes. The study did not claim to be the final authority on the question of a link, and suggested that more research was needed to resolve the conflicting findings between the three HMOs.

Several issues with the methodology of the study have already been expressed earlier in this document, and we will review and expand on them here. First, the inclusion of children in the study as young as one year of age could have significantly underreported the total cases of autism, given that the typical age of diagnosis is around four or five years of age.[1314]

Along those lines, the total number of autistic children identified in the study's population is lower than the general population as a whole. In HMOs A and B, both in California, 21 and 202 patients were diagnosed with autism, respectively. The size of the respective cohorts was 13,337 and 110,833, for a total of 223 cases in 124,170 children. That rate of autism works out to 0.18 percent of the population, or 18 per 10,000. Yet studies of autism in California reported that the rate for autism in California in the mid-1990s was 15 per 10,000 children and between 30 and 50 per 10,000 children, depending on the study.[1315 1316] Studies of other populations have also reported higher rates of autism in the United States in the mid-1990s than the data Verstraeten dealt with; a study of children in Atlanta found that 34 out of 10,000 children had autism.[1317]

These higher prevalence rates include Asperger's Syndrome and pervasive developmental disorder not otherwise specified (PDD-NOS), the two less severely affected of the three disorders then diagnostically recognized on the autism spectrum. ("Classic" autism is the most severe, third category.) The CDC researchers in the Verstraeten study did not include PDD-NOS in their analyses. If they had, the total number of autism cases (that is, autism spectrum disorder cases) would have been higher, possibly making the

CONFLICTS OF INTEREST IN POLICYMAKING AND REGULATION

relative risk ratios higher as well, and possibly making the results from HMOs A and B reach statistical significance.

Part of the reason for the low overall number of diagnosed autism cases could be that the researchers excluded cases that they said could have been misclassified. Around 60 percent of the ADD and associated ADHD cases were thus not counted in the analysis, and 20 percent of autism cases were eliminated, as they were not rendered by an in-network behavioral specialist.[1318] Many other exclusions were made on the basis of perinatal conditions or mothers who experienced any sort of complication during labor or pregnancy. In HMO B, the largest one, this methodological approach ultimately excluded 24 percent of children per low birth weight or other congenital, perinatal, or maternal complications. In a chapter for the 2011 textbook Autism Spectrum Disorders, University of California, Davis researcher Irva Hertz-Picciotto wrote that this aspect of the study "removed a disproportionate number [of children] with susceptibility to autism," which could have compromised the study's findings. Hertz-Picciotto called this a "considerable limitation" of the study, and wrote further:

> Low birth weight, anomalies, birth hypoxia and other perinatal conditions are risk factors for autism, suggesting that the children most at risk for autism were excluded. Hence population-based estimates of thimerosal effects [are] not possible from this analysis.[1319]

The fact that HMO A and C included much fewer children than HMO B, and that neurodevelopmental disorders could have been under- or overdiagnosed in the various HMOs, limited the statistical power of the study. The end result is that again, statistical significance for neurodevelopmental conditions was harder to attain. In a similar manner, Verstraeten split neurodevelopmental disorders into discrete, smaller categories such as ADD, tics, and speech and language delays, unlike he did in his earlier analyses, which also reduced the study's power, according to SafeMinds.

Furthermore, the Verstraeten study does not directly compare children who received Thimerosal to unexposed children. Instead, it compares children who had differences in Thimerosal exposure in increments of 12.5 micrograms, as well as children who were exposed to low, intermediate, and high levels of Thimerosal at one, three, and seven months of age. The study set a baseline not at 0 micrograms of Thimerosal exposure, but at 37.5 micrograms, which would statistically cause risk ratios to decrease.[1320]

An additional flaw with the Verstraeten study is the incongruity between the three HMOs. Harvard Pilgrim (HMO C) used a Costar diagnostic coding system rather than the International Classification of Diseases, Ninth Revision, Clinical Modification (ICD-9-CM) used at HMOs A and B. HMO B, it should be noted, coded differently from HMO A for speech and language disorders as well.[1321] HMO C, as previously discussed, also had questionable recordkeeping practices and went into bankruptcy.

In a December 2003 letter to *Pediatrics*, Neal Halsey and two colleagues from Johns Hopkins raised some of the above issues with regards to Verstraeten's study. They wrote:

The results differ somewhat from those presented to the Institute of Medicine (IOM) in 2001, where a statistically significant dose-response association was observed between thimerosal exposure by three months of age and neurodevelopmental delay assessed by combining several diagnostic categories. Such an analysis is reasonable since there is variability in coding of diagnoses for children with developmental delay and since a related compound, methylmercury, is known to be associated with multiple effects on neurological development. Analysis by separate diagnostic category may have substantially reduced the power to find important relationships. In addition, the selection criteria used in the published article appear to have been more lax than in the IOM presentation, as the latter was based on fewer outcomes.

Several important issues were not adequately described. Were all DTaP, Haemophilus influenzae type b, and hepatitis B vaccines assumed to contain the thimerosal preservative? Some vaccines were available that did not contain this preservative. Were diagnoses that were not made by a specialist (i.e. not validated) excluded from analyses? Primary care physicians are capable of diagnosing attention deficit disorder (ADD) without input from a subspecialist.[1322][1323][1324]

A special panel convened by the National Institute of Environmental Health Sciences (NIEHS) also pointed out weaknesses of the Verstraeten study among other criticisms of the VSD in general as a tool for addressing a potential association between Thimerosal and autism. The panel's report said of the Verstraeten study:

The design of a new study would have the additional benefit of enabling a reconsideration of some aspects of the original study design and the opportunity to collect additional data to evaluate issues such as diagnostic reliability and sensitivity. Of particular interest to the panel was the large proportion, about 25%, of births excluded from the analyses in the Verstraeten study. These exclusions were intended to decrease confounding. The panel noted that these children may represent a susceptible population whose removal from the analysis might have had the unintended consequence of reducing the ability to detect an effect of thimerosal.[1325]

Beyond these methodological issues, Verstraeten himself had a potentially significant conflict of interest. In July 2001, one year after the Simpsonwood meeting, Verstraeten accepted a job working for pharmaceutical company GlaxoSmithKline (GSK), a maker of Thimerosal-preserved vaccines.[1326] [1327] [1328] For the final study in 2003, Verstraeten was still identified as an employee of the CDC, and his subsequent employment with GSK was not declared in the text. Notably, Verstraeten actively solicited GSK employment for CDC scientists by sending an epidemiologist job posting via email in March 2004, for example.[1329] Other details of a continuing dialogue between Verstraeten and the CDC regarding his study after his departure, as well as his possible attempts to get inside information on vaccine safety trials, are not yet fully known, as the CDC is presently withholding nearly 400 pages of relevant correspondence, according to Brian S. Hooker, a research scientist at the Autism Healing Network mentioned previously.[1330]

Having left the CDC's employ, Verstraeten did not present the 2003 *Pediatrics* study himself to the 2004 IOM committee. Verstraeten has not offered public comment on the study, except in a letter to the editor of *Pediatrics* in 2004. In this letter, Verstraeten denied that his hiring by GSK in any way altered the eventual study, though he did acknowledge his involvement in the study's further analyses. Verstraeten wrote:

Did GSK hire me away to manipulate the data before publication? Definitely not. This suggestion could be viewed as simply silly, were it not that it offends the ethical integrity of both the company and myself. Although I have been involved in some of the discussions concerning additional analyses that were undertaken after my departure from the CDC, I did not perform any of these additional analyses myself, nor did I instigate them. GSK was at no point involved in any discussions I had with former CDC colleagues on the study, nor were details of these discussions ever discussed between myself and GSK. The company and I had a very clear deal from the very start of my employment that I would finalize my involvement in the study on my own time and keep this involvement entirely separated from my work at GSK.[1331]

In that letter, Verstraeten made clear that the study in no way rules out the possibility that vaccines cause autism. He also denied that the earlier analyses' results had been carefully and deliberately weakened. Verstraeten wrote:

Did the CDC water down the original results? It did not. This misconception comes from an erroneous perception of this screening study and other epidemiological studies. The perception is that an epidemiological study can have only 1 of

2 outcomes: either an association is found (or confirmed), or an association is refuted. Very often, however, there is a third interpretation: an association can neither be found nor refuted. Let's call the first 2 outcomes "positive" and "negative" and the third outcome "neutral."

In his letter, Verstraeten went on to explain that the initial results of his CDC screening study of Thimerosal-containing vaccines were indeed "positive," and "found an association between thimerosal and some neurodevelopmental outcomes." Verstraeten said that "this was the perception both independent scientists and anti-vaccine lobbyists had at the conclusion of the first phase of the study." However, it was "foreseen from the very start that any positive outcome would lead to a second phase." Given the "large potential public health impact" of the findings, Verstraeten and colleagues quickly sought "urgent validation" of their results in a second phase. This second phase, Verstraeten maintained, was not chosen with bias. He wrote:

Did the CDC purposefully select a second phase that would contradict the first phase? Certainly not. The push to urgently perform the second phase at health maintenance organization C came entirely from myself, because I felt that the first-phase results were too prone to potential biases to be the basis for important public health decisions. Health maintenance organization C was the only site known to myself and my coauthors that could rapidly provide sufficient data that would enable a check of the major findings of the first phase in a timely manner.

The data from HMO C did not suggest a correlation between Thimerosal-containing vaccine exposure and neurodevelopmental outcomes, as the first phase's data had. "Surprisingly, however," Verstraeten wrote, "the study is being interpreted now as negative by many." This interpretation is erroneous, Verstraeten went on to explain:

> The article does not state that we found evidence against an association, as a negative study would. It does state, on the contrary, that additional study is recommended, which is the conclusion to which a neutral study must come. Does a neutral outcome reduce the value of a study? It may make it less attractive to publishers and certainly to the press, but it in no way diminishes its scientific and public health merit. A neutral study carries a very distinct message: the investigators could neither confirm nor exclude an association, and therefore more study is required.[1332]

Despite the study's forthright neutrality emphasized by Verstraeten, his study has become one of the key arguments against a Thimerosal-autism link. Verstraeten has provided no further public comment to the knowledge of this book's contributors.

As conveyed in quotes from Simpsonwood and elsewhere, Verstraeten seems to have had a difficult time squaring his initial findings with the eventually published and allegedly manipulated results. In an email in July 2000 to Philippe Grandjean, the Danish researcher who published studies on mercury exposure in the Faroe Islands population, and some CDC colleagues and coauthors of his

2003 study, Verstraeten wrote, "I do not wish to be the advocate of the anti-vaccine lobby and sound like being convinced that thimerosal is or was harmful, but at least I feel we should use sound scientific argumentation and not let our standards be dictated by our desire to disprove an unpleasant theory." [1333] [1334]

Notes

[1313] Verstraeten T, Davis RL, DeStefano F, Lieu TA, Rhodes PH, Black SB, Shinefield H, Chen RT; Vaccine Safety Datalink Team. Safety of Thimerosal-containing vaccines: a two-phased study of computerized health maintenance organization databases. *Pediatrics*. 2003 Nov;112(5):1039-48.

[1314] http://www.cdc.gov/ncbddd/autism/data.html.

[1315] Croen LA, Grether JK, Hoogstrate J, Selvin S. The changing prevalence of autism in California. *J Autism Dev Disord*. 2002 Jun;32(3):207-15.

[1316] King MD, Bearman PS. Socioeconomic status and the increased prevalence of autism in California. *Am Sociol Rev*. 2011 Apr 1;76(2):320-346.

[1317] Yeargin-Allsopp M, Rice C, Karapurkar T, Doernberg N, Boyle C, Murphy C. Prevalence of autism in a US metropolitan area. *JAMA*. 2003 Jan 1;289(1):49-55.

[1318] National Academy of Science, Institute of Medicine, Immunization Safety Review Committee. *Thimerosal-Containing Vaccines and Neurodevelopmental Outcomes*. Public Meeting. Cambridge, Massachusetts. Monday, July 16, 2001.

[1319] Hertz-Picciotto I. Large Scale Epidemiologic Studies of Environmental Factors in Autism. *Autism Spectrum Disorders*. Amaral DG, Dawson G, Geschwind DH, eds. Oxford University Press, 2011.

[1320] Brian S. Hooker, correspondence with book researchers.

[1321] Verstraeten T, Davis RL, DeStefano F, Lieu TA, Rhodes PH, Black SB, Shinefield H, Chen RT. Safety of Thimerosal-containing vaccines: a two-phased study of computerized health maintenance organization databases. *Pediatrics*. 2003 Nov;112(5):1039-48.

[1322] http://pediatrics.aappublications.org/content/112/5/1039.abstract/reply#pediatrics_el_547.

[1323] http://www.jhsph.edu/faculty/directory/profile/3934/Salmon/Daniel.

[1324] http://www.jhsph.edu/faculty/directory/profile/1507/Moulton/Lawrence_H.

[1325] Department of Health and Human Services, National Institutes of Health. *Report of the Expert Panel to the National Institute of Environmental Health Science. Thimerosal Exposure in Pediatric Vaccines: Feasibility of Studies Using the Vaccine Safety Datalink*. August 24, 2006.

[1326] National Academy of Science, Institute of Medicine, Immunization Safety Review Committee. *Thimerosal-Containing Vaccines and Neurodevelopmental Outcomes*. Public Meeting. Cambridge, Massachusetts. Monday, July 16, 2001.

1327 Committee on Infectious Diseases and Committee on Environmental Health, American Academy of Pediatrics. Thimerosal in vaccines—an interim report to clinicians. *Pediatrics.* 1999 Sep;104(3 Pt 1):570-4.

1328 http://www.gsk.com/products/our-vaccines.html.

1329 Thomas Verstraeten, "Open position for epidemiologist at GSK Biologicals in Belgium," email to Robert Chen, Frank DeStefano, katrin@bellsouth.net, March 15, 2004.

1330 Brian S. Hooker, correspondence with book researchers.

1331 Verstraeten T. Thimerosal, the Centers for Disease Control and Prevention, and GlaxoSmithKline. *Pediatrics.* 2004 Apr;113(4):932.

1332 Verstraeten T. Thimerosal, the Centers for Disease Control and Prevention, and GlaxoSmithKline. *Pediatrics.* 2004 Apr;113(4):932.

1333 http://www.hsph.harvard.edu/philippe-grandjean/.

1334 Thomas Verstraeten, "RE: Thimerosal and neurologic outcomes," email to Philippe Grandjean, Robert Chen, Frank DeStefano, Robert Pless, Roger Bernier, Tom Clarkson, Pal Weihe, July 14, 2000.

Chapter 29:
CDC Interference and Intimidation in Thimerosal-Related Autism Research

A reader of this book might ask at this point why there has not been further analysis of Verstraeten's early data or other similar data sets. As part of the response after the Simpsonwood meeting, the CDC began taking what appear to be steps to block public access to the original Verstraeten data and the VSD files in general. The CDC has also suppressed research that is skeptical of Thimerosal's safety while encouraging other research that ultimately supports the agency's public assurances about the chemical.

Following the presentation of the early Verstraeten study data at the June 2000 ACIP meeting, shortly after the Simpsonwood conference, SafeMinds and other interested parties sought access to the raw VSD files in order to do their own independent analyses. The CDC responded that it would not grant access to the VSD to outside groups or individuals. The agency cited the rights and privacy of organizations involved in the database, adding that some HMOs threatened to leave the VSD for fear of lawsuits if patient records were released. The CDC did offer to work with the interested parties toward a solution, however. Among the back-and-forth that continued well into 2002, Congressman Burton wrote the CDC in July 2001 requesting the raw VSD data, his staff prepared a subpoena, and hearings were held.[1335]

In February 2002, the CDC relented, but insisted on a number of burdensome conditions for outside researchers to have to satisfy in order to access the VSD. The CDC proposed rules that the researchers must have institutional affiliations, must be working on funded, approved studies, and must submit detailed proposals for their research to the CDC, including a list of exact data files for review, hypotheses under study, and analytical methods. An additional obstacle was that interested researchers had to obtain permission to access data from the Institutional Review Boards of each managed care organization participating in the VSD. To access the requested data from the CDC, researchers had to travel to a designated facility in Maryland where CDC personnel could monitor the research activities, which were permitted at a single computer work terminal. No notes could be taken, and government programmers would supply printouts of the requested data runs.

Independent investigators Mark and David Geier eventually jumped through all these bureaucratic hurdles and more. In doing so, they encountered an extreme lack of cooperation from the

CDC in the process, as recounted in journalist David Kirby's book *Evidence of Harm* and elsewhere.[1336] Congressman Dave Weldon had to weigh in on the Geiers' behalf as well to secure the right to access the VSD in 2004. To date, the Geiers remain the only independent researchers to have accomplished this.[1337 1338 1339]

Despite being taxpayer-funded, the VSD has remained essentially inaccessible to the public. Part of this seems to relate to the fact that the CDC turned over data housing and administration of the VSD on September 20, 2002, through a $190 million contract to a third party, the American Association of Health Plans.[1340] Such an arrangement, critics have alleged, shields the data from "sunshine laws" like the Freedom of Information Act (FOIA), or even subpoena, by characterizing the data as proprietary to the HMOs that helped generate it.[1341] A PowerPoint presentation at a VSD team meeting in February 2002, held in Denver, points to these motives. Slides titled "Protecting Scientific Information" go on to read "Unpublished information being leaked to the public. . ." and "From FOIA, the congress, the courts. . . ."[1342]

Along with efforts to stymie the Geiers' research, the CDC also sought to discredit the Geiers' work in the eyes of the 2004 IOM panel. A review study prepared by Sarah Parker of Children's Hospital and University of Colorado Health Sciences Center and CDC employees was reviewed by the IOM prior to its September 2004 publication in, predictably, the journal *Pediatrics*.[1343] The Parker study, as mentioned in Chapter 25, cited weaknesses in the several then-available epidemiological studies from Europe, as well as the Verstraeten study. But the study went to extra lengths regarding the Geiers' work, making false and misleading statements.

The Parker paper stated that the Geiers could not possibly have arrived at accurate estimates of ethylmercury exposure for vaccinated children because the CDC Biological Surveillance Summaries with manufacturer-specific data—which the Geiers cited as their source—would not have been available to the Geiers. Frank DeStefano, project director of the VSD and a Verstraeten coauthor, learned in September 2003 that the Geiers had in fact received manufacturer-specific data from the CDC, as revealed in emails obtained via FOIA.[1344] DeStefano reviewed the Parker paper prior to January 15, 2004, yet did not offer any corrections on this point.[1345] The aspersion-casting statements regarding the Geiers' methods remained in the study text. The IOM panel, as described in the next chapter, went on to disregard the Geiers' epidemiological findings. In 2005, *Pediatrics* published an Erratum by Parker and her coauthors admitting—well after the IOM's 2004 report was released—that the Geiers did actually have the data.[1346]

With regards to the experience of researchers such as the Geiers looking into vaccine-autism links including Thimerosal and, separately, an immune reaction to the measles, mumps, and rubella (MMR) vaccine, Weldon had strong criticisms of the CDC's behavior. Speaking before an IOM committee meeting in February 2004, Weldon rebuked the CDC over its apparent muzzling of dissident scientists:

> I must begin by sharing how disappointed I am by the number of reports I continue to receive from researchers regarding their difficulties in pursuing answers to these questions. It is past time that individuals are persecuted for asking questions about vaccine safety—we have recognized error before

in the case of live polio, whole-cell pertussis, and rotavirus. I am repeatedly informed by researchers who encounter apathy from government officials charged with investigating these matters, difficulty in getting their papers published, and the loss of research grants. Some report overt discouragement, intimidation and threats, and have abandoned this field of research.

With specific reference to the VSD, Weldon said, "The CDC erected excessive barriers and has imposed severe limits on access to the data."[1347]

Adding to the irregularities, the CDC has told the Geiers and others that Verstraeten's original data sets were not maintained and that there is, accordingly, no way to replicate his original study.[1348] At a meeting of the IOM on August 23, 2004, about VSD data sharing, Melinda Wharton, acting deputy director of the National Immunization Program at the CDC, presented in PowerPoint that "many data sets from previous published VSD studies had not been archived in a standard manner" and she said that "those data sets may not allow all the re-analyses that one might want to do, or in fact may not be available at all."[1349] [1350] Kirby wrote that a contractor at this IOM meeting testified that "he was ordered to destroy data sets to 'protect privacy.'" The CDC claimed it had provided the Verstraeten data sets to the Geiers, but the Geiers said that the sets "contained no data and were 'totally unusable.'"[1351]

The CDC's "losing" of Verstraeten's original data sets, whether out of unintentional negligence or willful destruction, also appears to be illegal under federal statutes. Under the Public Health Service Act, section 300aa-25, which went into effect January 5, 1999, information regarding "vaccine-related illnesses, disabilities, injuries and conditions . . . shall be available to the public," excluding the information that "may identify an individual."[1352] In addition, the NIH and FDA have guidelines for scientific record-keeping and the retention of data, which would not appear to have been followed by the CDC with regards to Verstraeten data.[1353 1354] Finally, from a basic standpoint of due diligence, of course, preserving data would also allow for replication and subsequent review—an important element of any scientific study, let alone one that speaks to the health of a generation of children.

Study ideas that could help further settle the debate on a Thimerosal-autism link have not been funded or followed up on by the CDC and funding agencies. An example comes from United Press International (UPI), one of the few press organizations that has maintained skepticism regarding CDC's claims on vaccines. In the mid-2000s, senior editor Dan Olmsted wrote articles regarding the Amish of Lancaster County, Pennsylvania, and 30,000 homeschooled children in Chicago who were not vaccinated. In those populations, UPI reported a near-total absence of autism and other neurological illnesses associated with vaccines.[1355 1356] Despite calls from researchers such as Boyd Haley and the autism activist community, the CDC, NIH, and others have not seen it fit to develop or fund studies that could compare the rates of neurodevelopmental disorders in vaccinated American children to unvaccinated American children.[1357 1358 1359]

Another example of this chilling effect in academia concerns a research grant submitted to NIH in 2005 by Northeastern University scientist Richard Deth.[1360] He had applied for funds to study the effects of inflammation and heavy metals on methylation in autism, following up on previous research of his that suggested a Thimerosal-autism connection. In criticizing Deth's proposal, which was rejected, a reviewer of the grant cited language appearing then on an FDA web page. The language was drawn from the IOM's major 2004 report (a follow-up to the 2001 report, and discussed in the next chapter) that found no evidence of a link between autism and Thimerosal-containing vaccines.[1361 1362 1363]

In direct contrast to the apparent stifling of certain studies, the CDC has promoted and expedited studies that align with its pro-Thimerosal position. The CDC helped fund the 2003 Stehr-Green study exculpating Thimerosal, for example.[1364] Members of the CDC, including Verstraeten and Robert Chen, also consulted on and approved WHO funding for Elizabeth Miller's 2004 British study cited by the IOM in 2004, as revealed by emails obtained via FOIA.[1365 1366 1367 1368 1369]

In another example, on December 10, 2002, Jose Cordero, then the assistant surgeon general and director at the CDC's National Center on Birth Defects and Developmental Disabilities, sent a letter to the editor-in-chief of the journal *Pediatrics* urging him to publish Madsen's Danish study, which indeed the journal did in 2003. Cordero wrote:

> I am writing in support of an expedited review and consideration of the enclosed manuscript that examines the association between thimerosal, an ethyl mercury containing preservative, and autism. . . . I feel this is a very important study that deserves thoughtful consideration by the Journal. Its findings provide one strong piece of evidence that thimerosal is not causally linked to autism.[1370]

"It's quite unusual to have a CDC official endorse a study in that way," says Haley, who has published more than 130 papers in peer-reviewed journals.[1371] [1372] [1373] "I have never heard of it before."[1374] *JAMA* and *The Lancet*, as previously noted in this book, had already rejected the Madsen manuscript before Cordero wrote his letter. On December 5, 2006, Congressman Weldon sent a letter to the CDC's director, Julie Gerberding, inquiring about Cordero's actions, writing:

[The Madsen study] had just been rejected by two journals. The last thing it should have been subjected to was an expedited review. These actions by the CDC call into question the integrity and objectivity of the CDC's scientific investigations. We have an obligation to the taxpayers to examine this issue to determine whether or not this trust has been violated.[1375]

Cordero's decision to encourage the publication of research supporting the safety of Thimerosal by asking for its "expedited review" is again indicative of the CDC's failure to objectively address the Thimerosal-vaccine controversy.

Notes

[1335] Opening Statement, Chairman Dan Burton, Committee on Government Reform. *The Status of Research into Vaccine Safety and Autism.* June 19, 2002 *available at* http://www.whale.to/a/a.html.

[1336] Kirby D. *Evidence of Harm: Mercury in Vaccines and the Autism Epidemic: A Medical Controversy.* New York: St. Martin's Press, 2005.

[1337] http://www.iom.edu/~/media/Files/Activity%20Files/PublicHealth/ImmunizationSafety/IOMWeldonFinal2904.pdf.

[1338] United States. Mercury in medicine report. *Congressional Record.* Washington: GPO, May 21, 2003: 1011-1030.

[1339] Committee on the Review of the National Immunization Program's Research Procedures and Data Sharing Program, Board on Health Promotion and Disease Prevention, Institute of Medicine. *Vaccine Safety Research, Data Access, and Public Trust.* The National Academies Press. Washington, D.C. 2005 *available at* http://books.nap.edu/openbook.php?record_id=11234.

[1340] Centers for Disease Control and Prevention. Procurements and Grants Office. Public Notification of Award of Contract 200-2002-00732, American Association of Health Plans. September 20, 2002.

[1341] Brian S. Hooker, correspondence with book researchers.

[1342] VSD Team WebSite Security Issues. PowerPoint presentation. February 7, 2002.

[1343] http://www.ucdenver.edu/academics/colleges/medicalschool/departments/pediatrics/people/bios/Pages/parkerbio.aspx.

[1344] Frank DeStefano, "FW: Geier letter," email to Melinda Wharton, Penina Haber, Robert Chen, September 19, 2003.

[1345] Larry K. Pickering, letter to Sarah K. Parker, January 15, 2004.

[1346] Parker S, Todd J, Schwartz B, Pickering L. Thimerosal-containing vaccines and autistic spectrum disorder: a critical review of published original data. *Pediatrics.* 2005 Jan;115(1):200. Erratum for Pediatrics. 2004 Sep;114(3):793-804.

[1347] http://www.iom.edu/~/media/Files/Activity%20Files/PublicHealth/ImmunizationSafety/IOMWeldonFinal2904.pdf.

[1348] David Geier, correspondence with book researchers.

[1349] http://www.iom.edu/Activities/HealthServices/NIPDataSharing.aspx.

[1350] Melinda Wharton. *The Vaccine Safety Datalink (VSD) Data Sharing Program.* PowerPoint presentation to the IOM. August 23, 2004.

[1351] Kirby D. *Evidence of Harm: Mercury in Vaccines and the Autism Epidemic: A Medical Controversy.* New York: St. Martin's Press, 2005.

[1352] http://wonder.cdc.gov/wonder/help/vaers/42USC300aa-25.htm.

[1353] http://sourcebook.od.nih.gov/ethic-conduct/RECORDKEEPING.pdf.

[1354] http://sourcebook.od.nih.gov/ethic-conduct/Conduct%20Research%206-11-07.pdf.

[1355] http://www.upi.com/Health_News/2005/12/07/The-Age-of-Autism-A-pretty-big-secret/ UPI-68291133982531/.

[1356] http://www.upi.com/Health_News/2006/07/28/The-Age-of-Autism-Amish-bill-introduced/UPI-35321154110819/.

[1357] http://www.whale.to/vaccine/sch12.html.

[1358] http://www.ageofautism.com/2009/02/unvaccinated-children-madness.html.

[1359] http://safeminds.org/news/pressroom/safeminds-responds-IOM%20Report.html.

[1360] http://www.northeastern.edu/bouve/directory/faculty.php?name=Richard%20Deth.

[1361] NIH Center for Scientific Review. Application Number 1 R21 ES014640-01.

[1362] Richard Deth, correspondence with book researchers.

[1363] Immunization Safety Review Committee, Board on Health Promotion and Disease Prevention, Institute of Medicine. *Immunization Safety Review: Vaccines and Autism.* The National Academies Press. Washington, DC. May 2004.

[1364] Stehr-Green P, Tull P, Stellfeld M, Mortenson PB, Simpson D. Autism and thimerosal-containing vaccines: lack of consistent evidence for an association. *Am J Prev Med.* 2003 Aug;25(2):101-6.

[1365] Andrews N, Miller E, Grant A, Stowe J, Osborne V, Taylor B. Thimerosal exposure in infants and developmental disorders: a retrospective cohort study in the United Kingdom does not support a causal association. *Pediatrics.* 2004 Sep;114(3):584-91.

[1366] Elizabeth Miller, "RE: UK vaccine schedule and thimerosal exposure," email to Robert Chen and Thomas Verstraeten, June 26, 2001.

[1367] Elizabeth Miller, "thiomersal," email to Robert Chen and Nick Andrews, August 14, 2001.

[1368] Elizabeth Miller, "thiomersal," email to Robert Chen and Nick Andrews. October 18, 2001.

[1369] Elizabeth Miller, "RE:thiomersal," email to Robert Chen, November 8, 2001.

[1370] Jose Cordero, letter to Jerold F. Lucey, December 10, 2002.

[1371] http://www.novaccine.com/boyd_haley.asp.

[1372] http://www.ncbi.nlm.nih.gov/pubmed?term=Haley%20BE.

[1373] http://www.ncbi.nlm.nih.gov/pubmed?term=Haley%20B[Author]&cauthor=-true&cauthor_uid=7518829.

[1374] Robert F. Kennedy, Jr., telephone interview with Boyd Haley, April 9, 2005.

[1375] Dave Weldon, letter to Julie Gerberding, December 5, 2006.

Chapter 30:
The IOM 2004 Report and Response

In 2004, with Verstraeten's study now published and the four European epidemiological studies wrapping up, and further research stymied, as described in the last chapter, the CDC- and NIH-sponsored IOM Immunization Safety Review Committee convened again to issue another report. This last IOM report (of eight total addressing various aspects of vaccine safety), issued publicly on May 18, 2004, favored "rejection of a causal relationship between thimerosal-containing vaccines and autism."

The report went on to strongly recommend that no further studies should address the issue and that "available funding for autism research be channeled to the most promising areas."[1376] The quotes attributed to the committee's chairperson, Marie McCormick, in a press release that accompanied the report's issuance, were explicit in backing up the "no link" contention and cessation of vaccine-related inquiry:

The overwhelming evidence from several well-designed studies indicates that childhood vaccines are not associated with autism. . . . We strongly support ongoing research to discover the cause or causes of this devastating disorder. Resources would be used most effectively if they were directed toward those avenues of inquiry that offer the greatest promise for answers. Without supporting evidence, the vaccine hypothesis does not hold such promise.[1377]

In preparing its final report, however, this book contends that the IOM did not adequately assess the available literature regarding Thimerosal and neurological injury. At its February 9, 2004, public meeting, the IOM panel heard presentations from several scientists who had recently published studies or were working on important research relevant to the Thimerosal-autism question cited in this document.[1378] These researchers included Columbia University's Mady Hornig; Mark and David Geier; David Baskin, then at the Baylor College of Medicine; the University of Kentucky's Boyd Haley; and Jeff Bradstreet, who has worked with the Geiers and been active within the autism advocacy community.[1379 1380 1381 1382 1383 1384 1385 1386]

Yet the IOM committee refused to give weight to the pharmacological, clinical, and toxicological research presented by these and other scientists in its final report. Instead, the IOM committee relied almost entirely on epidemiological findings. As stated by the report:

The committee also concludes that the body of epidemiological evidence favors rejection of a causal relationship between thimerosal-containing vaccines and autism. The committee further finds that potential biological mechanisms for vaccine-induced autism that have been generated to date are theoretical only.[1387]

No transcript of the thirteen-member panel's 2004 deliberations is available. Yet it would appear that the panel deemed as acceptable only the CDC-affiliated epidemiological studies done in Europe and the heavily revised Verstraeten study, despite their many acknowledged flaws as described in an article by Parker in 2004, for instance, and in this document. Meanwhile, a total of six studies by the father-son Geier team were disqualified by the IOM committee for "serious methodological flaws" and "nontransparent" analytic methods, perhaps prompted by Parker's 2004 review study that slandered the Geiers' work.[1388]

The panel also did not hear all of the available evidence that was suggestive of Thimerosal having a connection to neurological damage. For example, the committee did not allow Richard Deth from Northeastern University to present his ongoing research, even though he had just published new evidence regarding Thimerosal in a respected journal two weeks prior to the February 9 meeting.[1389 1390] Deth's work, described in Part Three, pointed to the potent inhibition by Thimerosal of the epigenetic regulation of genes during early development. This work provided a direct explanation for the neurodevelopmental toxicity of Thimerosal.[1391]

Also, notably, when the IOM panel gathered again to review the Thimerosal issue, its focus had significantly narrowed. Rather than evaluating the potential link between Thimerosal and a range of neurodevelopmental disorders, the committee only addressed whether Thimerosal-containing vaccines might cause autism.

Narrowing the scope of their review allowed the IOM committee to ignore the significant body of literature suggesting a causal association between mercury exposure and a broader range of neurodevelopmental disorders, including attention deficit disorders and speech and language delay.

A second aspect of this narrowed focus is that, instead of assessing the evidence for "biological plausibility," as the first IOM panel had done and found that it could not rule out, the second panel focused on "biological mechanisms" for a relationship between Thimerosal exposure and autism. The biological mechanism evidence reviewed by the panel included, the report stated, "human, animal, and in vitro studies of biological or pathophysiological processes." However, according to Brian S. Hooker, the IOM failed to take into account nearly 140 studies pertinent to Thimerosal toxicity.[1392] Oddly, given the emphasis on biological mechanisms, the weight of evidence used by the panel to reject a Thimerosal-autism connection came down to epidemiological studies, which by their intrinsic nature do not speak directly to biological mechanisms. Furthermore, in 2004 the scientific community had yet to identify with any strong specificity potential biological mechanisms for the onset of autism; those posited since remain in need of significantly more research. As such, there were no valid biological mechanisms for the IOM to even consider. Ultimately, the focusing on biological mechanisms of autism alone was the trick used by the IOM, this book contends, to escape the "trap" described by Kaback during the IOM committee's January 2001 meeting.[1393]

When this book's author asked Stratton why the 2004 committee had focused on autism rather than neurodevelopmental disorders generally, as the Verstraeten study had done, she claimed that pending autism lawsuits were the committee's driving motivation. At that time, the government was defending more than 4,500 petitions submitted to the National Vaccine Injury Compensation Program (VICP, better known as the "Vaccine Court," discussed in Chapter 21) alleging that Thimerosal had caused autism.[1394] Stratton remarked, "Because that was sort of . . . what the court cases were about, that this would obviously be used ultimately . . . the government needed an answer on autism, so that's what we looked at." When I asked about the voluminous literature suggestive of Thimerosal's toxicity, and how I would be shocked if it were not injurious to infants, Stratton said:

> Clearly, mercury is very toxic. Clearly, ethylmercury is neurotoxic. Clearly, ethylmercury affects cell systems—animals, human cells—all those sorts of things, and clearly, when it was injected into newborn mice, they had weird behaviors . . . the point is, mercury is not good for you. Granted. Thimerosal probably, you know, I mean it can't be good for you, right? And certainly at some doses it's extremely bad for you. The question [we were charged with answering] is whether any of those animal or in-vitro studies make a connection to autism.[1395]

The release of the IOM's conclusions triggered strong reactions from the media and public. One committee member, Steven Goodman, of Johns Hopkins University at the time and now at Stanford, said in a 2004 article appearing in the *Southeast Missourian* that the final report's conclusions advocating no further research on a Thimerosal-autism connection were misconstrued:[1396]

First of all, we didn't dismiss anything. We simply stated the epidemiology evidence [viewed by the committee] favored no relationship, which is true. . . . What we did say is if you've got a fixed pot, don't spend huge amounts more on epidemiology. What we said was that resources would be better spent on understanding the biology.[1397]

Goodman also told this book's author:

Mercury is definitely a neurotoxin, absolutely. There's no question about that. We said that. The issue we addressed is, does it cause autism? There are plenty of reasons to take Thimerosal out of vaccines, plenty. . . . We made it clear in our report that it didn't close the book on [a Thimerosal-autism connection] because it can't, because of the nature of the studies. . . . The conclusion was that it favored no relationship, but it did not say that that verdict could not be reversed. . . . The [IOM] report didn't say more research should be done, it said we should gain a better understanding of autism so we can design better studies. That's what it said.[1398]

In a statement, Congressman Weldon characterized the IOM conclusions as "premature" and "hastily drawn." He wrote further:

In 2001 the IOM stated that it is "unclear whether ethylmercury [from vaccines] passes readily through the blood-brain barrier. . . ." The IOM recommended several biological and clinical studies to answer this question and whether this mercury could cause developmental problems. These studies were in large part never done. Yet IOM chose to ignore the need for this research and instead has focused its analysis on the data available today, most of which is statistical, but there is much more research that needs to be done before it can definitively be said that thimerosal does not contribute to NDDs [neurodevelopmental disorders]. Even today, the IOM cannot tell you with any degree of certainty what happens to ethylmercury once injected into an infant. Does it go to the brain? Does is [sic] cause developmental problems?

The IOM's scope of investigation was severely narrowed for this review. In 2001 the IOM considered thimerosal's relationship with nuerodevelopmental [sic] disorders as a whole, but here they only consider Autism. This raises suspicions that this IOM exercise might be more about drawing pre-designed conclusions aimed at restoring public confidence in vaccines rather than conducting a complete and thorough inquiry into whether or not thimerosal might cause neurodevelopmental disorders. Thomas Verstraeten, the author of one of the studies upon which the IOM relies, recently stated in an April 2004 letter to *Pediatrics*: "The bottom line is and has always been the same: an association between thimerosal and neurological outcomes could neither be confirmed nor refuted, and therefore, more study is required." It was after this study was published that the IOM scope was narrowed.

Unfortunately, the epidemiology studies that the IOM bases its findings on are not immune from conflicts or controversy. Many of the authors have conflicts of interest including funding from vaccine manufactures, employment by manufacturers, or conflicts in that they implemented vaccine policies that are now being investigated. Furthermore, the studies were designed to examine entire populations and would miss subgroups of genetically susceptible populations. Much like the infamous 1989 study by The National Institute of Child and Human Development (NICHD) which missed the link between folic acid deficiencies and neural tube defects, the epidemiology studies reviewed by the IOM in drawing today's findings, could easily have missed a link between thimerosal and NDDs. The IOM report is based on studies examining populations in the United Kingdom, Denmark, Sweden and the United States—all of whom have different vaccines, vaccine policies, and mercury exposures. Study results are only as reliable as the design of such studies. Relying on these studies to draw conclusions is shaky ground.[1399]

Furthermore, numerous vaccine safety, autism advocacy, and parental organizations criticized the IOM report's conclusions.[1400] SafeMinds issued a press release wherein its president, Lyn Redwood, said the following:

This committee and its report clearly chose to ignore groundbreaking scientific research on the mercury-autism link, and instead the IOM has issued a flawed, incomplete report that continues to put America's children at risk. The problem with this report begins with its violation of nearly every tenet of medical science. Respected researchers everywhere do not support the IOM belief that proof can be solely found in epidemiology. Yet, the IOM wants the public to buy into the absurd belief that this report, bought and paid for by the CDC, is complete, independent and trustworthy.[1401]

The National Vaccine Information Center in a press release declared that the IOM "played politics" with its report.[1402] The National Autism Association said in a statement that "the IOM panel dismissed strong clinical and epidemiological evidence presented during the hearings" described in this book from the researchers Baskin, Bradstreet, Geier and Geier, Haley, and Hornig.[1403]

Just two days after the IOM issued its report, the US Office of Special Counsel (OSC)—an independent investigative and prosecutorial agency that serves as a channel for whistleblowers—forwarded hundreds of specific complaints to the US Senate and House committees with oversight authority for HHS, requesting a congressional investigation. The OSC's special counsel, Scott Bloch, wrote in a letter to the committee chairmen that "there may be sufficient evidence to find a substantial likelihood of a substantial and specific danger to public health caused by the use of thimerosal/mercury in vaccines because of its inherent toxicity."[1404]

Ultimately, no appreciable action took place that brought about any sort of official reassessment of the IOM 2004 committee's conclusions. For more than eight years, the CDC has continued to present the 2004 panel's conclusions as the final word on the matter of Thimerosal and autism and neurological injury. Of note, the IOM did convene a separate panel of reviewers in 2005 to review how to improve access to the VSD for independent researchers, such as the Geiers, and improve public trust in internal CDC studies, such as Verstraeten's, based on the database. The February

17, 2005, report put forth numerous recommendations for the assurance of independence, transparency, and fairness of VSD research activities while protecting confidentiality.[1405] [1406] However, given the fact that the Geiers have not pursued additional VSD studies beyond previously accessed 1990s birth cohorts, nor have any other independent researchers been granted access to the VSD for Thimerosal-related studies, it would seem fair to say that the VSD remains essentially off-limits to external, public inquiry.[1407] [1408]

The CDC's unyielding stance on the Thimerosal issue, then, as now, has been effective, it would seem. The agency seems to remain very aware of the potential damage to its reputation and credibility that the Thimerosal issue continues to present. An internal CDC email from July 2012 obtained by Brian Hooker with regard to congressional investigations by Representatives Bill Posey (R-Florida) and Dan Burton (R-Indiana) speaks to this. The email, written by CDC employee Nancy Levine to Frank DeStefano director of the Immunization and Safety Office and others, relates a series of bullet points that need to be addressed in response to the congressional inquiry. Among other information, the CDC was to furnish Posey and Burton with "any correspondence or documents pertaining to autism and/or thimerosal between 1999 and June 22, 2012," as noted in one bullet point. A following bullet point stated, "Review all correspondences and documents to see if there is 'foreseeable harm' to the agency if they were released. Please 'flag' these documents and we will review them."[1409] It is not known at this time what documents were "flagged" and what happened to them.

A major reason why the CDC has succeeded at limiting debate and investigation into the Thimerosal issue has been the acquiescence of the media to the agency's official positions. As described by Dan Schulman, a senior editor at *Mother Jones*, in a piece for the *Columbia Journalism Review* seven months after the 2004 IOM report, "The perception that only distraught, activist parents and disreputable scientists back the thimerosal theory has seeped into the collective consciousness of the news media, which, in general, have been reluctant to cover the controversy."[1410][1411]

In the upcoming Part Five, we will examine some of these failings of the media in reporting on the Thimerosal controversy upon the IOM report release in 2004 and thereafter. But first, we will close Part Four with a chapter on the fast-developing situation of the "CDC Whistleblower," William Thompson, first mentioned in Chapter 7. Thompson's revelations provide some of the most convincing evidence of the CDC's obfuscation and obstruction regarding vaccines and neurodevelopmental injury, including autism.

Notes

[1376] Immunization Safety Review Committee, Board on Health Promotion and Disease Prevention, Institute of Medicine. *Immunization Safety Review: Vaccines and Autism.* The National Academies Press. Washington, DC. May 2004.

[1377] http://www8.nationalacademies.org/onpinews/newsitem.aspx?RecordID=10997.

[1378] Transcript, Immunization Safety Review Committee, Vaccines and Autism, February 9, 2004, National Academy of Sciences, Washington, DC. *available at* http://www.putchildrenfirst.org/media/6.16.pdf.

[1379] http://www.mailman.columbia.edu/our-faculty/profile?uni=mh2092.

[1380] Hornig M, Chian D, Lipkin WI. Neurotoxic effects of postnatal thimerosal are mouse strain dependent. *Mol Psychiatry.* 2004 Sep;9(9):833-45.

[1381] http://drdavidbaskin.com/hello-world/.

[1382] Baskin DS, Ngo H, Didenko VV. Thimerosal induces DNA breaks, caspase-3 activation, membrane damage, and cell death in cultured human neurons and fibroblasts. *Toxicol Sci.* 2003 Aug;74(2):361-8. Epub 2003 May 28.

[1383] http://www.chem.uky.edu/research/haley/.

[1384] Holmes AS, Blaxill MF, Haley BE. Reduced levels of mercury in first baby haircuts of autistic children. *Int J Toxic.* 2003;111(4):277-285.

[1385] http://www.icdrc.org/.

[1386] Bradstreet J, Geier DA, Kartzinel JJ, Adams JB, Geier MR. A case-control study of mercury burden in children with autistic spectrum disorders. *J Am Phys Surg.* 2003; 8: 76-79.

[1387] Immunization Safety Review Committee, Board on Health Promotion and Disease Prevention, Institute of Medicine. *Immunization Safety Review: Vaccines and Autism.* The National Academies Press. Washington, DC. May 2004.

[1388] Parker SK, Schwartz B, Todd J, Pickering LK. Thimerosal-containing vaccines and autistic spectrum disorder: a critical review of published original data. *Pediatrics.* 2004;114(3):793-804.

[1389] Waly M, Olteanu H, Banerjee R, Choi SW, Mason JB, Parker BS, Sukumar S, Shim S, Sharma A, Benzecry JM, Power-Charnitsky VA, Deth RC. Activation of methionine synthase by insulin-like growth factor-1 and dopamine: a target for neurodevelopmental toxins and thimerosal. *Mol Psychiatry.* 2004 Apr;9(4):358-70.

[1390] Richard Deth, correspondence with book researchers.

[1391] Robert F. Kennedy, Jr., telephone interview with Richard Deth, January 28, 2013.

[1392] Brian S. Hooker, correspondence with book researchers.

[1393] IOM Immunization Safety Review Committee January 2001 meeting, page 33.

[1394] http://www.hrsa.gov/vaccinecompensation/statisticsreports.html#Stats.

[1395] Robert F. Kennedy, Jr., telephone interview with Kathleen Stratton, April 28, 2005.

[1396] http://med.stanford.edu/profiles/Steven_Goodman/.

[1397] http://semissourian.rustcom.net/story/152176.html.

[1398] Robert F. Kennedy, Jr., telephone interview with Steven Goodman, May 4, 2005.

[1399] http://web.archive.org/web/20040805193937/http://www.house.gov/weldon/news/2004releases/IOMPR.pdf.

[1400] http://vaccineinfo.net/releases/IOM_vaccine_autism_report.htm.

[1401] http://www.safeminds.org/news/pressroom/press_releases/040518-PR10-BadIOMReport.pdf.

[1402] http://www.nvic.org/nvic-archives/pressrelease/iompolitics.aspx.

[1403] http://www.prnewswire.com/news-releases/national-autism-association-questions-iom-and-cdc-cover-up----how-far-will-they-go-to-protect-toxic-vaccines-74110397.html.

[1404] http://www.osc.gov/documents/press/2004/pr04_07.htm.

[1405] Committee on the Review of the National Immunization Program's Research Procedures and Data Sharing Program, Board on Health Promotion and Disease Prevention, Institute of Medicine. *Vaccine Safety Research, Data Access, and Public Trust.* The National Academies Press. Washington, DC. 2005. *available at* http://books.nap.edu/openbook.php?record id=11234.

[1406] http://www.iom.edu/Reports/2005/Vaccine-Safety-Research-Data-Access-and-Public-Trust.aspx.

[1407] http://www.ncbi.nlm.nih.gov/pubmed?term=geier%20vsd.

[1408] http://www.ncbi.nlm.nih.gov/pubmed?term=thimerosal%20vaccine%20safety%20data-link.

[1409] Nancy Levine, "FW: URGENT CONGRESSIONAL INQUIRY," email to Frank DeStefano, Eric Weintraub, Cindy Weinbaum, PerStephanie Thompson, July 27, 2012.

[1410] http://www.motherjones.com/authors/daniel-schulman.

[1411] http://web.archive.org/web/20071023194638/http://cjrarchives.org/issues/2005/6/schulman.asp.

Chapter 31: The "CDC Whistleblower," William Thompson

As briefly recounted earlier in this book, Brian S. Hooker recorded several phone conversations he had with the CDC's William Thompson in 2014. In these calls, Thompson disclosed at the very least unscientific, and arguably unethical, actions perpetrated by employees of the CDC with regard to vaccine safety studies.

Hooker consulted with lawyers and decided to release portions of the tapes later in 2014 because of their potentially profound importance to public health. Thompson, who had been unaware of the conversations being taped, did not authorize the release of their contents. Upon hearing of Hooker's plans to go public with some of the tape's information, Thompson sought and was granted whistleblower protection by the Obama Administration in August 2014. Thompson is now participating in an ongoing

Congressional investigation into the CDC's actions in this matter, led by Representative Posey.[1412][1413]

Hooker is a prominent figure in the vaccine-autism public controversy. He has provided documents and material support to the author and researchers of this book. At present, Hooker serves on the board of Focus For Health Foundation, an advocacy group.[1414] He became involved in the vaccine injury activist movement because has a son with autism. Hooker believes vaccinations his son received in 1998 and 1999 triggered the condition's onset. Following the IOM's report in 2004, Hooker has long tried to expose malfeasance within the CDC about its categorical denial of any link between vaccines and autism. A biochemist by training and now at Simpson University in California, Hooker has extensively reviewed the CDC's published studies claiming vaccines are safe, as well as extensive, non-published materials, such as emails and raw data, obtained via FOIAs.[1415][1416] Thompson, sympathetic to Hooker's situation based on his own experiences working for the CDC on vaccine safety, agreed to help.

Thompson is a seventeen-year employee of the CDC. He holds the position of senior scientist, has worked in the Immunization Safety Office and is currently employed at the National Center for Birth Defects and Developmental Disabilities.[1417] Thompson was an author on three CDC-funded studies evaluating Thimerosal-containing vaccines and neuropsychological outcomes in children aged seven to ten years. These studies were referenced and described in Chapter 7 of this book as Thompson 2007, Price 2010, and Barile 2012.

Before we proceed further, we'll take a moment to recall those studies' findings. As stated in its abstract, Thompson 2007 did "not support a causal association between early exposure to mercury from thimerosal-containing vaccines and immune globulins and deficits in neuropsychological functioning at the age of 7 to 10 years." The study reported some beneficial as well as detrimental associations in its subjects, the latter of which included motor and phonic tics as well as poorer performance on a measure of speech articulation.[1418] The Price 2010 study looked explicitly at autism. It found that "prenatal and early-life exposure to ethylmercury from thimerosal-containing vaccines and immunoglobulin preparations was not related to increased risk of ASDs."[1419] Barile 2012, meanwhile, reported "no statistically significant associations between thimerosal exposure from vaccines early in life" with "neuropsychological outcomes assessed at 7–10 years." The study did however note "a small, but statistically significant association between early thimerosal exposure and the presence of tics in boys."[1420]

In addition to these Thimerosal studies, Thompson took part in a 2004 *Pediatrics* study, not mentioned previously in this book, which evaluated the age of receipt of the MMR vaccine in children with and without autism. The study did not find meaningful differences in the time of MMR injection between the two groups.[1421]

Over their several conversations, Thompson provided Hooker with behind-the-scenes accounts of internal CDC deliberations over these several vaccine safety studies. Thompson described a pervasive culture of hostility and obfuscation within the CDC regarding objective analysis of any links between vaccines and injuries, in particular autism, partly in response to the Verstraeten study and its associated furor. Thompson said, referencing the Verstraeten study of 2004 in a May 2014 conversation with Hooker:

The CDC has not been transparent. We've missed ten years of research because the CDC is so paralyzed right now by anything related to autism. They're not doing what they should be doing because they're afraid to look for things that might be associated [with autism] . . . there's still a lot of shame with that.[1422]

In the same conversation, Thompson also shared his feelings over his having participated in the CDC's handling of the vaccine injury issue, saying "I'm completely ashamed of what I did . . . higher-ups wanted to do certain things and I went along with it."

Thompson was referring to numerous episodes where the initial data analyses were diluted to reduce the significance of negative outcomes correlated with Thimerosal exposure. The Barile 2012 study offered the strongest example of this manipulation. To try to lessen the interference Thompson had encountered from his CDC colleagues and superiors over his 2007 Thimerosal study, he asked a then-Georgia State University graduate student, John Barile (advised by another author on the paper, Gabriel P. Kuperminc) to help prepare a follow-up. This new research would further assess the tic association with Thimerosal exposure seen in Thompson's original 2007 study. Thompson said that he had said to Barile: "Because you guys are outside the CDC, we'll have more leverage . . . you will have fewer constraints than I will."[1423]

Accordingly, because the study was developed outside of the normal CDC channels, it did not at first show up on the radar of Thompson's superiors, who must "clear" a study before it publishes. Thompson said:

I would say every study that has ever come out on immunization safety, the people above know . . . If there's a significant finding, they know months in advance of it going into clearance. So, my paper [Barile 2012], I put into clearance without them knowing anything about it, and it caught people off guard.[1424]

Thompson explained that the study found very significant correlations between Thimerosal exposure and tics. The study's draft therefore "initially had pretty strong wording . . . about the association," Thompson said. The CDC would not let this drafted wording go out to a journal for review, so the study "sat in clearance for a year," Thompson said, "and people just hammered away at the paper and watered it down more and more and more."[1425]

In an unusual maneuver, the CDC even insisted on adding another author—Jonathan Mink, an expert on tics, from the University of Rochester Medical Center—during this long clearance process.[1426] "So we added him and every step of the way, we had to water down the discussion," said Thompson. "I've never been involved in a study like this before where I was asked to add a coauthor in the middle of clearance."[1427] When the CDC finally cleared the study, "you ended up with the final, cleared manuscript with just the most, you know, whitewashed discussion ever," Thompson said.[1428]

The manipulated study went to a journal for peer review. Three independent reviewers, Thompson said, highlighted the study's strange avoidance of discussion of the strong tic association evidenced in the data. "Three people who had no vested interest in the outcome of [the study asked] . . . 'Why aren't you talking about significant results in the paper?'" Thompson said.[1429] The study of course did eventually publish in 2012 and made no report of significant evidence of harm.

According to Thompson, the CDC also interfered in the Italian study it funded, Tozzi 2009, which assessed Thimerosal-containing vaccine exposure with neuropsychological outcomes.[1430] Thompson did not work on the study himself, but he had seen wording and analysis in a pre-published draft. Thompson told Hooker that Tozzi 2009 was the best of the three studies—meaning Thompson 2007 and Price 2010 (Barile 20012 used the same data set as Thompson 2007)—for its larger and more statistically rigorous population size. Tozzi 2009 had originally replicated the (watered-down) tic and language deficit results found in Thompson 2007. But between this replication and publication in *Pediatrics*, the study's initial associations essentially disappeared, with the study ultimately stating that "given the large number of statistical comparisons performed, the few associations found between thimerosal exposure and neuropsychological development might be attributable to chance." Thompson recalled thinking about the study's evolution: "It was like, what the heck happened? . . . How did it change so much?"[1431]

Overall, given these several studies regarding neurophysical and neurodevelopmental injury from vaccines, as well as Verstraeten's work, Thompson thinks there is clear evidence that Thimerosal-containing vaccine exposure can cause tics. "I do think that Thimerosal causes tics," Thompson told Hooker.[1432]

These tics, Thompson also said, likely speak to the possibility of broader neurological injury. "[Tics are] the canary in the coal mine . . . It's a manifestation of an exposure that may have had a lot of other effects such as verbal learning problems, which were

THIMEROSAL: LET THE SCIENCE SPEAK

also found in several studies."[1433] This broader neurological injury might well include autism. "I can say, tics are four times more prevalent in autism," Thompson told Hooker. "There is a biological, there is biologic plausibility right now, I really do believe there is, to say that Thimerosal causes autism-like symptoms."[1434]

In the separate, but related matter of Thompson's 2004 study assessing MMR vaccine exposure and autism, he talked to Hooker about the omission of a statistically significant association demonstrating higher autism risk in African American boys. Upon the advice of Hooker, Thompson secured a whistleblower attorney, Rick Morgan of Morgan Verkamp of Cincinnati, Ohio, a firm that specializes in Federal whistleblower cases. With regard to the 2004 MMR study, in a written statement through his attorney, Thompson said publically on August 27, 2014:

> I regret that my coauthors and I omitted statistically significant information in our 2004 article published in the Journal [sic] *Pediatrics*. The omitted data suggested that African American males who received the MMR vaccine before age 36 months were at increased risk for autism. Decisions were made regarding which findings to report after the data were collected, and I believe that the final study protocol was not followed.[1435]

Given the CDC's inability to objectively address immunization safety, Thompson and Hooker expressed agreement that an independent entity or scientists should conduct the necessary research. The CDC, according to Thompson, has vast, as-yet-untapped stores of data that could be brought to bear in scientifically seeking answers to the questions of vaccine safety, such as if Thimerosal can lead to autism. Thompson said:

> We are sitting on this gold mine. Here is the deal, the CDC is they're paralyzed. [sic] The whole system is paralyzed right now. And the whole branch is paralyzed and it's becoming more paralyzed. There's less and less and less being done as the place is coming to a grinding halt. Really, what we need is for Congress to come in and say give us the data and we're going to have an independent contractor do it and bring in the autism advocates and have them intimately involved in the study.[1436]

In a separate conversation, Thompson also espoused the idea of the how the National Transportation Safety Board (NTSB) investigates aviation accidents, rather than the airline's regulator, the Federal Aviation Administration (FAA). "The FAA is responsible for regulating all sorts of things, but then when an accident happens, you bring in the NTSB," said Thompson. "So, you would have the equivalent of an NTSB-like organization that would do vaccine safety studies independently."[1437]

Thompson's attorneys have handed over an extensive amount of CDC documents to Congressman Posey. A hearing may occur before either the House Oversight and Government Reform Committee or the Energy and Commerce Committee and which might involve a subpoena to Thompson to testify.[1438] "If forced to testify, I'm not going to lie," Thompson said to Hooker. "I basically have stopped lying."[1439]

Thompson also expressed that he is prepared for the personal consequences of going on the record with his experiences, commenting: "So I have to deal with a few months of hell if this becomes public. No big deal. I'm not having to deal with a child who is suffering day in and day out." In comments earlier in the same conversation with Hooker in May 2014, Thompson said: "I have great shame now when I meet families with kids with autism because I have been part of the problem."[1440]

We'll stop to note and reiterate here that Thompson is not at all "anti-vaccine," and nor are the authors of this book. In the written statement from his lawyer, Thompson was clear that vaccines are an overwhelming good:

> I want to be absolutely clear that I believe vaccines have saved and continue to save countless lives. I would never suggest that any parent avoid vaccinating children of any race. Vaccines prevent serious diseases, and the risks associated with their administration are vastly outweighed by their individual and societal benefits.[1441]

However, Thimerosal in no way has been demonstrated to make the vaccine supply any safer. And as the abundant evidence laid out in this book, from lab science to epidemiology to compromised public health agencies to the "Vaccine Court," would attest, Thimerosal has likely been responsible for a not insignificant number of neurological injuries, including autism, in the general populace.

A conversation between Hooker and Thompson touched on the public health threat still posed today by Thimerosal-preserved flu

CONFLICTS OF INTEREST IN POLICYMAKING AND REGULATION

vaccines, routinely administered to pregnant women. Thompson said, "In the United States the only vaccine [Thimerosal] is still in is for pregnant women . . . I don't know why they still give it to pregnant women, like that's the last person I would give mercury to."[1442]

Notes

[1412] http://www.mothering.com/articles/thimerosal-vaccines-autism-let-science-speak/.

[1413] http://dailycaller.com/2015/02/03/obama-admin-grants-immunity-to-cdc-scientist-that-fudged-vaccine-report-whistleblower-plans-to-testify-before-congress/.

[1414] http://www.marketwired.com/press-release/study-focus-autism-foundation-finds-cdc-whistleblower-reveals-widespread-manipulation-1939179.htm.

[1415] https://www.linkedin.com/pub/brian-hooker-ph-d-p-e/8/834/891.

[1416] http://simpsonu.edu/Pages/About/Connect/Faculty-Directory.htm.

[1417] http://www.morganverkamp.com/august-27-2014-press-release-statement-of-william-w-thompson-ph-d-regarding-the-2004-article-examining-the-possibility-of-a-relationship-between-mmr-vaccine-and-autism/.

[1418] Thompson WW, Price C, Goodson B, Shay DK, Benson P, Hinrichsen VL, Lewis E, Eriksen E, Ray P, Marcy SM, Dunn J, Jackson LA, Lieu TA, Black S, Stewart G, Weintraub ES, Davis RL, DeStefano F; Vaccine Safety Datalink Team. Early Thimerosal exposure and neuropsychological outcomes at 7 to 10 years. *N Engl J Med.* 2007; 357: 1281-1292.

[1419] Price CS, Thompson WW, Goodson B, Weintraub ES, Croen LA, Hinrichsen VL, Marcy M, Robertson A, Eriksen E, Lewis E, Bernal P, Shay D, Davis RL, DeStefano F. Prenatal and infant exposure to thimerosal from vaccines and immunoglobulins and risk of autism. *Pediatrics.* 2010 Oct;126(4):656-64. doi: 10.1542/peds.2010-0309. Epub 2010 Sep 13.

[1420] Barile JP, Kuperminc GP, Weintraub ES, Mink JW, Thompson WW. Thimerosal exposure in early life and neuropsychological outcomes 7-10 years later. *J Pediatr Psychol.* 2012 Jan-Feb;37(1):106-18. doi: 10.1093/jpepsy/jsr048. Epub 2011 Jul 23.

[1421] DeStefano F1, Bhasin TK, Thompson WW, Yeargin-Allsopp M, Boyle C. Age at first measles-mumps-rubella vaccination in children with autism and school-matched control subjects: a population-based study in metropolitan Atlanta. *Pediatrics.* 2004 Feb;113(2):259-66.

[1422] Transcript. Conversation between Brian Hooker and William Thompson. May 24, 2014. Not publicly available.

[1423] Transcript. Conversation between Brian Hooker and William Thompson. July 28, 2014. Not publicly available.

[1424] Transcript. Conversation between Brian Hooker and William Thompson. June 12, 2014. Not publicly available.

1425 Transcript. Conversation between Brian Hooker and William Thompson. July 28, 2014. Not publicly available.

1426 http://www.urmc.rochester.edu/people/23513877-jonathan-w-mink.

1427 Transcript. Conversation between Brian Hooker and William Thompson. May 24, 2014. Not publicly available.

1428 Transcript. Conversation between Brian Hooker and William Thompson. July 28, 2014. Not publicly available.

1429 Transcript. Conversation between Brian Hooker and William Thompson. July 28, 2014. Not publicly available.

1430 Tozzi AE, Bisiacchi P, Tarantino V, De Mei B, D'Elia L, Chiarotti F, Salmaso S. Neuropsychological performance 10 years after immunization in infancy with thimerosal-containing vaccines. Pediatrics. 2009 Feb;123(2):475-82.

1431 Transcript. Conversation between Brian Hooker and William Thompson. July 28, 2014. Not publicly available.

1432 Transcript. Conversation between Brian Hooker and William Thompson. May 24, 2014. Not publicly available.

1433 Transcript. Conversation between Brian Hooker and William Thompson. June 12, 2014. Not publicly available.

1434 Transcript. Conversation between Brian Hooker and William Thompson. May 24, 2014. Not publicly available.

1435 http://www.morganverkamp.com/august-27-2014-press-release-statement-of-william-w-thompson-ph-d-regarding-the-2004-article-examining-the-possibility-of-a-relationship-between-mmr-vaccine-and-autism/.

1436 Transcript. Conversation between Brian Hooker and William Thompson. May 24, 2014. Not publicly available.

1437 Transcript. Conversation between Brian Hooker and William Thompson. June 12, 2014. Not publicly available.

1438 http://www.mothering.com/articles/thimerosal-vaccines-autism-let-science-speak/.

1439 Transcript. Conversation between Brian Hooker and William Thompson. May 8, 2014. Not publicly available.

1440 Transcript. Conversation between Brian Hooker and William Thompson. May 24, 2014. Not publicly available.

1441 http://www.morganverkamp.com/august-27-2014-press-release-statement-of-william-w-thompson-ph-d-regarding-the-2004-article-examining-the-possibility-of-a-relationship-between-mmr-vaccine-and-autism/.

1442 Transcript. Conversation between Brian Hooker and William Thompson. May 8, 2014. Not publicly available.

PART FIVE:

FLAWS AND INTERFERENCE IN MEDIA COVERAGE

Chapter 32:
The Squashing of
Debate in the Media

Through the four previous parts, this book has presented substantial evidence questioning Thimerosal's safety and demonstrated the high likelihood that the chemical is responsible for widespread neurodevelopmental disorders, including autism. The studies most often cited in defense of Thimerosal's safety have grave or fatal flaws. Many of the individuals behind these studies also have serious conflicts of interest.

Despite this information, much of the media has come down firmly on the side of those who say Thimerosal does not pose a threat. People who have wished to express in print or broadcast media their concerns about the possible connections between Thimerosal and neurodevelopmental disorders have experienced censorship, unprofessionalism, hostility, and even vilification. In a remarkable admission in a *Reader's Digest* story in 2010, Health and Human Services (HHS) secretary Kathleen Sebelius acknowledged governmental efforts to suppress those who question official claims of vaccine safety, though HHS would later say it could not confirm the quote as being factual.[1443] According to the *Reader's Digest* story, Sebelius said:

> There are groups out there that insist that vaccines are responsible for a variety of problems despite all scientific evidence to the contrary. We have reached out to media outlets to try to get them to not give the views of these people equal weight in their reporting to what science has shown and continues to show about the safety of vaccines.[1444]

It is not known who HHS contacted, what was said, and whether the agency's wishes were followed. But this sort of "message management" has cropped up at other times. The publishing of William Thompson's 2007 study provides an example. As mentioned in Chapters 7 and 31, the Thompson study reported an association between Thimerosal exposure and tics, which had also been previously reported in Verstraeten's 2003 study and in Andrews's 2004 study. The Thompson study reported other negative outcomes related to speech articulation and language development. A reviewer within the CDC noted this prior to publication, writing to one of the paper's authors and other CDC employees in an internal email, "Although you are a bit tentative in your conclusions and Coleen [Boyle, a CDC official] suggests you could make it stronger, I think it is interesting that where there were negative effects, they are with some of the same outcomes as from other analyses (tics, articulation, suggesting overall speech and language disorders). Seems almost confirmatory."[1445]

The CDC did not encourage this sort of straightforwardness when it came to public comments, however. On September 26, Glen Nowak of the CDC's Office of Enterprise Communication wrote an email to various employees regarding "key media and communications plans" for the Thompson study's imminent release. One of the bullet points stated, "Our primary message emanates from the article—which is study [sic] does not support a causal association between early exposure to mercury from thimerosal-containing vaccines and immune globulins and deficits in neuropsychological functioning at age 7 to 10 years." Another bullet point described how the media might portray the study, to the evident chagrin of the CDC:

> We expect much interest and focus on the finding involving tics for a number of reasons—it is a negative association, it is the third time such an association has been reported in published research and advocacy groups will likely highlight. Further, I expect we will see some/many reporters and headline writers focus on it—one, media often focus on the unusual or negative outcomes and two, it lends itself to headlines like 'CDC finds link between mercury in vaccines and motor coordination in kids.' We will work to get media to focus on overall results, but we should expect many headlines and initial paragraphs of stories to focus on tics.[1446]

The CDC's appointed person to deal with the media inquiries on tics, Edwin Trevathan, then the director of the National Center on Birth Defects and Developmental Disabilities and now with Saint Louis University, apparently bristled at the message

391

massaging.[1447] He wrote back, "Glen. Do not ever speak for me again regarding what I will say without my approval on the specifics."[1448]

More often than not, though, it seems that the CDC has kept its message discipline in place. The occasional negative headline regarding the CDC and its complicity in the Thimerosal controversy has been largely drowned out by supportive, toeing-the-line coverage from major media. I have personally met extraordinary resistance in my own efforts to publicize the debate about Thimerosal and autism.

I first stepped into this hornet's nest in 2005 with an exposé, entitled "Deadly Immunity," that ran simultaneously in *Rolling Stone* magazine in the July 14, 2005 issue and online at *Salon*. The article covered much of what is presented in this book, laying out the scientific link between Thimerosal and childhood neurological disorders. This story also published, for the first time, the explosive excerpts from the transcripts of the CDC's June 2000 Simpsonwood conference with vaccine makers and government public health officials, included in this book.[1449] [1450] Both media publications "thoroughly" fact checked the article prior to its publication, according to *Rolling Stone*.[1451]

In the days following publication, government health agencies bombarded *Rolling Stone* and *Salon* with furious letters, and the article came under unrelenting scrutiny from major media outlets. As an initial example, ABC had asked for an exclusive right to broadcast a companion piece to my *Rolling Stone/Salon* article simultaneous to its publication. I spent days working with a team of enthusiastic reporters and technicians for the ABC story. Then, the day before the piece was to air, the senior producer, Jake Tapper, called me, distraught. "Corporate told us to shut it down," he said.

Tapper told me that it was the first time in his career that ABC officials had ordered him to kill a story.

When anti-Thimerosal activists sent a host of angry emails to the network, ABC changed its mind and promised to air the piece. Instead, following about a one-week delay, the broadcaster aired a re-cut version on July 22 that repeated vaccine industry talking points and faulted me, as a lawyer, for trying to address issues that, the broadcaster suggested, should best be left to doctors and scientists. "I'm putting my faith in the Institute of Medicine," ABC's medical editor Tim Johnson said during the piece.[1452] I saw with my own eyes how two pharmaceutical advertisements bracketed the segment.[1453] Afterward, Tapper did not answer or return my phone calls.

CBS also produced a story tied to the publication of "Deadly Immunity," which aired on July 14. The piece, reported by *CBS News* correspondent Sharyl Attkisson, who interviewed me on-air, fairly and accurately conveyed the controversy about Thimerosal.[1454] Behind the scenes, however, Attkisson told me over the phone in February 2011 that the story was among the worst experiences of her television career. Attkisson said to me that internally at CBS, there were attempts to alter her piece and change the context of my quotes. Attkisson has continued to fight for coverage of the issue but is frightened that her efforts might damage her job security. "I'm up against really strong, cult-like behavior," Attkisson told me. "I ask them to look at the science with me. They won't do it. They just say, 'There is no evidence. There is no basis for questioning Thimerosal's safety.'" She added, "You have to realize that the biggest chunk of advertising for the news departments in non-election years is pharmaceuticals."[1455]

By this point, in mid-2005, NBC, the third network comprising the "Big Three," had already come down on the side of the medical establishment regarding Thimerosal. A few months prior, NBC's Robert Bazell concluded his February 24, 2005, investigation by cautioning, "If we stop vaccinating our children, we run the risk of having these horrible diseases come back . . . and the evidence right now is that vaccines do not cause autism."[1456]

As the controversy swirled about "Deadly Immunity" in the summer of 2005, Rolling Stone's editors published a short commentary, "Kennedy Report Sparks Controversy," supporting my story. "What is most striking," the Rolling Stone commentary read, "is the lengths to which major media outlets have gone to disparage the story and to calm public fears—even in the face of the questionable science on the subject."[1457]

Ultimately, a total of six minor errors that had made it into the original article were discovered and corrected in the online versions of the story. None of those errors were even remotely material to the article's central propositions. Four were minor clarifications or corrections of inadvertent editing or punctuation errors and one was a wrong name applied to a congressional staffer. Rolling Stone agreed with me in my characterization of these mistakes, saying in the editors' commentary: "These [mistakes] ranged from inadvertently transposing a quote and confusing a drug license for a patent to relying on a figure that incorrectly calculated an infant's exposure to mercury over six months, rather than citing the even more dangerous amount injected on a single day . . . It is important to note, however, that none of the mistakes weaken the primary point of the story." In fact, as email record exchanges from the time show, most of the errors were made by Rolling Stone's and Salon's editors as they cut my 16,000-word submission to 4,700 words. The editors apologized to me and my research assistant, Brendan DeMelle, for the errors they had introduced into the copy.[1458]

The only error in my article to rise above the level of trivial nitpicking was the assertion that a six-month-old infant could receive a level of mercury from vaccines that was 187 times the EPA's limit for daily exposure. *Rolling Stone* and *Salon* hastily corrected that calculation to state that the child would only receive a dose 40 percent greater than EPA's daily maximum safe exposure. I was on a wilderness trip at the time, so both publications printed the errata without consulting me. When I returned, I argued that this correction was deceptive and should not be allowed to stand. Although the article's original calculation was slightly off, it was far closer to the truth than the correction.

Here is why: As covered previously in this book, the EPA's "RfD" guideline for mercury exposure is 0.1 microgram per kilogram of body weight per day.[1459] Using that guideline, the average 10 lb. two month old baby received 138 (not 187) times the EPA limit for mercury throughout the 1990s until approximately 2003 or 2004.

Incidentally, although 138 micrograms is considerably less than 187 micrograms, the 187 figure probably does not overstate the risk to the child. As we have covered in this book, the EPA's RfD is based on the risk of orally ingesting methylmercury, which multiple studies suggest is a poor stand-in for the ethylmercury in Thimerosal. To this day, I'm still not sure how *Rolling Stone* and *Salon* came up with their 40 percent figure, but after two weeks of my protests, the publications issued a clarification of their earlier, incorrect correction.[1460 1461]

Like the invective I received for writing "Deadly Immunity," the reactions against prominent media figures who have expressed skepticism regarding the CDC's assurances regarding Thimerosal's safety have been harsh. For example, when national radio host Don Imus questioned Thimerosal's safety on his popular show in early 2005, he was denounced by *Fox News* correspondent Steve Milloy. "A closer look at the facts," said Milloy, "reveals that while Thimerosal is safe, Imus unfortunately appears to be suffering from a case of Charlie McCarthy Syndrome, with his eco-crusader wife as the ventriloquist."[1462]

In general, a perception has emerged that those who disavow a Thimerosal-autism link are careful scientists, while those who suspect a link are not credible. A *Columbia Journalism Review* piece by Dan Schulman in October 2005 critiquing the American media's biased coverage of the Thimerosal issue had the following to say:

> The bulk of the scientific establishment denies the autism link, citing the conclusions of the IOM panel, and views believers as crackpots, conspiracy theorists, or zealots—a perspective many medical experts barely conceal in conversations with reporters. In an interview with Myron Levin of the *Los Angeles Times* after the publication of the IOM report, Dr. Stephen Cochi, the head of the CDC's national immunization program, dismissed supporters of the thimerosal theory as "junk scientists and charlatans." If so, then such universities as Harvard and Columbia, among others, employ charlatans—scientists who believe that a link between mercury exposure and autism is plausible.[1463]

Boyd Haley makes the point that even characterizing the "bulk of the scientific community" as deniers of a mercury-autism link might be overstating the case; those in the community who publicly disavow a link are usually associated with pro-Thimerosal groups such as the CDC. Many medical doctors do not take high-level courses in toxicology and biochemistry that would help inform a professional opinion on Thimerosal. More significantly, and on a practical basis, many physicians and researchers might simply recognize that wading into the controversy could damage their reputations and therefore stay above the fray.[1464]

The mainstream media has not succeeded or even shown interest in reporting on these opinions that are contrary to the orthodoxy. After the 2004 IOM report, major newspapers declared finality on the Thimerosal issue as well. The *Washington Post* went with a headline reading, "Experts Find No Vaccine-Autism Link," with the further qualifier that "Panel Says More Research on Possible Connection May Not Be Worthwhile."[1465]

Despite media reports repeatedly declaring the issue closed over the last decade, many Americans are still not convinced. A Harris Interactive/Health Day poll whose results were announced in early 2011 found that "a slim majority of Americans—52 percent—think vaccines don't cause autism."[1466] One would think that with almost half the population suspicious of a link, a genuine debate would be allowed to play itself out and that the chief concerns of the skeptics would be fairly addressed in major publications.

In recent years, this long trend of media silence or scorn toward the issue still shows few signs of breaking. The significant news of

Italian courts ruling in favor of plaintiffs claiming vaccine injuries in 2012 and 2014, for instance (discussed in Chapter 27), did not garner any appreciable domestic media coverage. Meanwhile, outlets in Italy and the United Kingdom reported and analyzed this news extensively, according to an article in *Age of Autism*.[1467]

The CDC whistleblower case of Thompson has garnered mainstream media attention, but through the now-established lens of those who question CDC orthodoxy lacking any credibility. Many blogs and informal online publications have carried news of Thompson's revelations about his 2004 MMR study, but larger outlets, such as *TIME*'s website, have dismissed them.[1468] [1469]

In his conversation with Hooker, Thompson acknowledged how breaking through the established media narrative of "vaccines do not cause autism" would be difficult. He suggested that concerned parties shift their focus, based on where research has been allowed to go—despite it eventually being watered down—on the association between Thimerosal exposure and tics, and not on autism directly.

> I just think there has to be a mantra. The mantra should be 'We know thimerosal causes tics.' That's been demonstrated. That's been demonstrated in the big studies. And just keep saying that, 'We know thimerosal causes tics,' because the CDC never said that thimerosal doesn't cause tics. The CDC always says thimerosal doesn't cause autism. You have to take it off that . . . I really do think it's a public relations campaign . . . I think as they teach you at the CDC, you have to stay on message. And the message I think to start getting out and then you wouldn't have the press jumping on you

saying 'well, vaccines don't cause autism.' If you said, 'yeah, that's true, but vaccines do cause tics.' And then eventually, eventually you could get the message over to 'oh tics are like 5 times as common among kids with autism' . . . Talk to people about how to market this fact that thimerosal causes tics. It's a marketing thing. It is all about marketing. And you have to learn, how do you get a message out. And I'm telling you, if you take autism out of it, you will get that message out.[1470]

Audiences that dismiss the Thimerosal-autism connection might be more receptive to the buried links between Thimerosal and tics, Thompson further suggested. Pregnant women, for example, still have their fetuses exposed to Thimerosal via multidose flu shots today; perhaps a new science-based argument would get their attention. Thompson said: "Once you get that message out, do you think a pregnant mother would take a vaccine that they knew caused tics? . . . Absolutely not! I would never give my wife a vaccine that I thought caused tics."[1471]

Changing the terms of the debate along these lines will remain extremely challenging, with the most trusted, big name media brands refusing to further consider the issue. One of the largest outlets of all, the *New York Times*, as the next chapter will discuss, has been among the most influential culprits in suppressing debate about the safety of vaccines in general and, our chief concern, those that contain Thimerosal.

Notes

1443 http://www.ageofautism.com/2011/09/kathleen-sebelius-throws-arthur-allen-under-the-bus.html.

1444 http://www.rd.com/health/wellness/h1n1-the-report-card/.

1445 Marshalyn Yeargin-Allsopp, "RE: Cleared Neurodevelopment Manuscript," email to Coleen Boyle, Robert L. Davis, Anne Schuchat, Melinda Wharton, February 12, 2007.

1446 Glen Nowak, "Update: New England Journal of Medicine Thimerosal-related article," email to Donna Garland, Edward Hunter, Miranda Katsoyannis, Anne Schuchat, Julie Gerberding, Bill Hall, Kristin Pope, Edwin Travathan, Katherine Galatas, John Iskander, Kathleen Toomey, PerStephanie Thompson, Charlis Thompson, William Thompson, William H. Gimson, Tanja Popovic, Lisa Lee, Kathy Skipper, Barbara S. Reynolds, David Daigle, Curtis Allen, Courtney Lenard, Maureen Culbertson, September 26, 2007.

1447 http://www.slu.edu/x40358.xml.

1448 Edwin Travathan, "Re: Update: New England Journal of Medicine Thimerosal-related article," email to Glen Nowak, Kathleen Toomey, Donna Garland, September 26, 2007.

1449 http://www.rollingstone.com/politics/news/deadly-immunity-20110209 .

1450 http://www.salon.com/2011/01/16/dangerous_immunity/.

1451 "Kennedy Report Sparks Controversy." [behind a subscription wall, but can be read at: http://www.globalresearch.ca/vaccinations-deadly-immunity/14510].

1452 "Kennedy Report Sparks Controversy." [behind a subscription wall, but can be read at: http://www.globalresearch.ca/vaccinations-deadly-immunity/14510].

1453 http://web.archive.org/web/20061211124818/http://www.huffingtonpost.com/2005/06/23/abc-vs-robert-f-kennedy_n_3071.html.

1454 http://www.cbsnews.com/stories/2005/07/14/eveningnews/main709269.shtml.

1455 Robert F. Kennedy, Jr., telephone interview with Sharyl Attkisson, February 24, 2011.

1456 http://www.nbcuniversalarchives.com/nbcuni/clip/5116260581_s08.do.

1457 "Kennedy Report Sparks Controversy." [behind a subscription wall, but can be read at: http://www.globalresearch.ca/vaccinations-deadly-immunity/14510.].

1458 http://www.robertfkennedyjr.com/articles/SalonRetraction_042415.html.

1459 http://www.epa.gov/hg/exposure.htm.

[1460] http://www.rollingstone.com/politics/news/deadly-immunity-20110209.

[1461] http://www.salon.com/2011/01/16/dangerous_immunity/.

[1462] http://www.foxnews.com/story/0,2933,152110,00.html.

[1463] http://web.archive.org/web/20071023194638/http://cjrarchives.org/issues/2005/6/schulman.asp.

[1464] Interview with Boyd Haley, January 27, 2013.

[1465] http://www.washingtonpost.com/wp-dyn/articles/A36703-2004May18.html.

[1466] http://www.harrisinteractive.com/NewsRoom/PressReleases/tabid/446/mid/1506/articleId/674/ctl/ReadCustom%20Default/Default.aspx.

[1467] http://www.ageofautism.com/2015/01/recent-italian-court-decisions-on-vaccines-and-autism.html.

[1468] https://www.google.com/?gws_rd=ssl#safe=off&q=cdc+whistleblower+william+thompson.

[1469] http://time.com/3208886/whistleblower-claims-cdc-covered-up-data-showing-vaccine-autism-link/.

[1470] Transcript. Conversation between Brian Hooker and William Thompson. May 8, 2014. Not publicly available.

[1471] Transcript. Conversation between Brian Hooker and William Thompson. May 8, 2014. Not publicly available.

Chapter 33:
The Role of the
New York Times

The *New York Times* (hereafter referred to as *NY Times*) is known as the "newspaper of record" in the United States, according to *Encyclopedia Britannica*; many readers of this book will have heard the term.[1472] The newspaper has received 114 Pulitzer Prizes as of this writing, far more than any other newspaper, and it is the third-ranked paper nationally by daily circulation and number-one in terms of online readership.[1473 1474 1475]

Such accolades, its global reach, and its generally superior reporting have won the *NY Times* its significant credibility. Yet the "Grey Lady" has enforced extremely biased message discipline regarding the Thimerosal-autism issue both in its news section and on its editorial page.

A typical example is a June 25, 2005, story titled "On Autism's Cause, It's Parents vs. Research," which ran a few weeks before the publication of my *Rolling Stone/Salon* piece.[1476] Autism activists held great hopes that the *NY Times*' prestige would finally force government officials to come clean about Thimerosal. The article's reporters, Gardiner Harris and Anahad O'Connor, encouraged those hopes. According to Dan Schulman in his *Columbia Journalism Review* piece, O'Connor told one mother of an autistic child in late January 2005 in an email:

> I'm thinking of a 2,000-word story, essentially saying that an array of studies over the years (the Institute of Medicine Report, I would think, being the most prominent) were [sic] intended to settle the issue of autism and vaccines once and for all. Yet it seems that the question is still very much open . . . and evidence for the case against vaccines has been mounting, despite many researchers' insistence that the issue is dead. I think, for now at least, I'd like to just present the evidence on both sides and let the readers decide.

The published story, however, was not at all evenhanded. Schulman of the *Columbia Journalism Review* shared the general consensus that the *NY Times*' published story was "one-sided," saying, "Several reporters I spoke with who have covered the Thimerosal controversy described the *NY Times* story as a smear, and called it a 'hit piece.'" According to Schulman:

> The story cast the thimerosal connection as a fringe theory, without scientific merit; held aloft by angry, desperate parents. The notion that supporters of the theory were disregarding irrefutable scientific findings was the underlying theme, drilled home several times.[1477]

The *NY Times* piece contained derisive passages about the Geiers and other researchers who have questioned government orthodoxy, yet respectfully offered quotes from IOM chairwoman Marie McCormick, such as, "It's really terrifying the scientific illiteracy that supports these suppositions."

Schulman wrote:

> Readers were left with little option but to believe that the case against thimerosal was scientifically unsound. . . . Omitted from the story was the work of Dr. Mady Hornig, a Columbia University epidemiologist; Richard Deth, a Northeastern University pharmacologist; Jill James, a professor of pediatrics at the University of Arkansas; and others whose work suggests that thimerosal may cause neurodevelopmental disorders in a subset of susceptible children (those who are not able to eliminate mercury from their body in the ways most people do). The story alluded to Boyd Haley, chairman of the department of chemistry at the University of Kentucky and an ally of thimerosal activists, in the same sentence as a Louisiana physician who believes "that God spoke to her through an 87-year-old priest and told her that vaccines caused autism"—leaving Haley, it would seem, guilty by association of lunacy.

The article proved controversial, and the *NY Times* received a massive response from readers. Schulman noted:

> As it turned out, the story had angered members of the epidemiology department at Columbia's Mailman School of

Public Health, including the department's chair, Dr. Ezra Susser. Since some of their work, including that of Dr. W. Ian Lipkin, a highly regarded neurologist, and Mady Hornig, explored the connection between environmental mercury exposure and autism, including exposure through thimerosal-carrying vaccines, they felt that they had been lumped into the category of scientific illiterates. Responding to the article in a June 28 letter to the *Times* (never published), signed by Susser, Lipkin, Hornig, and the epidemiologist Michaeline Bresnahan, the researchers wrote that "scientists pursuing research on mercury and autism are caricaturized as immune to the 'correct' interpretation of existing studies. Researchers rejecting a link are depicted as the sole voices of reason. . . . Whether mercury in any form (or any of several factors recently introduced to our environment) has anything to do with autism can and should be resolved with rigorous studies and respectful discourse, not moral indictments and denunciations."[1478]

Despite such criticisms of its coverage, the *NY Times* has been unyielding in its determination to shut down debate. The *NY Times* science writers are regarded as notoriously slanted within the autism community.[1479] [1480] My own personal experiences likewise support this view.

I was shocked when I brought a small group of research scientists and anti-Thimerosal activists, including Boyd Haley, Mady Hornig, and Sarah Bridges, to the editorial offices of the *NY Times* to meet with the science staff to discuss Thimerosal and the *NY Times*' allergy to covering the issue fairly. The tiny conference room quickly filled with senior editors from the editorial staff, the op-ed page, and the science section, including science editors Laura Chang and Erica Goode and reporters Gardiner Harris and Anahad O'Connor, who wrote the controversial article.[1481] [1482] [1483] There were so many people in the room that we ran out of seats, even with people crammed on couches and sitting on the backs of armchairs. I had never seen anything like it. They all seemed to be there to fortify each other's resistance to persuasion and to enforce message discipline. In contrast to many other experiences with the NY Times during my twenty-five years of environmental advocacy, I encountered a wall of resistance. The NY Times reporters and editors who met with us were grim, utterly impenetrable, openly rude, and dismissive to the scientists. The paper's staffers were unwilling to engage in rational debate, look at data, or listen to reason. They were altogether unwilling to hear rational criticism of the studies relied on by the CDC, or to look into the well-established conflicts of interest between the CDC and the vaccine producers.

Moreover, the newspaper has routinely turned its news and op-ed pages over to a strong supporter of the vaccine industry, Paul Offit, without disclosing his potential financial conflicts of interest.[1484] [1485] [1486] [1487] [1488] The NY Times has in effect given Offit and other Thimerosal apologists a bullhorn to repeat the federal government's and industry's talking points in its pages, a venue that has been almost entirely closed to those who question Thimerosal's safety. I've had more than a dozen editorials published in the NY Times, going back more than two decades, on a range of environmental and public health issues.[1489] But the paper refused to print a letter to the editor or a 2007 op-ed that I submitted about Thimerosal.

I maintained email exchanges with Clark Hoyt, the *NY Times* public editor from May 2007 until June 2010, in which I've chastised him in every manner that courtesy would allow for the paper's practice of closing the editorial page, the op-ed page, and the letters section to any dissenting views challenging the *NY Times*' frequent assurance that Thimerosal is safe.[1490] I reminded him of the parallels to the run-up to the Iraq War, when the *NY Times* abandoned independent reporting and accepted without proper vetting or investigation the claims of interested government officials—a lapse which the paper's editors subsequently felt compelled to publicly apologize for in 2004.[1491]

The *NY Times* is not the only major paper guilty of a bias against the Thimerosal debate. Regardless of the documentation I have produced, other papers have also refused to carry editorials I have written on the issue, as I'll explain in further detail in the next chapter.

Other individuals who have explored the connection between vaccines and neurodevelopmental disorders such as autism have similarly seen their reports stifled. When former *United Press International* (UPI) reporter Mark Benjamin wrote a comprehensive investigative report exposing conflicts of interests in the CDC vaccine program, Benjamin said that not a single American daily paper or mainstream news source would run the story.[1492 1493] Dan Olmsted, a former senior editor at UPI and a former assistant national editor of *USA Today*, has written dozens of stories on the topic.[1494] But, outside of the *Washington Times*, Olmsted told Schulman and us that he knows of no newspapers that have printed his stories, which instead are widely broadcast online.

According to author David Kirby, the *Huffington Post* has been pressured to not run his ASD-related stories.[1495 1496 1497]

There are other journalists who stand out for having pursued the "hot button" Thimerosal topic. One is Myron Levin, who worked at the *Los Angeles Times* until accepting a buyout in 2008.[1498] Another is Steve Wilson, who was the chief investigative reporter for Detroit's WXYZ Channel 7 television station until his contract was not renewed in 2010.[1499] Sharyl Attkisson, an investigative correspondent with CBS News who was mentioned in the previous chapter, has also from time to time reported on vaccine safety and a potential link to autism.[1500 1501 1502]

For the most part, however, Thimerosal and questionable vaccine safety stories have been hands-off for journalists. Schulman writes:

> Journalists agree that the thimerosal story is one of the most explosive they've ever encountered. . . . Some reporters who have portrayed this as an ongoing scientific controversy have been discouraged by colleagues and their superiors from pursuing the story. A reporter for a major media outlet, who did not want to be identified for fear of retribution, told me that covering the thimerosal controversy had been nearly "career-ending" and described butting heads with superiors who believed that the reporter's coverage—in treating the issue as a two-sided debate—legitimized a crackpot theory and risked influencing parents to stop vaccinating their children or to seek out experimental treatments for their autistic sons and daughters. The reporter has decided against pursuing stories on thimerosal, at least for the time being. "For some reason giving any sort of credence to the side that

says there's a legitimate question here—I don't know how it becomes this untouchable story, I mean that's what we do, so I don't understand why this story is more touchy than any story I've ever done."[1503]

Notes

[1472] http://www.britannica.com/EBchecked/topic/412546/The-New-York-Times.

[1473] http://topics.nytimes.com/top/reference/timestopics/organizations/n/newyorktimes_the/index.html.

[1474] http://abcas3.accessabc.com/ecirc/newstitlesearchus.asp.

[1475] http://www.comscore.com/Insights/Press_Releases/2012/9/comScore_Media_Metrix_Ranks_Top_50_US_Web_Properties_for_August_201.

[1476] http://www.nytimes.com/2005/06/25/science/25autism.html?pagewanted=all.

[1477] http://web.archive.org/web/20071023194638/http://cjrarchives.org/issues/2005/6/schulman.asp.

[1478] http://web.archive.org/web/20071023194638/http://cjrarchives.org/issues/2005/6/schulman.asp.

[1479] http://adventuresinautism.blogspot.com/2007/06/nyt-katie-denigrating-wrights.html.

[1480] http://www.ageofautism.com/2011/09/the-new-york-times-and-the-downplaying-of-the-autism-disaster.html.

[1481] http://www.nytimes.com/2006/05/12/business/media/12asktheeditors.html?pagewanted=all&_r=0.

[1482] http://topics.nytimes.com/topics/reference/timestopics/people/g/erica_goode/index.html.

[1483] http://www.opa.yale.edu/images/poynter/goode-bio.html.

[1484] http://www.nytimes.com/2009/10/12/opinion/12offit.html.

[1485] http://www.nytimes.com/2008/03/31/opinion/31offit.html?_r=0.

[1486] http://www.nytimes.com/2007/07/12/opinion/12Offit.html.

[1487] http://query.nytimes.com/search/sitesearch/#/%22paul+a.+offit%22/.

[1488] http://www.ageofautism.com/2011/01/counting-offits-millions-more-on-how-mercks-rotateq-vaccine-made-paul-offit-wealthy.html.

[1489] http://topics.nytimes.com/top/opinion/editorialsandoped/oped/contributors/?offset=0&s=newest&query=robert+f.+kennedy+jr&field=body&match=all.

[1490] http://topics.nytimes.com/topics/opinion/thepubliceditor/hoyt/index.html.

[1491] http://www.nytimes.com/2004/05/26/international/middleeast/26FTE_NOTE.html?ex=1400990400&en=94c17fcffad92ca9&ei=5007&partner=USERLAND.

1492 http://www.upi.com/Odd_News/2003/07/21/UPI-Investigates-The-vaccine-conflict/UPI-44221058841736/.

1493 http://www.huffingtonpost.com/mark-benjamin.

1494 http://www.ageofautism.com/2010/09/the-age-of-autism-mercury-medicine-and-a-man-made-epidemic-interviews.html.

1495 http://www.evidenceofharm.com/bio.htm.

1496 http://www.ebizmba.com/articles/political-websites.

1497 http://search.huffingtonpost.com/search?o_q=david+kirby&s_it=topsearchbox.search&q=david+kirby+autism+thimerosal.

1498 http://www.laobserved.com/archive/2008/03/times_reporters_note_to_t.php.

1499 http://www.detroityes.com/mb/showthread.php?4729-Steve-Wilson-Leaving-WXYZ-Channel-7.

1500 http://www.cbsnews.com/stories/2011/01/18/broadcasts/main524782.shtml;

1501 http://www.cogforlife.org/cbsnewsautism.pdf;

1502 http://www.cbsnews.com/8301-31727_162-20049118-10391695.html.

1503 http://web.archive.org/web/20071023194638/http:/cjrarchives.org/issues/2005/6/schulman.asp.

Chapter 34:
Salon's Retraction of "Deadly Immunity" and Press Censorship

My own experience has unfortunately continued to dovetail with these sentiments of the Thimerosal issue as a sort of "third rail" in the media environment. On Sunday, January 16, 2011, *Salon* joined in squashing legitimate debate on the Thimerosal topic by suddenly pulling my 2005 "Deadly Immunity" article from its website. *Salon* even took the unprecedented step of removing the article from its archives (though *Rolling Stone* stands by its version, which remains available online [behind a subscription wall], despite a rumor to the contrary).[1504 1505] No one at *Salon* ever cited a factual error that caused *Salon* to remove my piece. Instead, the editor-in-chief at the time, Kerry Laurman, in a short explanation published online that Sunday, made the odd claim that criticisms of and corrections to my piece "eroded any faith we had in the story's value" and that "we've grown to believe the best reader service is to delete the piece entirely."[1506] Joan Walsh, *Salon*'s editor-in-chief when "Deadly Immunity" was published and now an editor-at-large, wrote vaguely about how "the continued revelations of the flaws and even fraud tainting the science behind the connection [between vaccines and autism] make taking down the story the right thing to do."

Salon's founder and former editor-in-chief, David Talbot, is just as baffled and dismayed by the publication's actions in this matter as I am. Talbot explained his reaction in a letter to me on April 6, 2015:

> I was dismayed when I first heard that *Salon* had removed your article about the hazards of thimerosal from its web archives. As you know, I was no longer the editor of *Salon* when your article was published. And I am not an expert on the subject. But without taking a position on mercury preservatives in vaccines, I know enough about the debate—and about the pharmaceutical industry's general track record on putting profits before people, as well as the compromised nature of regulatory oversight in this country when it comes to powerful industries—to know that "disappearing" your article was not the proper decision.
>
> I founded *Salon* to be a fearless and independent publication—one that was open to a wide range of views, particularly those that were controversial or contested within the mainstream media. Removing your article from the *Salon* archives was a violation of that spirit and smacks of editorial cowardice. If I had been editor at the time, I would not have done so—and I would have offered you the opportunity to debate your critics in *Salon*'s pages.

In my day, *Salon* did not cave to pressure—and we risked corporate media scorn, advertising boycotts, threats of FBI investigations by powerful members of Congress, and even bomb scares because of our rigorous independence. Throwing a writer to the wolves when the heat got too hot was never the *Salon* way. It pains me, now that I'm on the sidelines, to ever see *Salon* wilt in the face of such pressure.[1507]

Salon's wilting in 2011 has seriously hampered further, reasoned discussion of the Thimerosal issue. My critics, along with newspaper editors and television producers, have cited *Salon*'s action as justification for their decision to not run my editorials, articles and letters to the editor, or to allow me to talk about vaccine safety on the air.

I have experienced this censorship, even outright insult, in particular while trying to get out word about this book. In the weeks prior to the August 2014 original publication of this book, many respected science writers, including Phil Plait of *Slate*, along with editor Laura Helmuth, who is also vice president of the National Association of Science Writers, Steven Salzberg at *Forbes*, and Jeffrey Kluger at *TIME*, all published scathing commentaries.[1508] [1509] [1510] [1511] [1512] [1513] [1514] [1515] The weird thing was that none of these writers ever read my book or talked to any of its studies' authors. At the time, we had no copies to send to reviewers.

Unwilling to wait to publish their critiques, and not being conversant with the science, these writers resorted to straight vilification. They called me a "conspiracy theorist," a "crackpot," "anti-science," "anti-vaccine," and so on. Since then, I've been attacked as for my "villainy" by the *New York Post* and have been referred to as a "notorious anti-vax celebrity crank."[1516] [1517]

Other outlets published highly personal attacks on me by vaccine industry insiders like Paul Offit and William Schaffner, posing as independent health experts.[1518] [1519] Schaffner diagnosed me as a psychologically troubled "true believer." As usual, neither writer identified his financial entanglements with the vaccine industry. Writer Keith Kloor, in a 2013 *Discover* blog post, said I'd "done as much as anyone to spread unwarranted fear and crazy conspiracy theories about vaccines," a claim he cited a year later in a profile of me in the *Washington Post Magazine*.[1520] [1521] *TIME*'s Kluger said I'd taken a "disreputable plunge into the world of anti-science."

This sort of smear campaign has closed the eyes and ears of journalists all over the country to my well-intentioned efforts to get us as a society to take a hard look at Thimerosal and get it out of all vaccines and medicines, period. I prepared an article to coincide with the publishing of this revised and updated version of *Thimerosal: Let the Science Speak* that you now hold. Ironically, the article was partially a jeremiad on press suppression of the Thimerosal issue. Opinion editors rejected the article at virtually all of the nation's leading papers and outlets, including *USA Today*, the *New York Times*, the *Wall Street Journal*, *Gannett*, the *Los Angeles Times*, the *Boston Globe*, the *Newark Star-Ledger*, the *New York Post*, the *Washington Post*, CNN's website, the *Bergen Record*, the *Chicago Tribune*, the *Chicago Sun-Times*, the *Houston Chronicle*, the *Dallas Morning News*, the *San Francisco Chronicle*, the *Sacramento Bee*, the *Atlanta Journal Constitution*, the *Miami Herald*, the *Austin American-Statesman*, the *News & Observer* in Raleigh, North Carolina, the *Star Tribune* in Minneapolis, Minnesota, as well as the so-called alternative press of *Salon*, *Slate* and the *Huffington Post*. Sadly, even *Mother Jones* has drank the Kool-Aid, so to speak. (Kudos go out to *Alternet* for having the courage to print my story.[1522])

Ultimately, a longer version of my article ran as a paid-for, full-page ad in *USA Today* the weekend of April 24–26, 2015. Readers of that ad, and this book, are reading information that every newspaper and every television news department in America does not want them to know.

Moving on, the next chapter will explore a book called *The Panic Virus*, a case study in how the media and media figures have failed to fairly report and examine the links between Thimerosal and autism.

Notes

1504 http://www.salon.com/about/inside_salon/2011/01/16/dangerous_immunity.

1505 http://www.rollingstone.com/politics/news/deadly-immunity-20110209.

1506 http://en.wikipedia.org/wiki/David_Talbot.

1507 David Talbot, letter to Robert F. Kennedy, Jr., April 6, 2015.

1508 http://www.slate.com/authors.phil_plait.html.

1509 http://www.slate.com/blogs/bad_astronomy/2014/07/21/robert_f_kennedy_jr_still_fighting_the_wrong_fight.html.

1510 http://www.nasw.org/nasw-officers-executive-board-and-staff.

1511 http://www.slate.com/articles/health_and_science/medical_examiner/2013/06/robert_f_kennedy_jr_vaccine_conspiracy_theory_scientists_and_journalists.html.

1512 http://www.forbes.com/sites/stevensalzberg/.

1513 http://www.forbes.com/sites/stevensalzberg/2014/07/20/robert-kennedys-dangerous-anti vaccine activism/.

1514 https://twitter.com/jeffreykluger.

1515 http://time.com/3012797/vaccine-rfk-jr-thimerosal/.

1516 http://nypost.com/2015/03/27/rfk-jr-s-vaccine-villainy/.

1517 http://www.slate.com/articles/health_and_science/medical_examiner/2015/04/california_anti_vaccine_movement_politics_wealth_bob_sears_and_robert_f.html.

1518 http://acsh.org/2014/07/robert-f-kennedy-promotes-dangerous-unscientific-position-thimerosal/.

1519 http://www.medpagetoday.com/Pediatrics/Vaccines/46926.

1520 http://blogs.discovermagazine.com/collideascape/2013/06/01/is-robert-f-kennedy-jr-anti-science/#.VUqGsZNRKRJ.

1521 http://www.washingtonpost.com/lifestyle/magazine/robert-kennedy-jrs-belief-in-autism-vaccine-connection-and-its-political-peril/2014/07/16/f21c01ee-f70b-11e3-a606-946fd632f9f1_story.html.

1522 http://www.alternet.org/personal-health/thimerosal-let-science-speak.

Chapter 35:
Seth Mnookin's *The Panic Virus*: A Flawed Account of Thimerosal and Autism

Salon partly based its concerns for its readers regarding the reaction of my article on a new 2011 book by Seth Mnookin, whom *Salon*'s then-editor-in-chief, Lauerman, claimed as "a personal friend and a friend of this publication, one who wrote for us during his early days as a writer."[1523] Mnookin's book, *The Panic Virus: A True Story of Medicine, Science, and Fear*, is a curious creation. A front cover blurb proclaims the book "a nonfiction story worthy of Michael Crichton."[1524] The late Michael Crichton was a best-selling novelist and well-known global warming denier who spoke out against climate scientists and even helped convince President

George W. Bush not to take any action.[1525] [1526] In an unintended irony, Mnookin could now be said to be performing the same service for the vaccine industry that Crichton performed for the fossil fuel industry.

Mnookin's book heaps invective on what he describes as the "anti-vaccine" movement while showcasing the government's and industry's talking points.[1527] Like the rest of the mainstream media, Mnookin accepts as a given the claims by CDC and the vaccine industry that, as the CDC says on its website, "there is no convincing evidence of harm caused by the low doses of thimerosal in vaccines."[1528] Mnookin accuses parents who are seeking greater vaccine safety, government-industry transparency, and vaccination choice of "paranoia"; author David Kirby of "spreading misinformation"; and activist and actress Jenny McCarthy of peddling "gibberish."[1529] Mnookin goes on to vilify the Thimerosal-induced autism theory as "a bit of chicanery barely worthy of a boardwalk three-card monte [sic; Monte] dealer."[1530] He charges me with being part of a "conspiracy of dunces."[1531] His only substantive complaint leveled against me is that I used quotations in my "Deadly Immunity" article from the CDC and government public health officials at the Simpsonwood meeting out of context, yet the lengthy excerpts Mnookin cites from the edited Simpsonwood transcript prove exactly the opposite.[1532]

To a high degree, Mnookin's coverage of the vaccines and autism issue comes across as misogynistic. Historically, from approximately the 1950s through the 1970s, autism had been falsely blamed on uncaring, emotionally frigid "refrigerator mothers."[1533] Mnookin, in line with the *NY Times* article described previously, in an analogous manner characterizes the Thimerosal disagreement as a clash between serious scientists and hysterical mothers. The mostly male, white-coated scientist "experts" are the heroes of Mnookin's tale, and the mostly female parents searching for answers and accountability for their children with autism are the borderline-irrational villains. Mnookin describes one mother, Lyn Redwood, who maintained an online mailing list devoted to mercury and autism, as being "armed with only the fervency of her beliefs."[1534] He then mockingly titles a chapter "Jenny McCarthy's Mommy Instinct," in reference to an Oprah Winfrey interview wherein McCarthy used the term in talking about how she discovered a diet that ameliorated some of her autistic son's symptoms.

Despite this patronizing portrayal, the controversy is far from a clash between mothers and scientists; it is a dispute within the scientific community pitting government and vaccine industry officials against a large number of independent researchers and a mountain of data casting doubt on assertions of vaccine safety. My experience with autism activists—most of whom are indeed women—is inconsistent with Mnookin's and others' patronizing assessments.

Over the past several years, I have met or communicated with several hundred of these women. Instead of a desperate mob of irrational hysterics, I've found these anti-Thimerosal activists to be calm, grounded, and patient for the most part. As a group, they are highly educated. Many of them are doctors, nurses, schoolteachers, pharmacists, psychologists, PhDs, and other professionals. Many of them approached the link skeptically and only through dispassionate and diligent investigation became convinced that Thimerosal-preserved vaccines seriously damaged their children's or grandchildren's brains. As a group, they have sat through hundreds of meetings and scientific conferences, and studied hundreds of research papers and results from medical tests. They have networked with each other at meetings and across the Internet through email, Facebook, Twitter, and other means. Along the way, they have endured the mockery and abuse heaped on them by the vaccine industry and public health authorities and casual dismissal by the *NY Times* and other mainstream media outlets, as well as their recent vilification by Mnookin.

Mnookin expresses bewilderment that the parents seemingly most susceptible to vaccine skepticism are among the most highly educated Americans. He observes:

> There's been a dramatic rise in the number of communities where vaccination rates have fallen below the 90 to 95 percent threshold needed to maintain herd immunity. An overwhelming percentage of those are left-leaning, well educated enclaves demographically similar to the neighborhood in which I live. The city that's gotten the most attention as of late is Ashland, Oregon, which is home to a nationally renowned Shakespeare festival and the Ashland Independent Film Festival and has a vaccine exemption rate of around 30 percent, which is the highest in the country. Just north of San Francisco, Marin County, which has the fifth-highest average-per-capita income in the United States, has an exemption rate more than three times that of the rest of California.[1535]

At the end of the book, Mnookin dismisses those who disagree with his evaluation and rejection of a Thimerosal–neurodevelopmental disorder connection as being "swept up in a wave of self-righteous hysteria."[1536] In essence, Mnookin's *The Panic Virus* spends 300 pages or so of text trying to explain why smart people who have studied the science disagree with its author, who it is not clear has done the same.

In the few instances when Mnookin does address the scientific evidence and literature, the author gets things wrong. Mnookin states, for example, that Thimerosal seemed "ideally suited" for the role of a vaccine preservative because "it was inexpensive to manufacture, side-effect-free, and lethal to a broad range of microbes without undermining the potency of the vaccine it was mixed with."[1537] Thimerosal's history is marked by numerous case reports of topical and other side effects in humans, as well as harm to animals and cells in culture, as described in previous chapters.

Many other errors appear in Mnookin's book, some small, some very significant. At various places in the text, Mnookin states without citation the dubious theory that ethylmercury in Thimerosal is neither as persistent in the body nor as toxic as the methylmercury that is regulated by state and federal seafood advisories. Mnookin writes, "Vaccinologists also knew that ethylmercury—the form present in vaccines—was less toxic than methylmercury," and later, "As it turns out, ethylmercury half life ranges from ten to twenty days in children and is as short as seven days in infants while methylmercury's half life is around seventy days."[1538 1539] As shown in Chapter 4 of this book, in studies such as those by Magos in 1985, Harry in 2004, Burbacher in 2005, and Pichichero in 2008, the relative toxicity of ethylmercury compared to methylmercury and the true rates at which it leaves the body are not settled issues.[1540 1541 1542 1543]

Another significant lapse occurs early in the book, when Mnookin informs the reader that "after reading hundreds of academic papers and thousands of pages of court transcripts," he had "arrived at the conclusion that there was no evidence supporting a link between childhood inoculations and developmental disorders."[1544] This statement ignores the dozens of studies cited in this white paper, as well as the thousands of injuries that the 1986 National Vaccine Injury Compensation Program (VICP), discussed back in Part Three, has acknowledged and settled.[1545] The compensated cases have involved encephalopathy, seizures, and developmental disorders such as speech and language disorder, mental retardation, and—although not conceded for directly—autism spectrum disorders.[1546]

Mnookin misreports other information regarding the VICP along these lines. Halfway through the book, Mnookin asserts that the "court had addressed claims for more than a dozen different purported injuries. Autism was not one of them. It wasn't just that the disorder was not listed as a table injury and hadn't shown up in the VAERS reports that served as an early warning system for vaccine reactions—it hadn't even been the subject of any significant discussions."[1547] To review, the "table" is the VICP's Vaccine Injury Table, which lists and explains compensable injuries and conditions presumed to be caused by certain vaccines. Since its creation in 1988 and through several modifications, the last of which occurred in 2011, the table has indeed never listed "autism" as an "illness, disability, injury or condition covered."[1548][1549] Yet a significant number of cases with publicly available decisions and other proceedings have included descriptions of the injured child as having "autistic characteristics" or "tendencies," and in other cases "autism" or an "autism spectrum disorder." An early example of this is the 1990 case, *Sorensen v. Secretary of Health and Human Services*, indicating that autism has long been indirectly compensated by the VICP.[1550] Furthermore, the Vaccine Adverse Event Reporting System (VAERS) Mnookin refers to had in fact received dozens of reports of autism by 1999, as reported in articles by Emily Jane Woo in 2004 and David and Mark Geier in 2006 and elsewhere.[1551 1552]

Other errors are minor but perhaps indicative of a lack of attention to detail. For example, Leo Kanner's seminal 1943 paper on autism, a case study of eight boys and three girls, is described as a study of "eleven young boys."[1553 1554] And while finding fault with Thimerosal's critics, Mnookin, like the rest of the mainstream press, does not probe the conflicts of interest between federal agencies and researchers publishing against a Thimerosal-autism link. Mnookin often quotes Paul Offit, whose conflicts have been mentioned previously. Mnookin also describes McGill University psychiatry professor Eric Fombonne's testifying in Vaccine Court against a petitioner.[1555 1556] In studies he has coauthored, Fombonne has had to provide a conflict-of-interest statement noting the fees he has collected for advising vaccine manufacturers in addition to serving as an expert witness for these companies in Thimerosal-related legislation.[1557 1558]

For all the passes given and mistakes committed, even Mnookin acknowledges that the European studies relied on by the IOM are flawed. Mnookin quotes Vanderbilt Department of Preventive Medicine chair William Schaffner, who said that the European studies are "imperfect," but together they formed "a whole mosaic of studies . . . that all add up to this theme: thimerosal is not the culprit."[1559]

Echoed by the media, such categorical statements from the medical establishment, even when logically weak as in the case of Schaffner's—amounting to "one false study is false, but a collection of false studies must be true"—tend to marginalize those who question the public health establishment's verities. There are many past examples, though, when scientifically and societally blasphemous positions have over time proven to be correct and life-saving.

Notes

[1523] http://www.salon.com/2011/01/16/seth_mnookin_panic_virus_autism/.

[1524] http://www.amazon.com/Panic-Virus-Story-Medicine-Science/dp/1439158649/ref=ntt_at_ep_dpi_1%23reader_1439158649#reader_1439158649.

[1525] http://www.michaelcrichton.net/aboutmichaelcrichton-biography.html.

[1526] http://thinkprogress.org/climate/2008/11/05/203302/michael-crichton-worlds-most-famous-global-warming-denier-dies/?mobile=nc.

[1527] Mnookin S. *The Panic Virus: A True Story of Medicine, Science, and Fear.* Simon and Schuster. New York, New York. 2011.

[1528] http://www.cdc.gov/vaccinesafety/Concerns/thimerosal/index.html.

[1529] *The Panic Virus*, pages 199, 218, 270.

[1530] *The Panic Virus*, page 296.

[1531] *The Panic Virus*, page 221.

[1532] *The Panic Virus*, pages 223-227.

[1533] http://en.wikipedia.org/wiki/Refrigerator_mother_theory.

[1534] *The Panic Virus*, page 140.

[1535] *The Panic Virus*, pages 304-305.

[1536] *The Panic Virus*, page 308.

[1537] *The Panic Virus*, page 119.

[1538] *The Panic Virus*, page 122.

[1539] *The Panic Virus*, page 159.

[1540] Magos L, Brown AW, Sparrow S, Bailey E, Snowden RT, Skipp WR. The comparative toxicology of ethyl- and methylmercury. *Arch Toxicol.* 1985 Sep; 57(4):260-7. PMID: 4091651.

[1541] Harry GJ, Harris MW, Burka LT. Mercury concentrations in brain and kidney following ethylmercury, methylmercury and Thimerosal administration to neonatal mice. *Toxicol Lett.* 2004 Dec 30;154(3):183-9.

[1542] Burbacher T, Shen D, Liberato N, Grant K, Cernichiari E, Clarkson T. Comparison of blood and brain mercury levels in infant monkeys exposed to methylmercury or vaccines containing thimerosal. *Environ Health Perspect.* 2005; 113(8):1015-1021.

[1543] Pichichero ME, Gentile A, Giglio N, Umido V, Clarkson T, Cernichiari E, Zareba G, Gotelli C, Gotelli M, Yan L, Treanor J. Mercury levels in newborns and infants after receipt of thimerosal-containing vaccines. *Pediatrics*. 2008 Feb;121(2):e208-14.

[1544] *The Panic Virus*, pages 11-12.

[1545] www.hrsa.gov/vaccinecompensation/statisticsreports.html.

[1546] Holland M, Conte L, Krakow R, Colin L. Unanswered questions from the vaccine injury compensation program: a review of compensated cases of vaccine-induced brain injury. *Pace Envtl. L. Rev.* 2011;28:480.

[1547] *The Panic Virus*, page 179.

[1548] http://www.hrsa.gov/vaccinecompensation/vaccinetable.html.

[1549] http://www.gao.gov/new.items/he00008.pdf.

[1550] Holland M, Conte L, Krakow R, Colin L. Unanswered questions from the vaccine injury compensation program: a review of compensated cases of vaccine-induced brain injury. *Pace Envtl. L. Rev.* 2011; 28:480.

[1551] Woo EJ, Ball R, Bostrom A, Shadomy SV, Ball LK, Evans G, Braun M. Vaccine risk perception among reporters of autism after vaccination: vaccine adverse event reporting system 1990-2001. *Am J Public Health*. 2004 Jun;94(6):990-5.

[1552] Geier DA, Geier MR. An assessment of downward trends in neurodevelopmental disorders in the United States following removal of Thimerosal from childhood vaccines. *Med Sci Monit*. 2006 Jun;12(6):CR231-9. Epub 2006 May 29.

[1553] Kanner L. Autistic disturbances of affective contact. *Nerv Child* 1943; 2: 217-250.

[1554] *The Panic Virus*, page 76.

[1555] http://muhc.ca/research/researcher/eric-fombonne-md.

[1556] *The Panic Virus*, page 290.

[1557] Smeeth L, Cook C, Fombonne E, Heavey L, Rodrigues LC, Smith PG, Hall AJ. MMR vaccination and pervasive developmental disorders: a case-control study. *Lancet*. 2004 Sep 11-17;364(9438):963-9.

[1558] Fombonne E, Zakarian R, Bennett A, Meng L, McLean-Heywood D. Pervasive developmental disorders in Montreal, Quebec, Canada: prevalence and links with immunizations. *Pediatrics*. 2006 Jul;118(1):e139-50.

[1559] *The Panic Virus*, page 167.

Chapter 36: Historical Comparisons between Thimerosal and Other Revealed Threats

Why has the mainstream press disengaged in a genuine debate on Thimerosal and accepted government orthodoxies, despite ample evidence questioning Thimerosal's safety?

There are many possible explanations. In an increasingly competitive media environment in which many staffs have had to downsize, overworked reporters might not have the time, inclination, or expertise to read complex scientific studies and follow a long chain of developments.[1560] Schulman in his previously cited *Columbia Journalism Review* article opines on this aspect of the Thimerosal controversy:

Pursuing this story is unattractive for other reasons, too. The issue is exceedingly complex and easily oversimplified. "It took me two and a half years and four hundred pages to tell this story, and I'm sure I made some mistakes," David Kirby told me, adding that the complexity convinced him to write a book.

A web of relationships between science reporters and the public health officials whom they trust and depend on could also cloud the former's news judgment. Steve Wilson, mentioned in Chapter 33, spoke with Schulman about this dynamic:

> The fact that the bulk of the public health establishment dismisses the thimerosal theory is also daunting, particularly for science reporters who rely on the same pool of medical experts and health officials regularly. "They depend on these people in this symbiotic relationship that they have," said Steve Wilson, an investigative reporter for the local ABC affiliate in Detroit, WXYZ, whose three-part series on thimerosal won an Emmy. "They've come to trust them and respect them and to believe when they tell them, 'Look, you're barking up the wrong tree here; these parents are just looking for somebody to blame.'"[1561]

It would appear that the defense of Thimerosal's safety by the medical establishment has indeed proven highly successful in tamping down deeper investigation into the vaccine industry. Another key factor could be that major pharmaceutical companies, the makers of vaccines, are among the biggest advertisers in the United States. According to the trade publication *Advertising Age*, twelve pharmaceutical companies made it into the top one hundred national advertisers by dollar amount of purchased ads in 2011.[1562] As an example of the relationship between major media and pharmaceutical companies, from January through September 2004, the Big Three networks' nightly news programs garnered almost a third of their advertising revenue ($110 million out of $376 million) from prescription drug ads, according to TNS Media Intelligence/CMR and reported in the *NY Times*.[1563]

The unfortunate dynamics of the Thimerosal controversy are not without historical precedent or literary allusion. Henrik Ibsen's 1882 play *An Enemy of the People* is noteworthy in this respect. It tells the story of a doctor in southern Norway who discovers that his town's magnificent new public baths are actually sickening visitors who flock to them. Discharges from local tanneries have infected the spas with bacteria. When the doctor tries to go public with the information, government officials, their eventual allies in the "liberal-minded independent press," and other financially interested parties move to muzzle him. The doctor is deprived of his medical practice, vilified, and branded "an enemy of the people" by the townsfolk.[1564]

Ibsen's fictional doctor experienced what has come to be known as the "Semmelweis reflex." This is a metaphor for the reflex-like rejection of new evidence that contradicts an established belief system or paradigm. The term describes the aggressive, knee-jerk rejection by the press, the medical community, and allied financial interests in the face of new scientific information suggesting that established medical practices are actually harming public health.

The real-life plight of Ignaz Semmelweis, a Hungarian physician, inspired the term. He was working as an assistant to the professor of the maternity clinic at the Vienna General Hospital in Austria in 1847, where around 10 percent of women died from puerperal fever. Based on a theory that cleanliness could have some positive impact, Semmelweis introduced the practice of hand-washing for interns after they completed autopsies. The rate of fatal puerperal fever infections dropped to around 1 to 2 percent.[1565]

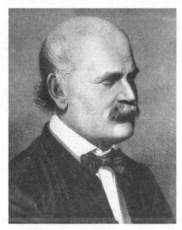

Ignaz Semmelweis. Credit: public domain

Rather than building a statue to Semmelweis, the medical community, unwilling to admit its culpability in the injury to so many patients, harassed the doctor and expelled him from the medical profession. Some of his colleagues tricked him into visiting a mental institution in 1865, where he was involuntarily committed and subsequently died two weeks later.[1566] Right around this time in the 19th century, although Semmelweis would never know, the validity of his ideas was being confirmed through Louis Pasteur's germ theory of disease and Joseph Lister's work on hospital sanitation.[1567] [1568] [1569]

Modern analogs abound. Herbert Needleman of the University of Pittsburgh endured the Semmelweis reflex as he worked to reveal the brain-killing toxicity of lead in the 1980s.[1570] Needleman published a groundbreaking study in 1979 in the *New England Journal of Medicine* showing that children with high levels of lead in their teeth scored significantly lower than their low-lead peers on an intelligence test, on auditory and speech processing, and on an attention measure. Deficits in classroom performance also increased in a dose-response fashion to the levels of lead detected in children's teeth.[1571] Instead of being hailed for his findings, Needleman came under fire from the lead industry. A 2005 study that interviewed Needleman described the situation as thus:

> Needleman became the focus of the lead industry's ire. Beginning in the early 1980s, the industry's attacks on his research and use of public relations firms and scientific consultants to undermine his credibility became a classic example of how an industry seeks to shape science and call into question the credibility of those whose research threatens it. Industry consultants demanded that the Environmental Protection Agency and, later, the Office of Scientific Integrity at the National Institutes of Health, investigate Needleman's work. And then, in 1991, under pressure from industry consultants, the University of Pittsburgh formed a committee to evaluate the integrity of his lead studies.
>
> Ultimately the federal government and the university found no basis for questioning Needleman's integrity or

the results of his research. But the impact of the industry's actions affected both Needleman's academic life and the field of lead research. On the one hand, the industry explicitly showed the power it had to disrupt researchers' lives if they dared to question the safety of its products. On the other hand, Needleman's experience galvanized a generation of researchers who were profoundly influenced by the implications of his studies.[1572]

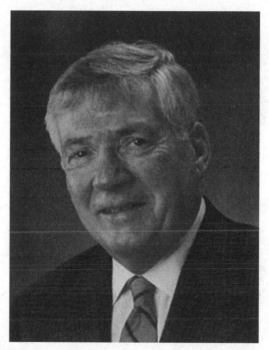

Herbert Needleman. Credit: Brown University, http://www.brown.edu/
Administration/News_Bureau/2005-06/05-110.html

Rachel Carson ran the same gauntlet in the early 1960s when she told the truth about the dangerous pesticide DDT, which the medical community promoted as a treatment against body lice and in fighting malaria.[1573][1574] Chemical manufacturers joined by government officials and medical professionals led by the American Medical Association vilified Carson.[1575][1576][1577] Trade journals and the popular media attacked her as a "hysterical woman," and also derided Carson as a "spinster" and for being unscientific. Criticisms of her book appeared in reviews and articles in *Time*, *Life*, *Newsweek*, *The Saturday Evening Post*, *US News and World Report*, and even *Sports Illustrated*.[1578][1579]

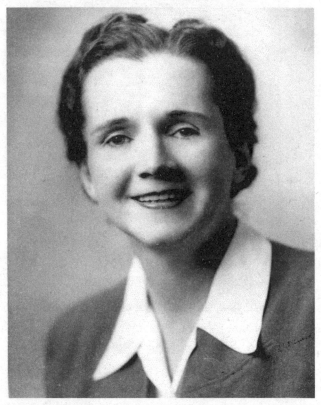

Rachel Carson. Credit: public domain

The experience of British physician and epidemiologist Alice Stewart offers a near-perfect analogy to the public health community's intransigence in the current Thimerosal debate. In the 1940s, Stewart was one of the rare women in her profession and the youngest fellow ever elected at the time to the Royal College of Physicians.[1580] She began investigating the high occurrences of childhood cancers in affluent families, a puzzling phenomenon given that many diseases correlated with poverty. Stewart published a paper in *The Lancet* in 1956 offering strong evidence that the common practice of giving X-rays to pregnant women was behind many of the cancers that would later afflict their young children.[1581] According to Margaret Heffernan, author of *Willful Blindness*, Stewart's finding "flew in the face of conventional wisdom" regarding the contemporary enthusiasm for the new technology of X-rays, as well as "doctors' idea of themselves, which was as people who helped patients." Instead of heeding the science, a coalition of government nuclear promoters and the nuclear industry allied with the US and British medical establishments in attacking Stewart. Stewart, who died in 2002 at the age of ninety-five, never again received another major research grant in England.[1582] It took twenty-five years after Stewart's paper was published for the medical establishment to finally accept her findings, replicated thereafter by other scientists, and recommend abandoning the practice of X-raying expectant women.[1583] [1584]

The example that could be the most pertinent to Thimerosal is that of the mercury compound Calomel, discussed briefly in Parts One and Three. From the late 1800s to the 1930s in the United States, and still until 1954 in the United Kingdom, Calomel was used as an ingredient in infant teething powders, as well as in worming preparations and other medications. Despite scientific literature in the mid- to late 1940s connecting Calomel-containing tooth powders to acrodynia, or pink disease, in children, some in the medical community strongly defended its use, which continued for many years.

It has been commented that the history of acquired autism may perhaps end like the cases of acrodynia, where the withdrawal of the causal substance, Calomel, led to the virtual disappearance of the disease. Only 1 in every 500 children exposed to Calomel developed pink disease, reaffirming the concept that specific genetic vulnerabilities exist among subsets of children who are susceptible to mercury's damage.[1585]

In a 1997 paper, the late Ann Dally of the Wellcome Institute for the History of Medicine described why it took as long as it did for reality to sink in for the medical establishment, particularly in the United Kingdom:[1586]

> The resistance to the evidence of mercury poisoning is typical of resistance to new medical knowledge and declined only when the opponents and s[k]eptics grew old and disappeared from the scene. . . . [John] Zahorsky [who commented on the similarity between pink disease and mercury poisoning in 1922] did not investigate the idea that some children were particularly susceptible to mercury but instead he dismissed rather than pursued his new idea of possible mercury poisoning and suggested a theory that was more in tune with current fashion. This may be because new and unfashionable ideas are harder to investigate than variations on current themes. . . . Unfashionable ideas, even when they turn out to be valid, are notoriously ignored.[1587]

Notes

[1560] http://adage.com/article/media/internet-media-employment-fuels-digital-job-growth/237440.

[1561] http://web.archive.org/web/20071023194638/http:/cjrarchives.org/issues/2005/6/schulman.asp.

[1562] http://247wallst.com/2012/07/13/the-ten-largest-advertisers-in-america/.

[1563] http://www.nytimes.com/2004/12/21/business/media/21adco.html?_r=0.

[1564] Ibsen, Henrik. *An Enemy of the People.* Translated by R. Farquharson Sharp. 1882.

[1565] http://semmelweis.org/about/dr-semmelweis-biography/.

[1566] http://en.wikipedia.org/wiki/Ignaz_Semmelweis.

[1567] http://www.britannica.com/EBchecked/topic/230610/germ-theory.

[1568] http://web.mit.edu/invent/iow/pasteur.html.

[1569] http://www.britannica.com/EBchecked/topic/343342/Joseph-Lister-Baron-Lister.

[1570] http://www.psychiatry.pitt.edu/person/herbert-needleman-md.

[1571] Needleman HL, Gunnoe C, Leviton A, Reed R, Peresie H, Maher C, Barrett P. Deficits in psychologic and classroom performance of children with elevated dentine lead levels. *N Engl J Med.* 1979 Mar 29;300(13):689-95.

[1572] Needleman H. Standing up to the lead industry: an interview with Herbert Needleman. Interview by David Rosner and Gerald Markowitz. *Public Health Rep.* 2005 May-Jun;120(3):330-7.

[1573] http://www.epa.gov/pbt/pubs/ddt.htm.

[1574] http://www.cdc.gov/biomonitoring/DDT_BiomonitoringSummary.html.

[1575] Sideris L, Dean Moore K, eds. *Rachel Carson: Legacy and Challenge.* New York: State University of New York Press; 2008.

[1576] http://e360.yale.edu/feature/fifty_years_after_rachel_carsons_silent_spring_assacult_on_science_continues/2544/.

[1577] http://clinton2.nara.gov/WH/EOP/OVP/24hours/carson.html.

[1578] http://www.environmentandsociety.org/exhibitions/silent-spring/personal-attacks-rachel-carson.

[1579] http://www.fws.gov/rachelcarson/toolkit/Public%20Servant/index.html.

[1580] http://www.rcplondon.ac.uk/.

[1581] Giles D, Hewitt D, Stewart A, Webb J. Malignant disease in childhood and diagnostic irradiation in utero. *Lancet*. 1956 Sep 1;271(6940):447.

[1582] http://iicph.org/alicestewartobit.

[1583] http://www.mheffernan.com/book-wb-summary.shtml.

[1584] http://www.nytimes.com/2002/07/04/world/alice-stewart-95-linked-x-rays-to-diseases.html.

[1585] Shandley K, Austin DW. Ancestry of pink disease (infantile acrodynia) identified as a risk factor for autism spectrum disorders. *J Toxicol Environ Health A*. 2011;74(18):1185-94.

[1586] http://www.guardian.co.uk/news/2007/jun/01/guardianobituaries.obituaries1.

[1587] Dally A. The rise and fall of pink disease. *Soc Hist Med*. 1997; 10: 291-304.

CONCLUSIONS AND RECOMMENDATIONS

This book has strived to comprehensively demonstrate how Thimerosal is dangerous to human health. Significant evidence shows that exposure to the mercury-containing chemical could be responsible for many neurodevelopmental disorder cases. In this manner, increased levels of Thimerosal in vaccines might have greatly contributed to the shocking rise in neurodevelopmental disorders, including autism, seen since the early 1990s. Accordingly, Thimerosal should be immediately removed from all remaining vaccines.

Readers of this book are expected to maintain a healthy skepticism regarding a connection between Thimerosal and brain injury. New studies continue to be published every few weeks that fill in more pieces of the puzzle, adding to the substantial existing evidence. Yet absolutely proving a mercury-autism connection may remain as elusive as proving the link between carbon and global warming, or cigarettes and cancer, the latter being a controversy that raged for forty years despite the wide acceptance of causation in the late 1950s.[1588 1589]

The contributors to this book therefore hope that a convincing argument has nevertheless been made for the elimination of Thimerosal on the grounds of prudent public policy. Continuing to wait for more research is not a reasonable option at this point. If the suffering of affected individuals and their families is not basis enough for policy makers to take action against Thimerosal, despite their lingering doubts, they should consider the cost to society. A March 2012 study by Autism Speaks, with guidance and technical assistance from the World Health Organization, estimated the annual economic costs in the United States from autism alone to be a staggering $137 billion. This estimate was based on a prevalence of 1 in 110, a figure that has recently gone up still further to 1 in 68.[1590] [1591] [1592] [1593] The toxicity of Thimerosal, whatever links it may or may not have to any particular disease or condition, should be more than enough to justify doing whatever it takes to eliminate it from all vaccines.

We hereby restate the recommendations as put forth in the Executive Summary:

- The immediate removal of Thimerosal from all vaccines globally, which has precedent in the United States (except for flu vaccines) with the post-1999 AAP/USPHS statement phaseout.
- The reevaluation of the cost-effectiveness of multidose vials considering reports of 60 percent wastage and missed vaccination opportunities because of the reluctance of health care workers to open multidose vials to vaccinate only a few children.
- The consideration of switching to single-dose vials, the use of 2-PE as an alternative preservative, and research into new and different preservative options.

Relegating Thimerosal to history's proverbial dustbin should also help boost confidence in vaccines in general. Although childhood vaccination rates for most vaccines in the United States fortunately remain high—at or above national goals of 90 percent, according to the CDC—widespread anxiety about vaccine safety is well documented.[1594][1595] A 2011 survey found that less than a quarter of parents had "no concerns" about childhood vaccines, while 30 percent expressed concern about vaccines causing autism, and about a quarter were concerned about vaccine ingredients.[1596]

Such attitudes would be expected to fuel the continuing problem of voluntary vaccine regimen compliance in various communities. It has been widely reported that parts of California, Colorado, Montana, Oregon, and Washington, among other states, have dangerously low vaccination rates. The rates have sometimes dipped below 80 percent, threatening the "herd immunity" that provides a measure of protection to nonimmune individuals.[1597] Nearly 90 percent of the huge spike in measles cases nationwide in 2011 struck unvaccinated people, and some in the media have fingered low vaccination rates for an epidemic of whooping cough in Washington in 2012.[1598][1599]

Ensuring that the vaccine program in the United States and around the world remains a success depends on assuaging fears while making every effort to avoid the "collateral damage" of vaccine-related injuries. The Institute of Medicine (IOM), the same institution that published the 2004 report that effectively shut down further research regarding a potential Thimerosal-autism link, sounded a rather different note in a recent report. Published just last May, the report commented that "all aspects of the vaccine schedule are currently under-studied with regards to potential adverse events," including adjuvants (such as aluminum) and preservatives (such as Thimerosal).[1600]

Given the continuing concern from so many corners regarding Thimerosal, its immediate outright elimination makes eminent sense.

Notes

[1588] Cummings KM, Brown A, O'Connor R. The cigarette controversy. *Cancer Epidemiol Biomarkers Prev.* 2007 Jun;16(6):1070-6.

[1589] Milberger S, Davis RM, Douglas CE, Beasley JK, Burns D, Houston T, Shopland D. Tobacco manufacturers' defence against plaintiffs' claims of cancer causation: throwing mud at the wall and hoping some of it will stick. *Tob Control.* 2006 Dec;15 Suppl 4:iv17-26.

[1590] http://www.autismspeaks.org/science/science-news/%E2%80%98costs-autism%E2%80%99-summit.

[1591] http://www.autismspeaks.org/science/science-news/autism%E2%80%99s-costs-nation-reach-137-billion-year.

[1592] http://www.cdc.gov/media/releases/2012/t0329_Autism_Telebriefing.html.

[1593] http://www.cdc.gov/mmwr/preview/mmwrhtml/ss6302a1.htm?s_cid=ss6302a1_w.

[1594] http://health.usnews.com/health-news/news/articles/2012/09/06/childhood-vaccination-rates-remain-high-cdc-says.

[1595] http://www.who.int/immunization_monitoring/data/usa.pdf.

[1596] Kennedy A, Lavail K, Nowak G, Basket M, Landry S. Confidence about vaccines in the United States: understanding parents' perceptions. *Health Aff (Millwood).* 2011 Jun;30(6):1151-9.

[1597] http://online.wsj.com/article/SB10001424052702303863404577284001227981464.html

[1598] http://www.cdc.gov/media/releases/2012/t0719_pertussis_epidemic.html.

[1599] http://www.forbes.com/sites/stevensalzberg/2012/07/23/anti-vaccine-movement-causes-the-worst-whooping-cough-epidemic-in-70-years/.

[1600] Martin Kulldorff. *Study Designs for the Safety Evaluation of Different Childhood Immunization Schedules.* Prepared for the Institute of Medicine, Committee on Assessment of Studies of Health Outcomes Related to the Recommended Childhood Immunization Schedule. May 14, 2012 *available at* http://www.iom.edu/~/media/Files/Activity%20Files/PublicHealth/ChildhoodImmunization/Commissioned%20Paper/Report-Webpost.pdf.